RADIOGRAPHIC IMAGING

A PRACTICAL APPROACH

RADIOGRAPHIC IMAGING

A PRACTICAL APPROACH

Derrick P. Roberts
Nigel L. Smith

Technical Manager and Training Manager,
Diagnostic Imaging Systems Division,
Agfa-Gevaert Ltd, Brentford, Middlesex

Churchill Livingstone

EDINBURGH LONDON MELBOURNE AND NEW YORK 1988

CHURCHILL LIVINGSTONE
Medical Division of Longman Group UK Limited

Distributed in the United States of America by Churchill
Livingstone Inc., 1560 Broadway, New York, N.Y. 10036,
and by associated companies, branches and
representatives throughout the world.

First published 1988
  Reprinted 1990

ISBN 0-443-03061-8

British Library Cataloguing in Publication Data
Roberts, Derrick P.
   Radiographic imaging: a practical approach.
   1. Diagnosis, Radioscopic
   I. Title II. Smith, Nigel L.
   616.07'57   RC78

Library of Congress Cataloging in Publication Data
Roberts, Derrick P.
   Radiographic imaging: a practical approach/Derrick P. Roberts,
Nigel L. Smith.
      p.   cm.
   Includes index.
   ISBN 0–443–03061–8
   1. Diagnostic imaging. I. Smith, Nigel L. II. Title.
   [DNLM: 1. Radiography. 2. Technology, Radiologic.   WN 200 R643r]
RC78.7D53R63 1988
616.07'57—dc19   87–27636

Produced by Longman Singapore Publishers (Pte) Ltd.
Printed in Singapore

Preface

It is often argued that radiography is more art than science. Whilst the argument has never been settled, it is indisputable that a great deal of radiography requires a practical approach.

This book has been written to satisfy the need for more practical knowledge in the imaging sciences. To this end every chapter, wherever possible, connects the theory with the practice.

The book is aimed at students in the field of diagnostic imaging, from graduate and postgraduate radiographic students to trainee radiologists. The book can be of use as a reference within the imaging department and as a manual of photographic quality assurance and fault finding which is easy to understand and read.

Particular attention has been paid to the subject areas where our experience has indicated most of the common misconceptions occur. The science of imaging is too complex a subject to be covered by one book. If further information is required in specialised areas, the reader is referred to other experts in the field.

It should be added that the interpretations expressed in this book are our own and may conflict with the long-standing opinions of others.

D. P. Roberts
N. L. Smith

Acknowledgements

The authors would like to acknowledge the witting, and sometimes unwitting, help offered by a large number of friends and colleagues. Whenever numbers of people of the same vocation meet, inevitably the conversation resorts to 'shop'. We cannot acknowledge the help of the many who talked 'shop', but we can list a few. To those we have missed, we apologise.

All of the following at D.I.S. Division, Agfa-Gevaert, Mortsel, Belgium have contributed greatly in one way or another in personal communications or in liberal supplies of help and literature: Dr R. Bollen, Mr F. Crick, Mr J. Lambrechts, Mr H. Pattyn, Dr A. Suys, Mr M. Vrielink, Mr R. Van de Wouwer and Mr J. Van de Wyngaert.

For their assistance in the areas particularly connected with image quality, we are grateful to Dr Borcke and Mr W. Merkle at D.I.S. Division, Agfa-Gevaert, Munich, West Germany.

The following from D.I.S. Division, Agfa-Gevaert, Brentford, Great Britain have all contributed in the supply of information and moral support for the project: Mr D. W. P. Croucher, Mr R. Howard, Mr H. H. Kimmins, Mrs J. Meehan, Mr G. Mountford and Mrs A. Ranelli.

Special thanks are extended to Miss S. J. Roberts, who typed the Queen illustration; Miss M. C. Roberts and Miss A. E. Roberts, who now both know a lot more about photography.

Mention must also be made of the hundreds of students without whom our lives would have been much easier, but not as much fun.

And finally, our thanks to our wives for their support — and a 5 year endless supply of coffee!

D. P. R.
N. L. S.

This book is dedicated to our wives:

Kath Roberts
Jenny Smith

without whose support this book would not have been possible.

Contents

1

Film materials

Introduction

The literal translation of photography is *photo + graphos*, to write with light. If this definition is taken to the extreme then the inventors of photography were probably the Chinese about 3000 years ago. They possessed a light-sensitive material that transferred the images of leaves on to the surfaces of pots and vases. In the more conventional sense photography has been with us since the beginning of the 1800s with the Frenchman Joseph N. Niépce responsible for many of the early developments. Arguably, the father of modern photography is the Englishman William Henry Fox Talbot who, in 1841, developed the calotype process which was the first example of a negative/positive approach to image production (i.e. the original scene is recorded as a negative image then reproduced by 'printing' as a positive print).

Other developments quickly followed, for example, the wet collodion process, the demonstration of three colour additive synthesis by Clerk Maxwell in 1861 and three colour subtractive synthesis in 1868 by Ducos du Hallron.

Since these early days photography has been given to the masses by the development of the camera, the bulk production of film and the ready availability of processing. It has also stepped out of the visible spectrum, material now being available for the recording of infrared rays at one end and X-rays and gamma rays at the other.

The main aim of this chapter is to discuss the structures of film, basic film types and the manufacturing process; however, emulsion technology is a quickly developing area and by the time this book reaches print no doubt many developments and advances will have been made.

ELECTROMAGNETIC SPECTRUM

For a full description of the electromagnetic spectrum the reader is referred to any good physics text book. The following is intended to act as revision of the basic principles and only contains sufficient information to enable understanding of the rest of the text.

By definition the electromagnetic spectrum is 'the range of frequencies over which electromagnetic radiation can be propagated' (Penguin dictionary of physics 1979). It ranges from the low frequencies that are associated with radio waves, to cosmic rays that have higher and higher frequencies. Figure 1.1 shows the electromagnetic spectrum with its common divisions and sub-divisions. In general we are concerned with the frequencies between 10^{12} Hz and 10^{22} Hz, but in many cases, as in the chapter on screens, for example, discussion will take place in terms of wavelengths in nanometers (nanometer $= 10^{-9}$ m).

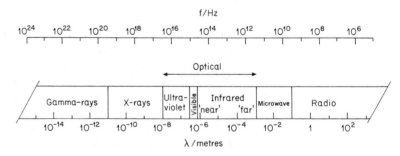

Fig. 1.1 The electromagnetic spectrum.

Electromagnetic radiation

Electromagnetic radiation is radiation consisting of waves of energy that are caused by the acceleration of charged particles. They consist of electric and magnetic fields that are propagated at right angles to each other and to the direction of propagation. The vibration causing the waves is sinusoidal and, unlike sound waves for example, electromagnetic waves require no supporting medium for their transfer. In free space (i.e. a vacuum) they travel at a uniform velocity of 2.997925×10^8 m/s (which is approximately 186 282 miles/s). The nature of electromagnetic radiation depends on its frequency (f) and its velocity (c), the relationship being that

$$c = f \lambda$$

where λ is the wavelength (Fig. 1.2).

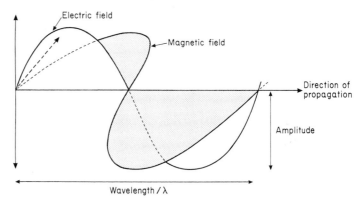

Fig. 1.2 Electromagnetic radiation.

It would probably all be quite simple if it ended here, but unfortunately when observed phenomena are being explained it is necessary to use either the *wave* concept of electromagnetic radiation or the *particle* concept of electromagnetic radiation (i.e. quantum theory). This is due to the fact that phenomena such as reflection, refraction and interference can be explained using wave theory while other phenomena, such as the photoelectric effect and absorption, require an explanation in terms of particles.

The basis of the wave theory has already been discussed. It is based on the premise that electromagnetic radiation is propagated in the form of sinusoidal waves consisting of an electric field with its associated magnetic field at right angles to it and also at right angles to the direction of propagation. Figure 1.2 illustrates this and the 'cardinal' points of the sinusoidal wave, such as amplitude, wavelength, etc. Since all electromagnetic radiations have the same velocity it follows that the frequency is inversely proportional to the wavelength. Wavelength may vary from miles, as in certain radio waves, to billionths of a metre, as in X-rays.

Particle theory

The particle theory of electromagnetic radiation is the basis of the concept of quantum physics. It applies particularly to 'waves' of short wavelength and high velocity which can be considered as consisting of a stream of particles, or quanta, each having a discrete amount of energy (alternatively, these quanta may be known as photons). The amount of energy (E) carried in this discrete parcel is described by the formula:

$$E = hf$$

where:
  E = energy
  h = Planck's constant
  f = frequency of the radiation

Planck's constant has been determined by experiment to be 4.13×10^{-18} keV/s or 6.626196×10^{-34} Js.

As the velocity of the particle in this case is constant, if the frequency of the radiation is doubled the energy of the photon is also doubled.

Throughout the text the principle used to describe physical processes will be the particle theory. On some occasions, however, use will be made of the wave theory, but this will be largely when dealing with optics.

Visible spectrum

Figure 1.1 shows that the visible spectrum occupies only a minute portion of the whole range of the electromagnetic spectrum. It is called the visible spectrum because it is the range of wavelengths within which the unaided human eye perceives wavelength changes as an alteration in colour. The extent of this spectrum is from approximately 400–700 nanometers (nm) and is a gradual change in colour from violet (400 nm) through to red (700 nm approx.), encompassing all the colours of the rainbow. Traditionally it is conveniently divided into seven colours, as illustrated in Figure 1.3, but it must be remembered that no sharp delineation occurs between each of the stated colours. There is some sensitivity of the eye to wavelengths outside the 'normal' range, down to about 380 nm (just ultraviolet) at the shorter wavelengths and up to about 780 nm (just infrared) at the longer wavelengths.

The value of the longest wavelengths to which the eye is sensitive is dependent on the 'brightness' of the 'object'. It can be extended up to 900 nm if a very high-power light source is used, but this is an extreme example.

Conventional photography is mainly concerned with a film's response to the visible spectrum and conveniently divides the spectrum up into three areas or bands: 400–500 nm, blue violet; 500–600 nm, green; 600–700 nm, red. This is only an approximate division, but for many practical purposes it holds true. In radiography our concern is not only with the visible spectrum but also with the effects of ultraviolet, X- and gamma rays on the film. This is frequently

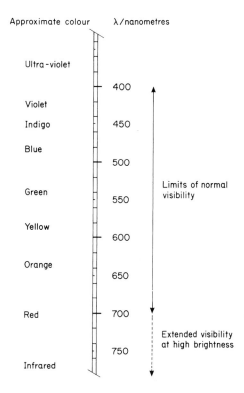

Fig. 1.3 The visible spectrum.

further complicated by the fact that most images are built up by a combination of differing effects depending on the different parts of the electromagnetic spectrum to which the film is exposed, e.g. a conventional film and X-ray intensifying screen produce an image that is made up partly of the effects of blue/green light exposing the film and partly of the effects of direct X-ray exposure.

Each of these effects and any effects they may have on each other must be considered if an accurate assessment of how the image has been formed is to be made.

Further discussion of the visible spectrum will be made as and when required in the following chapters. The reader is referred to the index if further information is required.

Summary

1. Photography in the conventional sense has its roots in the calotype process invented by Fox Talbot in 1841.

2. The electromagnetic spectrum is the range of frequencies over which electromagnetic radiation can be propagated. Figure 1.1 illustrates this spectrum and its divisions.

3. Electromagnetic radiation has two field components that are at right angles to each other (Fig. 1.2). These are the electric field and

the magnetic field; both move at right angles to their direction of propagation and require no supporting medium for their transfer. These properties can be described by either wave theory or particle (quantum) theory.

4. A large proportion of photographic theory is concerned with the effects of the visible spectrum. It extends from approximately 400–700 nm and is a gradual change in colour from violet through to red (see Fig. 1.3).

STRUCTURE OF THE FILM EMULSION

The film emulsion is the basic 'sensitive material' used to record the image. It is a suspension of a suitable light-sensitive salt (i.e. the silver halides) within a gelatine binder. Conventionally this suspension is coated on a supporting medium called the base, and is also subject to other coatings in order to protect it from damage. There are many ways of coating the base in order to produce a film with particular characteristics, but in order not to unduly confuse the discussion on the emulsion, the specifics of commonly available film types are considered in the next section (see Basic film types, p. 22). It is perhaps surprising to note that even with advances in computerised data storage techniques, film emulsion is still the most common way to provide the so-called 'hard copy' for the radiologist or physician.

Silver halides

Many light-sensitive materials are known but only very few possess the characteristics that are necessary for use in a photographic emulsion. The principal materials in use are the silver halides, metallic crystalline solids formed by reacting a suitable silver compound with one of the group of elements known as the halogens. There are four halogens, but only three produce a combination with silver that is useful in the photographic emulsions.

The three 'useful' halides are:

silver bromide (AgBr)
silver iodide (AgI)
silver chloride (AgCl)

All three have a natural spectral sensitivity that ends in the 'blue' part of the visible spectrum at approximately 480 nm, i.e. they are not sensitive to light with wavelengths longer than about 480 nm. Also, the pure form of each of the three halides is of no use photographically, as they are all unable to form a usable latent image (see Ch. 3, Photochemistry). It is only the presence of the gelatine and other impurities deliberately added during manufacture which introduce imperfections to the crystal structure and enable a useful image to form.

Silver bromide (AgBr)

Silver bromide is the most used silver halide in emulsion manufacture. When used on its own it has a 'cut-off' sensitivity of approximately 480 nm and a 'peak' sensitivity at approximately 430 nm. The 'cut-off' sensitivity is the wavelength above which the film is not sensitive, whilst the 'peak' sensitivity is the wavelength to which the film is most sensitive (Fig. 1.4).

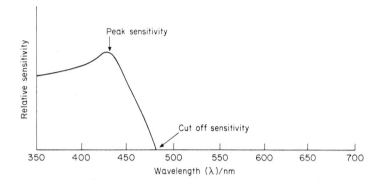

Fig. 1.4 Spectrogram showing the sensitivity of silver bromide (AgBr).

Practical emulsions are rarely pure silver bromide (with some notable exceptions, see *tabular grains*, p. 14) but are usually mixed with a small percentage of silver iodide. This small amount, of the order of 2–4%, has the effect of increasing the speed of the emulsion (i.e. its sensitivity) and altering its spectral sensitivity. Figure 1.5 shows the relevant spectrogram. The mixing of the silver iodide and bromide should mean that we refer to these emulsion as iodobromide emulsions; however, as the proportion of silver iodide is so low, common usage has resulted in X-ray emulsions being termed silver bromide only. It should be noted that a mix of two halides produces grains that contain both halides in the same structure but not in the same proportion in all grains, i.e. not separate grains of the individual halides.

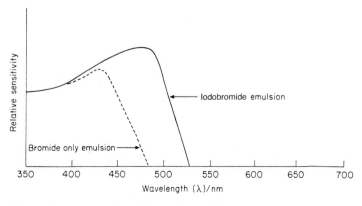

Fig. 1.5 Spectral sensitivity of an idobromide emulsion.

Silver chloride (AgCl)

Silver chloride has a low inherent sensitivity when compared to silver bromide and this disadvantage precludes its use in X-ray-type emulsions. It has, however, an advantage for certain applications in that it possesses very rapid development and fixing properties.

Silver iodide (AgI)

Silver iodide is only used in combination with either silver bromide or chloride. When used in combination with silver bromide it increases its sensitivity and marginally extends its spectral response (see Figs 1.4, 1.5). It is the effect that AgI has on speed that makes it particularly useful in X-ray emulsions. Unfortunately AgI has two important disadvantages: firstly, the presence of iodide in the emulsion significantly extends the time taken for the film to fix; secondly, it possesses certain chemical characteristics, irrelevant here, which preclude its use without either silver bromide or chloride. Having said that there is an increase in fixing time due to the AgI, it is only fair to point out that this is of little practical significance as most automatic processors adequately fix the film in approximately 22 seconds.

Spectral sensitivity

The spectral sensitivity of the emulsion is the range of wavelengths of the electromagnetic spectrum to which the emulsion will respond. Alternatively it may be considered as the range of wavelengths that the emulsion will record as a latent image (whether that latent image is useful or not is irrelevant). Response of an emulsion is usually represented graphically by a spectrogram. It is a plot of a suitable measure of sensitivity against wavelength expressed as nanometers (Fig. 1.6).

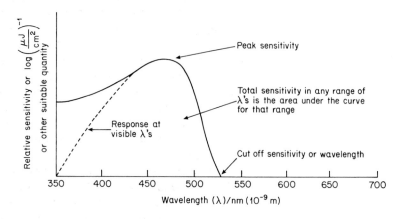

Fig. 1.6 Typical spectrogram and 'cardinal' points.

The sensitivity measure may range from something as vague as relative sensitivity to something as explicit as log X,

where x $= \left(\dfrac{\mu J}{cm^2}\right)^{-1}$

There seems to be no standard starting point for the wavelength scale and it appears to be chosen to suit the emulsion being illustrated. However, most films used in radiology use a starting point of 300 nm. Other significant parts of the spectrogram are *peak sensitivity* and *cut-off sensitivity*.

Peak sensitivity is the wavelength or range of wavelengths at which the emulsion exhibits its highest response, i.e. the wavelength to which it is most sensitive.

Cut-off sensitivity is the wavelength beyond which the film is no longer sensitive.

The spectral sensitivity of film emulsions can be conveniently divided into three sections:

- Monochromatic emulsions
- Orthochromatic emulsions
- Panchromatic emulsions.

Each of these divisions describes the range of wavelengths to which the emulsion will respond. Before considering each in detail we must first take a brief look at the generalities.

SPECTRAL SENSITISING

When used on their own, silver bromide emulsions have their cut-off sensitivity at approximately 480 nm. This is only marginally improved by adding silver iodide (see Figs 1.4, 1.5). In simple terms this means that silver bromide is sensitive only to blue light, the other colours of the spectrum making no contribution to image production. In practice this limitation of an emulsion's ability to respond only to a small range of visible wavelengths has certain advantages and disadvantages; for example, limiting the spectral sensitivity of a film allows it to be handled using suitable safelights and therefore makes processing and loading the film into cassettes much easier. Alternatively, it limits the amount of information the film may record, but again this depends on the 'spectral nature' of the 'object' that film is exposed to. It is easy to see that this is a complex problem. A general rule that seems to hold true is that the film should be able to record the whole of the spectral output of the object it is trying to image.

Extending the natural sensitivity of the silver halides is achieved by adding a suitable dye to the emulsion. This principle was discovered in 1873 by Vogel, who managed to extend spectral sensitivity into the green part of the spectrum. Other dyes, which extended spectral response into the red and infrared, followed. The use of dyes in this way is termed spectral sensitising, dye sensitising, colour sensitising or even optical sensitising.

Dyes that can achieve this feat are called colour sensitisers. The use of the word 'dye' is not an accident, as the materials used are literally coloured dyes. These 'dyes' are added to the emulsion during manufacture and are designed to cover the surface of the silver bromide crystal. The amount of dye required is very small, of the order of only one molecule thick over the whole surface of the grain. This 'monolayer' may occasionally be extended to three or more molecules thick in exceptional circumstances.

In an unsensitised emulsion the silver bromide crystal has the ability to absorb all wavelengths up to 480 nm (blue). This absorption then releases free electrons into the crystal structure forming the latent image (see Ch. 3, Photochemistry), and longer wavelengths pass through the crystal with no effect. In a sensitised emulsion the layer of dye surrounding the crystal allows the shorter 'blue' wavelengths into the crystal but absorbs, say, the longer 'green' wavelengths and converts these into electrons which then contribute to latent image formation.

Two important points emerge from this discussion. Firstly, absorption of wavelengths longer than about 480 nm is achieved at the surface of the crystal by the use of dyes in layers that may be only one molecule thick; secondly, the sensitivity of a 'dyed' emulsion is always *additional* to the parent crystal's inherent sensitivity. Finally, it is important not to confuse spectral sensitising with the production of a 'coloured picture'.

This section has been concerned with a monochrome (i.e. black and white) material's ability to detect colour changes in a subject and register these changes as an alteration in shades of grey, *not* in the production of a true 'colour image' which is a complex topic beyond the scope of this book.

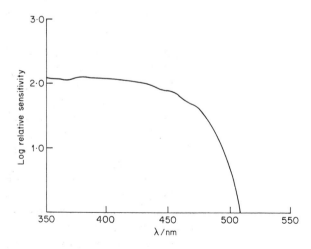

Fig. 1.7 Spectrogram of typical monochromatic screen-type X-ray emulsion.

Monochromatic emulsions

Monochromatic emulsions are variously known as blue sensitive, non-colour sensitive or blind emulsions, as well as other variations of these terms. 'Blind' is a term often used by manufacturers, as the emulsion cannot 'see' any colours of longer wavelength than blue. Figure 1.7 is a typical spectrogram for a monochromatic screen-type X-ray film. These emulsions are generally composed of globular grains (see Grain technology, p. 13) and are particularly useful in calcium tungstate, blue-emitting rare earth and ultraviolet-emitting screen systems. Their use in ultraviolet screens is particularly marked due to the low degree of crossover produced when using these systems. For references on screens, see Chapter 5.

Orthochromatic emulsions

Orthochromatic emulsions are those emulsions that have a spectral sensitivity up to and including the 'green' part of the visible spectrum.

The term orthochromatic is in fact a misnomer, as literally it means 'correct colour' and was used by the developers of these emulsions as they believed they had an emulsion sensitive to all the spectrum.

The extension of the spectral response, as compared to mono-chromatic emulsions, is achieved by spectral sensitising, using dye sensitising agents. These dyes allow the green parts of the visible spectrum to be absorbed at the surface of the silver halide grain and thus contribute to image formation (see also Spectral sensitising, p. 9, and Grain technology, p. 13). Up to now the discussion has been rather vague, using the term 'green part of the visible spectrum'. This has been deliberate, as modern orthochromatic emulsions can be sub-divided into:

- Short orthochromatic,
- Medium orthochromatic, and
- Long orthochromatic.

The three are differentiated by the exact position of their spectral cut-off sensitivity, and peak sensitivity is achieved by careful selection of the sensitising dye. In turn this governs the portion of the 'green' part of the spectrum that will be absorbed. Figure 1.8 is a spectrogram illustrating typical responses of short, medium and long orthochromatic emulsions. These are *not* of particular film types but illustrate general principles. Details of particular films are available from manufacturers.

Uses of film with orthochromatic characteristics are numerous, e.g. green-emitting rare earth screens, monitor photography, photofluorography, certain ciné films, etc. Its use is indicated whenever the 'object' to be imaged contains a high proportion of light from the green part of the visible spectrum.

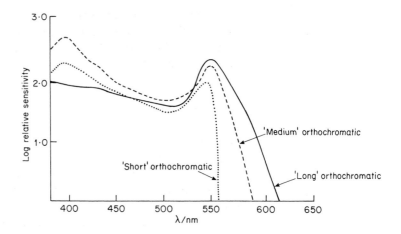

Fig. 1.8 Spectrogram showing examples of short, medium and long orthochromatic emulsions.

Panchromatic emulsions

Panchromatic materials have a spectral sensitivity that covers all the wavelengths of the visible spectrum. Again, as with orthochromatic materials, they are sensitised to wavelengths longer than blue light by the use of dye sensitising agents.

The use of these materials in radiography has been limited by the fact that they are not particularly 'user friendly', in that they must be handled in complete darkness until processed. This feature is not very popular with most darkroom technicians. Additionally there is no particular advantage from a technical view, as most present imaging techniques would benefit little from the use of these emulsions. Figure 1.9 is a typical spectrogram of a panchromatic material. Most of these films are differentiated by variations in the position of their long wave cut-off sensitivity.

For the sake of completeness, it must be mentioned that spectral sensitivity can be extended into the infrared part of the spectrum, to

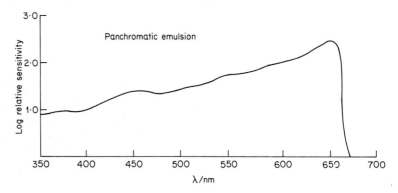

Fig. 1.9 Spectrogram showing typical panchromatic emulsion.

approximately 1200 nm. These materials are of particular use in aerial photography, scientific and technical photography, medical photography and the production of special effects. Technical difficulties encountered in the use of these films negate their common use.

GRAIN TECHNOLOGY

The subject of grain technology has assumed significant importance in recent times, especially with the move towards the greater use of orthochromatic-type emulsions in general radiography. This is an area of quick advances and no doubt some of the following will be out of date in some respects even before it is published.

As far as radiography is concerned, we can divide grain technology into two sections:

- Globular grains and
- Tabular grains.

Globular grains

In blue sensitive or monochromatic systems, globular grains are always used. This is because in the wavelengths up to blue, the light-absorbing ability of the grain depends only on its volume. If the emulsion needs to have a higher speed, i.e. an increased sensitivity, then research shows that the silver bromide grains should be a compact spherical shape, hence the name globular (Fig. 1.10). The spherical shape provides a high volume to give good absorption without producing excessive unsharpness in relation to film speed. The surface area of the grain has no effect on the amount of light absorbed.

If it is necessary to extend the spectral sensitivity of a globular grain into the green or red part of the visible spectrum then a dye sensitising agent must be used. This is a layer of coloured dye that is absorbed into the surface of the silver bromide crystal. It may be up to a maximum of 3 molecules thick, but normally a monolayer is sufficient. The dye absorbs light of wavelengths longer than blue and

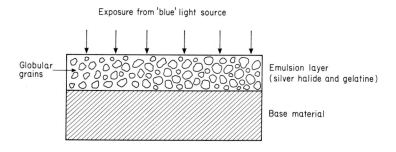

Fig. 1.10 Diagrammatic representation of globular grains.

releases the absorbed photons as electrons that can contribute to image formation. The extension of the spectral sensitivity in this way depends on the colour of the dye and is a 'surface' phenomenon, i.e. the dye sensitising agent is adsorbed at the surface of the grain and the wavelengths longer than blue are absorbed by the dye and therefore also at the surface. It is apparent that the ideal grain to maximise this effect would be one of little or no volume but which would present maximum surface area to the incoming light photons and therefore enhance absorption.

Tabular grains

These are grains of a particular shape that are used exclusively in sensitised emulsions. In radiography, orthochromatic sensitising of tabular grains is used in screen film technology. These grains can be divided into two main types:

- T-Mat emulsions and
- Structured Twins.

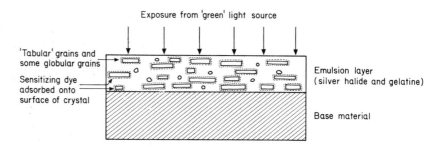

Fig. 1.11 Diagrammatic representation of tabular grains.

Tabular grains have a 'table top'-like structure (Fig. 1.11), which provides a very large surface area but has a small volume. They are therefore particularly suitable for sensitisation as they present a large surface area to the dye and increase the amount of absorption possible.

Tabular grains are not particularly new; they have been known since about 1963, and have been used in high resolution colour films for many years. They are particularly impressive in that they produce a high speed emulsion with very high resolution and relatively low silver coating weights.

T-Mat emulsions

T-Mat is a registered trademark of Kodak Limited, who were first to introduce this form of technology into X-ray-type emulsions. A T-Mat emulsion is a tabular grain emulsion of a specific type (Fig. 1.12). In

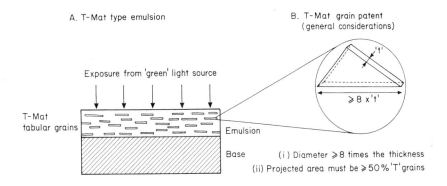

A. T-Mat type emulsion

B. T-Mat grain patent
(general considerations)

Exposure from 'green' light source

T-Mat
tabular grains

Emulsion

Base

't'

$\geqslant 8 \times$ 't'

(i) Diameter $\geqslant 8$ times the thickness
(ii) Projected area must be $\geqslant 50\%$ 'T' grains

Fig. 1.12 Diagrammatic representation of (A) T-Mat emulsion; (B) T-Mat silver bromide grain.

a conventional tabular grain emulsion there is always a small proportion of grains that are not flat. T-Mat technology makes an emulsion in which nearly all the grains are identical and extremely flat. The patent for T-Mat then goes on to specify surface diameter/thickness ratios for the individual silver bromide grains. Interestingly, these are silver bromide only emulsions and this situation somewhat limits the ability of the crystal to absorb the dye sensitising agent.

There are some distinct advantages to this technology, particularly in the area of sharpness. The gain in sharpness is primarily due to a decrease in the amount of crossover, which can be as high as 75% in orthochromatic emulsions, to about 37%. This is simply because the flatter grains have a greater capacity to absorb light than spherical grains (Fig. 1.13). However, the gain in sharpness produces a marked increase in 'graininess' which is very easily visible.

Note: Crossover is a feature of duplitised emulsions in which light from one screen exposes not only the emulsion closest to it but passes through the base and exposes the emulsion furthest away (see Ch. 5, Intensifying screens).

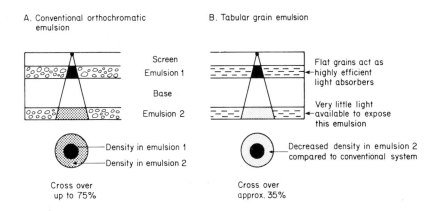

A. Conventional orthochromatic
emulsion

B. Tabular grain emulsion

Screen
Emulsion 1
Base
Emulsion 2

Flat grains act as
highly efficient
light absorbers

Very little light
available to expose
this emulsion

Density in emulsion 1
Density in emulsion 2

Decreased density in emulsion 2
compared to conventional system

Cross over
up to 75%

Cross over
approx. 35%

Fig. 1.13 Crossover in (A) conventional orthochromatic and (B) tabular grain emulsions.

Structured twin emulsions

'ST' or Structured Twin is a trademark of Agfa-Gevaert Limited. As with T-Mat, it is a form of tabular grain technology, but in this case the increase in the surface area of the crystal is achieved by using two tabular-type grains in combination, hence the name Structured Twin. Close examination of the exact crystal structure of 'T' and 'ST' grains will reveal major differences between the two. However, both technologies have the same approach, producing a crystal that has a large surface area compared to its volume, and conferring sensitivity by dye sensitisation. 'ST' grains are more 'conventional', being a mix of silver bromide and iodide, and this improves the ability of the crystal to absorb more dye into its surface.

Again, the main advantage is to improve sharpness by reducing crossover. Figure 1.14 is a diagrammatic representation of a Structured Twin-type grain and a conventional 'T' grain. The differences are obvious.

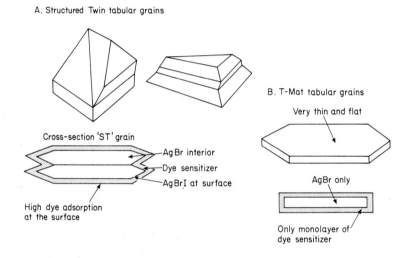

Fig. 1.14 Diagrammatic representation of (A) Structured Twin tabular grains; (B) T — Mat tabular grains.

Advantages of tabular grains

The advantages of tabular grains are potentially significant. However, in order to realise some of these advantages a radical re-think of attitudes towards films and processing would be required. The following is a list of some of the possible advantages. Only a few are immediately available, and only some will find their way into the X-ray department.

1. Increased resolution; when compared to a film of conventional grain technology with the same speed. This is mainly due to reduction in crossover.

2. Reduction in silver coating weights; making the crystals thinner and flatter reduces the amount of silver used in manufacture. This does not affect sensitivity, as green light absorption now takes place in the dye layer at the surface of the crystal. Blue light is absorbed in the volume of the crystal, but this is almost irrelevant when using green-emitting rare earth screens.

3. Suitable for 45 s processing; this is mainly due to the reduction in silver coating weights, coupled with the facts that it is easier to harden the film (in fact it may be possible to totally harden the film in manufacture) and it simplifies developer chemistry. This is only speculative at the present time, as to convert the whole of radiographic processing to this system would be a formidable task.

Disadvantages of tabular grains.

1. Higher graininess; this is mainly due to the better imaging of quantum mottle, rather than to an increase in true film grain. Almost entirely due to the reduction in crossover.

2. Lower silver recovery; due to the reduction in silver coating weights as detailed in the list of advantages.

Other grain technology

Many manufacturers are experimenting with other kinds of grain technology; a detailed discussion of these would fill a book in its own right. In an attempt to illustrate this, the following is a list of high resolution films and the particular grain technology claimed:

- ST grains: Structured Twin tabular grains (Agfa-Gevaert)
- T-Mat: Homogeneous tabular grains (Kodak)
- SMG grains: Surface Modified grains (Fuji)
- CLG grains: Concentrated Latent image grains (Fuji)
- HMG grains: High ortho Mono-dispersed grains (Konica)

This is not intended to be a complete list, but illustrates the efforts being made to advance grain technology.

Grain size and distribution

Grain size and distribution are governed during manufacture when the emulsion is undergoing the first (or Ostwald) ripening stage of production. Here the crystals grow to the required size, correct distribution is achieved and this fixes the emulsion speed, contrast and graininess characteristics.

In the not-too-distant past it was possible to be quite specific as to what effects grain size and distribution would have on contrast and speed. However, with the advent of the dye sensitised tabular-type grains this delineation into separate groupings has become less relevant. The good news is that the generalities still apply, especially when considering globular grain emulsion.

Contrast

The degree of contrast produced depends on grain size distribution, i.e. the range of grain sizes. An emulsion that has a wide range of grain sizes produces a film that has a low film contrast. This is because, as the film is sensitive to a wide range of exposures, it therefore has high exposure latitude and by the rules of sensitometry must have low film contrast. At a crystalline level this is because the larger crystals are most sensitive and the smaller crystals least sensitive to exposure. The sensitivity of intermediate sizes varies accordingly. Therefore a wide range of grain sizes implies a wide sensitivity to exposure and, because of the above argument, a low contrast film. It follows that a small range of grain sizes produces a film with high contrast and, in the limit, a film with only one grain size produces virtually no grey scale but very high contrast.

In practice the production of emulsions with a narrow range of grain sizes is quite difficult and these films are useful only in highly specialised situations.

Speed

The speed of an emulsion is governed by its average grain size. In general the larger the average grain size the more sensitive the film and the greater its speed. The reverse is also true. With dye sensitised emulsions this general rule is somewhat more complicated. Consider two emulsions, both with the same average grain size and general crystal shape. If one emulsion is monochromatic and the other orthochromatic in its spectral response and both are exposed to a light source containing the whole of the visible spectrum, then the orthochromatic film will apparently have a higher speed. This is simply because it is capable of recording more of the wavelengths of the light exposing it as an image. These features open up some interesting possibilities; for example, an orthochromatic film can have a lower silver coating weight than its monochromatic alternative and still have the same speed class (assuming the correct screens are used), or a smaller average grain size but again the same speed class. It must be remembered, however, that other factors may become more relevant, in terms of the the final image quality, as radiographic systems become more complex.

Finally, the production of high speed emulsions with large grain sizes usually results in the simultaneous growth of other grains of smaller sizes. Inevitably this means that fast film tends towards low contrast and slower film towards high contrast.

Graininess

The subject of graininess is a complex topic which comprises many variables. As far as the film emulsion is concerned, the silver halide crystals are responsible for what is called 'true film grain'. True film grain is not visible to the naked eye; even the largest crystals are very small, being only about 1 micron in diameter ($1\mu = 10^{-6}$ m). However, a grainy pattern can usually be detected with little or no magnification. This is due to the fact that the grains are spatially distributed not only in area but also in depth, giving the appearance of being clumped together and forming random density variations in areas that should appear as an homogenous density. Grains may also be actually clumped together (i.e. in physical contact) due to techniques of manufacture or as a result of processing.

The rule of thumb usually applied to film grain is to say that, the faster the film the larger the grains and the greater degree of graininess. In practice this proves to be quite accurate, but certainly as far as film and screen combinations are concerned by far the largest contributing factor to graininess is quantum mottle. A more complete insight into graininess is given in Chapter 7, Image quality.

GELATINE

Gelatine has been used as an emulsion binder for well over 100 years. It succeeded a substance known as collodion, which was a mixture of gun-cotton, ether and alcohol. The reason for the change to gelatine is complex, and beyond the scope of this book. However, it was a well-known fact that some of the photographers using collodion became addicted to the ether and alcohol vapour.

Gelatine is a complex common protein deriving its name from the Latin *gelata*, i.e. 'formation in water'. The common misconception is that it is produced from horses' hooves, muscle tissue or blood. It is not. Commercial manufacture is based on white fibrous connective tissue, or more correctly collagen fibres, the principal sources of which are cartilage, skin and ossein (the protein matrix of bone).

Collagen is converted into gelatine by the process known as hydrolysis (which is the chemical decomposition of a substance by water). During this conversion the water destroys the cross-linking of the collagen, and this produces the gelatine polymer (Fig. 1.15).

No definite structure or size has been determined for the gelatine molecule since it is a mixture of degradation products. However, its general form is thought to be:

$$(NH_2\ CH_2\ COOH)_n$$

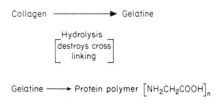

Fig. 1.15 The production of gelatine.

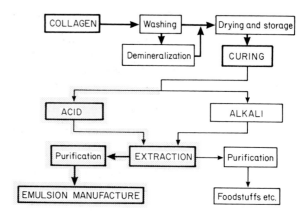

Fig. 1.16 The manufacture of gelatine.

Commercial manufacture

A detailed knowledge of the manufacture of gelatine is not necessary. Figure 1.16 is an abbreviated flow diagram of the various stages involved. Photographically, it is the curing process that has the first important effect on the nature of the emulsion. It is here that the *isoelectric point* of the emulsion is determined and this has profound consequences on the film's final characteristics.

Isoelectric point (IEP)

The isoelectric point of an emulsion is very significant in determining certain important characteristics. It depends on the type of gelatine and is defined as 'the pH value at which a substance or system is electrically neutral'.

Acid cure gelatine has a low isoelectric point, being electrically neutral at a typical value of pH 4.85, whilst alkali cure has a high isoelectric point at approximately 7.8 pH (Fig. 1.17). From a photographic point of view, the isoelectric point effectively:

- Determines how easily products are removed from the emulsion
- Affects the degree of hardening.

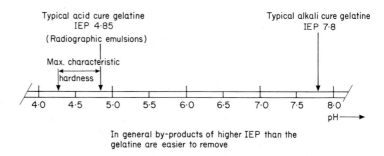

Fig. 1.17 Diagrammatic representation of isoelectric points (IEP).

At its isoelectric point, gelatine has the following properties:

- Minimum solubility
- Minimum viscosity
- Minimum conductivity
- Minimum swelling.

The isoelectric point can be altered by the addition of suitable contaminants, thus allowing fine control of the factors listed above. Emulsions can therefore have a variable range of properties to suit very specialised applications.

One of the principal factors affecting the choice of an emulsion's IEP is the IEP of the by-products of processing that need to be removed. In general, if the by-products have a higher IEP than the emulsion, the products are easier to remove. In the case of conventional X-ray-type emulsions, an IEP of approximately 4.8 is usual as the majority of by-products requiring removal have IEPs greater than this value. It follows that gelatine used in the manufacture of these products should be of the acid cure variety (see Fig. 1.17).

Finally, not only is the IEP of the emulsion significant, but the IEP of the supercoat (see p. 25) is also important. Medical X-ray films are conventionally low IEP emulsions with a low IEP supercoat due to the reasons outlined in the previous paragraph. However, this is not always the case, as on some occasions a high IEP supercoat can be advantageous (although the reasons for this are beyond the scope of this book). It should be noted that isoelectric points do not only apply to film emulsions but are important in a wide variety of applications not related to the photographic process.

Function of gelatine

Photographically the function of gelatine can be divided into two sections:

- Physical properties
- Photographic properties.

Physical properties

1. Gelatine absorbs the water present in processing and can go from a sol to a gel and the reverse an infinite number of times. In the act of changing from a sol to a gel the gelatine swells, opens its molecular structure, and allows easy penetration of the processing solutions.

2. Gelatine keeps the silver bromide in suspension and assists in keeping the individual crystals separate from each other. This reduces the amount of grain clumping.

3. Gelatine binds the emulsion to the film base. A thin layer of pure material is often included as part of the manufacturing process to literally 'glue' the emulsion to the base (see Substratum, p. 24).

4. Gelatine provides a growth medium during emulsion manufacture allowing the silver halide crystals to develop to the required size.

Photographic properties

1. Gelatine provides impurities of sulphur which give active points of silver sulphide (Ag_2S) within the crystal structure. These points deepen electron traps and consume certain photo by-products (see Latent image formation, p. 78). The amount of impurity added is carefully controlled during manufacture in order to produce an emulsion with the desired characteristics.

2. Gelatine allows and encourages the production of electron traps due to the formation of crystal defects. Electron traps are vital during the formation of the latent image and without them there would be no photography as we know it (see Latent image formation, p. 78).

3. During exposure some of the silver bromide is split into its component ions ($Ag^+ + Br^-$). Gelatine helps prevent the recombination of the bromine ions after their release by exposure.

$$AgBr \rightleftharpoons Ag^+ + Br^-$$

Gelatine reduces the rate of the back reaction and prevents the effects of exposure becoming undone; i.e. it reduces latent image fade.

Age fog

Discussion of age fog at this point may seem inappropriate. However, the advantage of gelatine providing sulphur impurities also has a disadvantage in that it increases the amount of fog formed on unexposed film, even if all storage factors are ideal.

Age fog is due to the increase in the amount of silver sulphide in the emulsion with storage. This increase renders the silver bromide crystal more susceptible to development. Some silver sulphide is 'built in' to the crystal so it is suitable for latent image formation; the rest comes from the colloidal sulphur (present in the emulsion gelatine) combining with either free interstitial silver ions or actual crystal lattice ions.

BASIC FILM TYPES

Introduction

There is a wide variety of film types available to suit many different needs, ranging from the astronomer to the amateur photographer. In radiography there is still a significant choice of film types but the basic structures of the films found in the X-ray department fall into three basic categories:

- Duplitised

- Single-coated
- Double-coated.

The specifics of each type will be discussed in some detail in the sections that follow. However, it is sufficient to say now that duplitised films have the emulsion layer on both sides of the film base, single-coated films have an emulsion layer on only one side of the film base, and double-coated films have two emulsion layers but both are on the same side of the film base (in this case they are usually different emulsion types). Triple-coated films do exist, the best example of these being conventional colour print and slide films typically used in 35 mm cameras.

Duplitised films

These are films with emulsion coated on both sides of the film base. The general structure and typical dimensions are shown in Figure 1.18. This represents a screen-type film. As can be seen, it is composed of various layers each with a particular function.

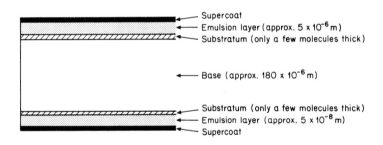

Fig. 1.18 Duplitised film: cross-sectional structure and dimensions.

The base

This acts as a supporting medium for the other layers and may be one of several materials, such as glass, cellulose triacetate or paper. However, *all* X-ray films are coated on a 'polyester base' (or, to be more technically accurate, polyethylene teraphthalate). Polyester has many advantages that encourage its use:

- Dimensional stability
- Optical clarity
- Waterproof
- High tensile strength
- Flexible
- Chemical 'memory'
- Inert to processing chemicals
- Conforms to non-flammability regulations (i.e. is a safety base).

All these factors combine to produce a material that is particularly suitable for automatic roller processing at high temperatures, indeed it was the introduction of polyester base that cured many of the problems associated with early roller processors.

The base is either completely colourless or, more usually, tinted various shades of blue according to the particular use the film is designed for. The degree of tinting depends on dye type and other complex factors, but all dyes used are the subject of very heavy patent protection by manufacturers. Blue tinting has the advantage of improving apparent perceptibility when the film is viewed with an intense white (6500 K) light source, but it has a tendency to reduce grey scale rendition (especially important in recording ultrasound techniques). It is fair to say that personal preference plays a large part in the choice of a blue or clear base material, some observers preferring blue base even for images requiring wide grey scale.

Of the many advantages of polyester, some are worthy of particular note. The combination of high dimensional stability (size charge $\simeq$ < 0.002% per °C) and low water absorption combine with other factors to give a processing size change of $\pm$ 0.03% (approx.). This low value reduces problems with the differing expansion and contraction rates of the emulsion and base causing curling and cracking.

High tensile strength with associated good flexibility allows the base to be made thinner (thus reducing parallax errors) and to be transported through roller processing successfully. The 'chemical memory' means the film 'remembers' that it was made flat. Films with acetate-type bases do not possess this 'memory'. Consequently if a flat acetate base film is rolled (e.g. as in roller processing) it tends to take on a curved profile, whilst polyester film does not. This is a particular advantage during high temperature roller processing.

Finally, it is as well to note that polyester base is an oil-related product and is subject to all the vagaries of fluctuations in oil price. It is, therefore, not necessarily less costly than its alternatives.

Substratum

Also known as the subbing layer, this is an adhesive layer that literally sticks the emulsion to the base. The choice of substance for this function primarily depends on the nature of the base material. If the base is of the acetate type then it is a very thin, almost monolayer of gelatine; however, polyester base is not so easy and poses some considerable problems.

The single main problem is finding a material that has adhesive qualities and also an affinity for both the natural gelatine organic polymer and the man-made 'polyester' polymer. In the early days of polyester base this was somewhat problematic, but the problems were soon overcome by rapid advances in technology. Actual details of materials in use are not available for publication at this time.

Emulsion

The specific details of the film's emulsion have been fully considered earlier in this chapter. It is sufficient to state here that the emulsion is a mixture of gelatine and one of, or a mixture of, the silver halides of bromine, chlorine and iodine.

The shapes of the crystals in this suspension may range from globular to tabular grains, according to the use the emulsion will be put to, and there may be present dye sensitising agents in order to control the spectral sensitivity characteristics of the film. X-ray films are principally silver bromide emulsions.

Supercoat

This is a thin layer of clear, specially hardened gelatine that is coated onto the top surface of the emulsion. Its purpose is to protect the emulsion from mechanical damage and provide the required surface characteristics.

The most usual mechanical damage is abrasion marks due to mishandling and roller transportation in processing; this is minimised by making the supercoat as smooth and as hard as possible. However, it must not be too smooth, as a certain amount of 'roughness' is required to enable the film to transport through roller processors and automated film-handling systems. Likewise it must not be too hard, as this could make the penetration of the processing chemistry more difficult and extend processing times. A suitable compromise is therefore made between all significant factors.

Screen-type duplitised films

With all the information available from manufacturers it seems, at first, that numerous different film types are available. Closer examination reveals that, in the case of screen-type duplitised films, availability can conveniently be divided into three sections, with only subtle variations in basic characteristics between different manufacturers' products within each section.

- 'Conventional' or standard contrast type
- Half speed type
- 'Latitude' type

Each of these may be available in either monochromatic or orthochromatic spectral sensitivities (depending on the screen type with which it is to be used; see Ch. 5, Intensifying screens), as well as conventional or advanced technology grain emulsions. The variation in characteristics between each of the divisions provides the facility to choose the best possible combination of film and screen to enable an image of the highest possible diagnostic content to be produced, with regard to other significant factors such as dose, etc. The advantage to the patient is obvious.

'Standard contrast'-type emulsions

Standard contrast-type emulsions are so called for historical reasons: films with these general contrast characteristics were originally the

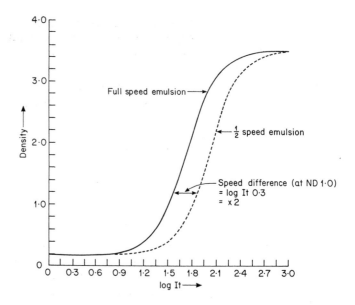

Fig. 1.19 Characteristic curves of conventional and 'half speed'-type emulsions.

most often-used. It is comparison with this type that has resulted in the names of the other two, i.e. half speed and 'L'.

The features of 'conventional' emulsions are best considered by examining their sensitometric characteristics (Fig. 1.19), and then comparing the other two types to this base line. To ensure that the comparison is fair, it is assumed that each film is exposed to a light source of spectral emission that corresponds to the film's sensitivity, the same source is used in each case, and that each film receives identical processing.

Figure 1.19 shows a typical characteristic curve for a standard contrast-type emulsion:

- Base + fog = 0.18;
- Average gradient ($\bar{G}$) = 2.6
- Maximum density (D max) = 3.5–4.0, and
- Speed = log It 1.53 (at net density 1.0).

These values are not representative of any specific emulsion, but illustrate the general case.

Half speed-type emulsions

As the name implies, these films have approximately half the speed of their conventional counterparts. The reduction in speed generally improves the image quality but increases the dose to the patient. However, the use of half speed film with high speed rare earth screens to produce a certain 'speed class' (i.e. the speed of film and screen in combination) seems to produce improved image quality when compared to a 'conventional' film and screens in the same speed class. The use of such a film greatly increases the range of film/screen combinations available to suit differing situations. Unfortunately, making the choice of which combination to use is not simple.

The reduction in speed is achieved by reducing the silver coating weight of the emulsion (although it is not reduced by one-half, as the relationship between speed and coating weight is not that simple). Again, Figure 1.19 shows the essential characteristics. All factors are similar except the speed, which is decreased to log It 1.83.

Finally, it is as well to note that half speed emulsions are available in standard contrast and/or latitude ('L')-type emulsion coatings.

Latitude or 'L'-type emulsions

These emulsions were specifically introduced to improve the detail seen in the peripheral areas of the chest radiograph. With standard contrast emulsions, detail tends to be lost in these areas as they are at the upper limit of the useful density range, and of high subject contrast due to the air acting as a negative contrast agent.

In an 'L'-type emulsion, the silver halide grain size distribution within a particular size range is so arranged that at higher densities, the gradient of the characteristic curve decreases. This decreases the subject contrast enhancement and increases the latitude (i.e. increases grey scale) in high density areas (Fig. 1.20). Thus a film of high perceptibility in both high and low density areas can be made.

When applied to a chest radiograph, this means that the detail available should be similar over all the areas of the lung fields.

An obvious spin-off of this is that it also increases the film latitude and therefore the exposure latitude of the whole emulsion.

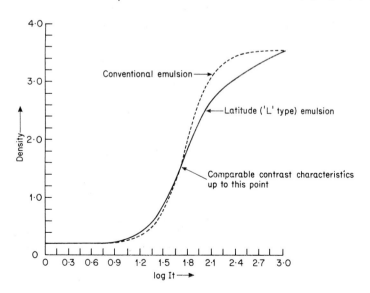

Fig. 1.20 Characteristic curve of a latitude ('L')-type emulsion (compared to a conventional emulsion).

Marketing of these film types has therefore concentrated on this wide latitude and the fact that this leads to fewer repeat examinations, especially in situations where exposure assessment is difficult (e.g. theatre). However, the visual appearance of this kind of emulsion is not to the liking of some radiologists and clinicians, and this emulsion has proved to be simply another addition to the types available.

Figure 1.20 is a typical characteristic curve of an 'L' emulsion. All the essential features are the same as for a standard contrast film (or half speed film, if that is being considered) except for the average gradient, which is reduced to $\bar{G} = 2.2$. The average gradient can be misleading here, as at lower densities the curve has a gradient similar to a conventional emulsion, whereas at higher densities it is somewhat less than the average. The reader is advised to study Figure 1.20 carefully.

Resolution

Resolution values of screen-type emulsions are of no practical significance, as the limiting factor is not the film but the screen with which the film is being used. Therefore system resolution is used in preference. For a 200 class rare earth system with 'conventional' film, a typical value at 10% MTF would be 6 lp mm^{-1}.

In general, within a speed class using the same film, rare earth screens have higher resolutions compared to calcium tungstate screens. Increasing speed class usually means decreasing resolution.

In all cases the resolution capabilities of the film greatly exceed that of the screens.

Reciprocity failure

This is a feature of very short exposure times at high intensities, and very long times at low intensities, not producing the density expected. It is always a problem when light is the principal image producer and therefore affects all film/screen systems.

In general it is not a problem if exposure times are kept between 0.003s and 3s. A fuller description of reciprocity failure is given in Chapter 5, Intensifying screens.

Advantages of duplitisation

Increased film speed

Doubling the amount of emulsion available to expose must increase the 'sensitivity' of the system. This is especially so when a duplitised film is used between a pair of intensifying screens. If a single screen with a single-coated film is exposed to an X-ray beam, about 10% of the beam will be converted into useful exposure on the film, and 90% will be wasted. If another screen and emulsion are provided, a further 10% of that 90% can be made useful and contribute to the image, therefore providing a second emulsion and screen approximately doubles the sensitivity of the system (the figures here are highly generalised but illustrate the point).

This increase in film speed has many advantages, the principal ones being:

- Reduces dose to the patient
- Reduces kinetic unsharpness (due to decreased exposure times)
- Reduces geometric unsharpness (e.g. smaller focal spots)
- Reduces potential dose to staff.

Increased contrast

In simple terms, contrast is the difference in density between two adjacent areas on the film. A duplitised film will always have the potential to have higher contrast than single-coated film of the same coating weight, because higher density differences are possible with the same exposure due to the presence of a higher level of available density-producing silver halide. Thus density differences are always potentially greater from duplitised than from single-coated materials.

Disadvantages of duplitisation

The largest single disadvantage of duplitisation is the increase in photographic unsharpness due to the parallax effect. Consider the build-up of an image of a narrow slit in the emulsion (Fig. 1.21). When viewed perpendicular to the plane of the film, the images are perfectly superimposed and appear as one. However, because the two images are spatially separated, if they are viewed at an angle the

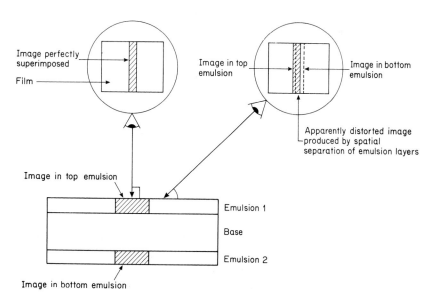

Fig. 1.21 Image distortion due to parallax.

edges of the image will appear unsharp as the two images are slightly displaced from each other, i.e. they look 'blurred'. The effect of this 'blurring' is very limited as the distances between the emulsion layers are very small, and in any case other unsharpness factors are more significant.

Under certain conditions, though, it can become a problem, for example in the days of manual processing films were often viewed in their 'wet' state and a provisional diagnosis made. This was always followed up by a report when the films were dry, due to the fact that the parallax unsharpness caused by the wet swollen emulsion was unacceptable.

Other duplitised emulsions

In any attempt to generalise it is inevitable that certain items will not conveniently fit into the proposed categories. It is the same in this case. In an attempt to be as complete as possible, the following are film emulsions which are available but are not in such common use as the ones previously discussed.

Contrast or 'C' type emulsions

This type is very popular with certain physicians, particularly in the USA. It is a *very* low contrast mono- or orthochromatic emulsion with fog and speed characteristics similar to standard contrast films. Particularly designed for chest radiography, it has wide grey scale rendition that makes the film appear to be lacking in detail, especially to the untrained observer. Again the subjective choice of the radiologist or clinician is of great importance.

High speed emulsions

As the name suggests, these are high speed films. They produce (approximately) an 800 speed class when used with regular screens (this would be 200 with standard speed films) and are advanced grain technology emulsions. This is necessary in order to maintain high resolution at high speeds, therefore they are orthochromatic in spectral sensitivity. All high speed tabular grain emulsions tend to have higher contrast than their conventional counterparts.

FILM FORMATS AND PACKAGING

Films are available in a vast array of sizes and different packaging to suit virtually all possible situations. In Europe, metric sizes are used almost exclusively (but see Ch. 8, Monitor photography), whilst imperial sizes still predominate in the USA. The following is a list of the most often-used metric sizes available from manufacturers:

18 × 24 cm

24 × 30 cm
30 × 40 cm
15 × 30 cm
35.5 × 35.5 cm
35.5 × 43 cm.

Most manufacturers will cut to a specified size, providing the volume required is high enough to justify the cost. However, these are special orders and may take some considerable time to be available. A quick glance at any manufacturer's price/product list will reveal a considerable number of readily available sizes that will probably mean a special order is unnecessary. (For example, Agfa-Gevaert CURIX RP1 is available in 26 different 'cut' film sizes and 4 roll sizes up to 50 m long, which is indeed a wide choice.)

Packing

Film is usually supplied in boxes of 25, 50, 100 and 500 sheets and either FW, AFW or NIF wrapped.

FW stands for folder wrapped. In this packing each sheet of film is individually wrapped in a folded sheet of photographic quality paper. This is to reduce abrasion marks on the surface of the film, which may occur as the films rub against each other during transportation, removal from the film hopper and during loading into the cassette. Folder wrapping also acts as protection against finger marking.

AFW stands for alternate folder wrapped, i.e. every other film in the box has its own separate cover of paper. The paper used is one of the most pure that can be made and must be free of any contaminant that may adversely affect the emulsion. Particularly problematic is the presence of very low level radioactive material which as it decays 'exposes' the film, producing a mottled appearance after processing.

A particularly bad outbreak of 'paper mottle' occurred in the early 1970's in paper supplied from an originally pure source. It was eventually traced to very low level contamination in the water supply to a particular paper mill. Large amounts of film were affected, at some considerable cost to the manufacturers. Since this 'accident', manufacturers have tried to move towards NIF packing, with considerable success. This removes the chance of 'mottle' and reduces packing costs.

NIF stands for non-interleaving folders. The film is not protected from its neighbours in any way, but scratch marks on the surface of the film are virtually non-existent. This is due to two factors; firstly, improved hardening of the supercoat protecting the film, and secondly the trend towards hermetically sealed vacuum/partial vacuum packs of foil or plastic. These packs hold the sheets of film firmly together in a single package, eliminating movement between adjacent sheets during transportation. Occasionally severe mishandling can cause film movement and produce localised abrasion marks that appear as a 'bird's nest' of high density scratches. Not surprisingly, this is called transport abrasion, and is best seen using a magnifying glass after processing.

The film is further protected by placing the foil or plastic bag in a strong outer box of high quality card. Some manufacturers include a lead strip that completely encompasses the box or internal packing. This enables the user of the film to tell easily if it has accidentally been exposed to ionising radiation. The strip shows on the film as an area of low density below the general fog density on a film processed straight from the packet.

An additional advantage to hermetically sealed packaging is the fact that the relative humidity of the atmosphere during storage is less critical. The film is effectively enclosed in its own microclimate at the ideal moisture content to ensure maximum storage without an adverse effect on base + fog level — however, other factors may become more significant (see Ch. 2, Sensitometry).

Not every film size is available in FW or AFW, but most are sold in NIF packing. Film packed in 500s is a so-called 'econopack' and is usually subdivided into 4 × 125s within one large external pack. It is obviously most useful where a particular size has a high volume turnover, and normally has a cost advantage over smaller boxes (say 5 × 100) for the same amount.

DIRECT EXPOSURE DUPLITISED FILMS

These films can be divided into two types, those specifically designed for medical use and those for industrial use. Their general structure is the same as screen-type duplitised film (see Fig. 1.18). Films for medical use usually come in their own individual envelope with no need to reload into a cassette; films for industrial use come in a multitude of different packings to suit varying applications.

The main differences, when compared to screen-type emulsions, are:

1. *Higher resolution.* In direct exposure emulsions, resolution is principally limited by average AgBr grain size, unlike screen film in which it is limited by the particular screen in which the film is used. In industrial film, average grain size is between about 0.23–1.7 μ depending on speed. This gives resolution values of approximately 200 lp mm^{-1}.

2. *Higher silver coating weight.* As the film is entirely dependant on X-rays or gamma rays for image production, it follows that density is built up by direct absorption of these rays by the AgBr in the emulsion.

To increase the sensitivity of the emulsion, a higher silver coating weight is used; this increases the chance of the X-rays or gamma rays being absorbed. Typically, silver coating weights will be four times that of a screen film.

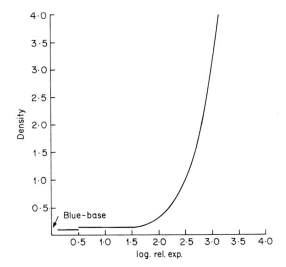

Fig. 1.22 Typical characteristic curve of industrial X-ray film.

3. *Lower speed.* When exposed in the conditions for which the film is designed their speed will be slower. However, film speed in practice is a relative concept and in any case industrial emulsions use a different speed point than medical screen films (see Ch. 2, Sensitometry). Therefore any comparison between systems must be carried out with care.

4. *Higher maximum density.* Due to the fact that these emulsions have a higher silver weight, a higher maximum density is also possible. Typically this would be around density 6–7.

5. *Higher contrast.* The average gradient of the characteristic curve measured between net density 1.5 and 3.5 would typically be a value of about 5.0, depending on processing, and represents a film with very high contrast when compared to a medical screen film ($\bar{G} = 2.5$ approx.). Figure 1.22 shows a typical characteristic curve of an industrial film.

The use of direct exposure films in medical radiography has declined in recent years, due to the development of high resolution rare earth screen techniques which have the advantage of low patient dose but excellent image quality.

SINGLE-COATED EMULSIONS

Structure

The general structure of a single-coated film is shown in Figure 1.23. As can be seen, it has an emulsion layer on only one side of the base. The basic features of the structures on this side of the film are as previously discussed, although the emulsion layer will probably have

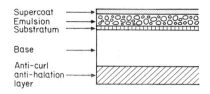

Fig. 1.23 Cross-section through a single-coated emulsion.

a lower silver coating weight and be spectrally sensitised to wavelengths above 510 nm (blue), depending on its use. The non-emulsion side has some very significant features.

Anti-curl backing

This has the function, just as its name suggests, of preventing the film curling during processing and allows the film to stay flat after processing. Curling occurs due to the differential expansion of the emulsion caused by water absorption from the processing solutions. The base, however, is waterproof and dimensionally stable and therefore stays the same size. As the emulsion is attached to the base by the subbing layer, the film curls with the emulsion side out (somewhat similar in principle to a heated bi-metallic strip). To prevent this, another layer of gelatine is coated on the non-emulsion side. This expands to the same degree as the emulsion layer, equalising the stresses and ensuring that the film stays flat.

Anti-halation layer

This is a coloured dye included in the gelatine of the anti-curl backing. In preventing *halation* it improves the resolution of the film. Halation, as shown in Figure 1.24, is caused by the reflection of light

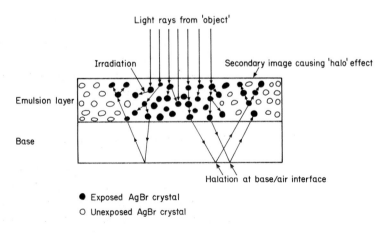

Fig. 1.24 Diagrammatic representation of halation and irradiation.

(which has already passed through the emulsion) at the boundary of the base with the air. If the angle of incidence is greater than the critical angle, the light may be reflected back and re-expose the emulsion layer. This produces a 'halo' unsharpness effect that reduces resolution. The density of the unsharp area is less than that of the true image.

The dyes used in anti-halo layers are the subject of stringent patent protection by manufacturers, and are designed to absorb light that passes through the base and into the anti-curl/halation layer. Their principle of operation is based on the colour complimentary process which, in simple terms, means if a certain colour light is passed through the correct colour filter, total absorption will take place and no light will pass through. In this context, therefore, halation cannot take place.

The anti-halo dye must be removed in processing, otherwise correct viewing of the image is not possible (due to light absorption from the viewing box). This is achieved in the fixing bath and requires no special alteration to the chemistry. However, removal of the dye takes considerably more 'energy' out of the fixer than the exposed AgBr does, resulting in the need for higher fixer replenishment rates in processors that are using large volumes of single-coated emulsions.

Irradiation

This produces an effect similar to that of halation and is caused by the lateral scatter of light within the emulsion layer. The reflection makes developable AgBr crystals that are outside the true edge of the image, producing a 'halo'-type effect after processing. As this is produced within the emulsion layer, the anti-halo backing will not prevent this effect (see Fig. 1.24).

Identification of emulsion side

Because of the factors considered in the previous section it is vital to be able to determine accurately the emulsion side of the film. This is to ensure that it is loaded into the cassette the correct way round, so it faces the 'object' to be imaged, e.g. so it always faces the TV monitor in a multiformat camera, or the screen in a single screen mammographic technique.

Identification of the emulsion side is achieved by the manufacturer cutting a small notch out of the edge of the film. When this notch is positioned in the top right or bottom left corner, the emulsion is facing the person handling the film. Contrary to popular opinion, it is not possible to determine accurately the emulsion side by trying to judge which side is matt or shiny, or by 'tasting' the corner of the film.

FILMS FOR SPECIALISED USE

The general structural features of films to be found in the X-ray department have already been discussed. Virtually all these films fall into the duplitised or single-coated emulsion catagories. In the following section, specific details of film characteristics according to their use is presented. It should be noted that a full understanding of these details requires some knowledge of sensitometry; the reader is referred to Chapter 2.

Monitor photography

Use

Imaging the video output from CT, MRI, and ultrasound units and other similar modalities, usually via a multiformat or other camera system (see Ch. 8, Monitor photography)

Example film

Agfa-Gevaert SCOPIX CR2B

Film type

Single-coated with anti-halo/curl backing

Base + fog

Density 0.15

Average gradient

$\bar{G}$ 1.4–2.0, depending on processing conditions

Speed

Dependent on processing and $\bar{G}$ required

D max

Density 2.6 approx.

Spectral sensitivity

Short orthochromatic. Peak sensitivity 540 nm approx. Cut-off sensitivity 560 nm approx.

Resolution

130 lp mm^{-1} approx.

Film formats

5 in. × 4 in. up to 35 cm × 43 cm, to suit imaging camera in use

Special features

Available in blue or clear base and high or low contrast for use in ultrasound, etc.

Cine radiography

Use

Cine recording of the output phosphor of a specialised image intensifier (usually in cardiography/cardiology departments)

Example film

Agfa-Gevaert SCOPIX RPIS

Film type

Single-coated

Base + fog level

Density 0.13

Average gradient

$\bar{G}$ 1.2–1.7. Variable to suit personal preference of cardiologist

Speed

Dependent on processing temperature and on $\bar{G}$ required

D max

2.5 Approx.

Spectral sensitivity

Long orthochromatic (see Fig. 1.8). Peak 550 nm. Cut-off 610 nm approx.

Resolution

At 10% MTF, 130 lp mm^{-1} approx.

Film formats

35 mm × 90 m rolls emulsion coated inside, 35 mm × 180 m rolls emulsion coated inside or outside. Cut and perforated to DIN standard 15501; negative perforation short pitch, and conforms to ANSI P.H. 2293

Special features

Also suitable for other applications of intensifier photography and photofluorography. Stable reciprocity characteristics at exposures between 0.001–1.0s

Image intensifier photography and photofluorography

Use

Recording the output phosphor of image intensifiers, especially those used for barium and associated techniques and mass mini-radiography

Example film

Agfa-Gevaert SCOPIX RPIS

Film type

Single-coated with anti-halo/anti-curl backing

Base + fog level

Density 0.15 approx.

Average gradient

Variable, depending on processing time and temperature, but usually between $\bar{G} = 2.0$ and $\bar{G} = 3.2$

Speed

Dependent on processing temperature and $\bar{G}$ required

D max

2.5 approx.

Spectral sensitivity

Short orthochromatic (see Fig. 1.8). Peak sensitivity 540 nm. Cut-off sensitivity 570 nm approx.

Resolution

At 10% MTF, 100 lp mm^{-1} approx.

Film formats

Available as sheet film (100 × 100 mm) or roll film, 70 mm × 45 m; 90 mm × 30 m; 105 mm × 45 m

Special features

Variable contrast to suit individual radiologist choice and stable reciprocity characteristics between 0.001–1.0s exposure.

Copy or duplicating film

Use

Producing exact copies in terms of size and density reproduction, by direct contact printing

Example film

Agfa-Gevaert Curix duplicating film

Film type

Pre-solarized single-coated with anti-halo/anti-curl backing

Base + fog level

Not appropriate for pre-solarized film

Average gradient

$\bar{G}$ = 1.0–1.5 but depends on spectral emission of exposing light source

Speed

Adjusted to suit most copiers on the market

D max

Density 2.5 approx.

Spectral sensitivity

Monochromatic but with peak sensitivity very much in the ultra-violet region of the spectrum, at 350 nm approx.

Resolution

Limited by the resolution of the original to be copied

Film formats

Available as sheet film, usually in a whole range of sizes from 35 × 43 cm to 18 × 24 cm

Special features

A pre-solarized film is unusual in that an increase in exposure received results in a decrease in density. The average gradient should be as close to 1 as possible, to ensure accurate reproduction of the 'object film's' density range (see Ch. 2 Sensitometry).

Holographic emulsions

A complete description of the characteristics of holographic emulsions is beyond the scope of this book; however, the essential features are as follows.

Holography involves the recording of interference patterns that have dimensions usually of the order of magnitude of the wavelength of light used for exposure, i.e. 10^{-9} m. This obviously involves film emulsions of extremely high resolution, but high speed is also required to allow short exposure times. However, as high speed and high resolution are not compatible properties, a compromise is made. The nature of the subject will determine whether high speed or high resolution is the most desirable property and a whole range of films is available to suit particular applications. In addition, different spectral sensitivities are essential to match the wavelength emission of the laser in use.

A typical holographic emulsion would be Agfa-Gevaert 10 E 75 Holotest material. This has high sensitivity, grain size of approximately 90 nm, resolution of 3000 lp mm^{-1} and is to be used with red light lasers.

SAFELIGHTS

Safe lights are a specialised application of optical filters. Their function is to provide a high level of 'darkroom' illumination without any detrimental effect on the sensitive material (film) that is being handled. They thus provide the darkroom worker with a more acceptable environment than working in complete darkness, although this is still sometimes necessary.

Safelights used in radiographic darkrooms come in two types, but both depend on the same principle of operation.

Principles of operation

Their basis of operation is the selective optical filtering of a white light source in such a manner that the film material being handled is subject only to wavelengths to which it is not sensitive.

The performance of a particular filter can be assessed by plotting the percentage of light transmitted through the filter at selected wavelengths throughout the visible spectrum; alternatively, due to the relationship between transmittance and density (see Ch. 2, Sensitometry), by plotting filter density at particular wavelengths. Because in practice film sensitivity and safelight performance are linked, it is traditional to superimpose the film spectrogram onto the safelight transmittance properties, as Figure 1.25 illustrates. This allows the user to see at a glance if any wavelength of the light transmitted is close to the spectral sensitivity of the film. The manufacturer will almost always recommend a suitable safelight for a particular film, but failing this a rough rule of thumb is: for monochromatic emulsions an orange safelight, for orthochromatic a dark red safelight, and

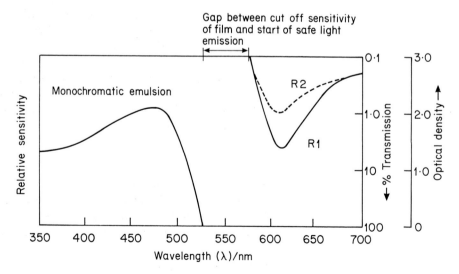

Fig. 1.25 Safelight transmission features versus film spectral sensitivity, showing a 'safe' combination with two different safelight filters: Agfa-Gevaert Rl and R2.

for panchromatic total darkness — but as ever, generalisations can be dangerous.

Factors affecting safelight peformance

The main factors affecting safelight performance are:

- Distance from the darkroom bench
- Wattage of the bulb
- Number and position of safelights
- Spectral emission features of the filters
- Safe handling time
- White light leakage.

Distance and bulb wattage

The recommended distance between the safelight and the working bench depends principally on the wattage of the bulb in the safelight. The higher the wattage, the further away it needs to be 'safe' (inverse square law applies).

For a direct ('beehive')-type safelight with a 25 W pearl tungsten filament bulb, the recommended closest distance is 1.2 m (4 feet); this may be reduced to 0.6 m (2 feet) if a 15 W bulb is used. In an indirect safelight, i.e. one that depends entirely on reflection from the walls and ceiling of the darkroom to provide illumination, bulb wattage may be up to 60 W, but careful testing must be carried out to ensure safety.

Number and position

The number of safelights governs the overall illumination of the dark-room. Darkrooms should not be 'dark'; they should have sufficient 'safe light' to be able to work without undue difficulty, commensurate with keeping the fog level on the film to a minimum. One indirect light for every 6 m^2 of ceiling area at a height of 2 m above floor level should be sufficient to provide a good general level of illumination. Specific areas of the bench can be specially illuminated by using a 'direct'-type safelight. Too many and/or badly positioned safe lights can have a significant effect on the base + fog level of the film, and can therefore influence image quality.

Spectral emission

The specific details are covered in principles of operation (above). However, the problem arises from 'mismatching' the spectral emission of the safelight with the sensitivity of the film, e.g. an orange safelight with an orthochromatic film emulsion.

White light leakage

A cracked or damaged filter or housing may be leaking minute amounts of white light, totally invisible to the naked eye but easily 'seen' by the film. At low intensity levels this would be more than sufficient to raise the base + fog level to an unacceptable degree.

Safe handling time

This is the length of time the film may be handled in normal safelight conditions without an increase in the base + fog level. In a general darkroom this should be approximately 45 seconds. All the factors listed above can affect this, therefore routine testing of the safe handling time should be undertaken. A test for this is included in Chapter 2, Sensitometry.

MANUFACTURING PROCESS

The manufacture of film is a complex physical and chemical process. A detailed understanding is not necessary, but a brief outline of the stages involved may help in the appreciation of topics such as photochemistry and sensitometry.

As stated previously, X-ray emulsions are mainly composed of silver bromide so we will now consider the manufacture of this material.

Silver bromide is produced in the following reaction:

$$AgNO_3 + KBr = AgBr + KNO_3$$

	(excess)		(insoluble)	(soluble)
silver nitrate	+	potassium bromide	= silver bromide	+ potassium nitrate

Emulsion manufacture can now be divided into seven stages:

- Emulsification
- Physical ripening
- Shredding
- Washing
- Chemical ripening
- Doctoring
- Coating.

These stages and the various imputs and extractions are illustrated in Figure 1.26. Many of these stages are under complex computer control to ensure accurate mixing and maintenance of temperatures, etc. Obviously all these processes must be carried out in complete darkness.

Emulsification

A mixture of gelatine and KBr is made in a large stainless steel vat to which is added the $AgNO_3$ solution, thus forming AgBr crystals. Continuous violent stirring ensures even mixing of the additives.

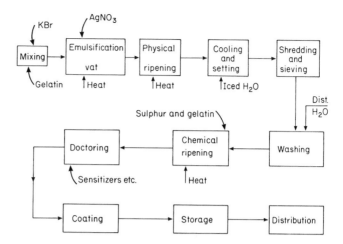

Fig. 1.26 Block diagram of the manufacturing process.

The temperature of the mixture and the rate of addition of the $AgNO_3$ solution determines the sizes of crystal produced, and varying the rate of addition has a strong effect on the contrast of the final emulsion.

Physical ripening

In this process the emulsion is stirred at a fixed temperature for a fixed length of time. This allows two processes to take place:

- Coalescence
- Ostwald ripening.

Both these processes allow an increase in the grain size of the mixture, causing an increase in sensitivity of the emulsion. Ostwald ripening is the more important of the enlargement stages, as it allows large grains to grow at the expense of the small grains. Many factors influence this stage of manufacture including temperature, pH, concentration, time of ripening and the amount of agitation.

At the correct moment the emulsion is allowed to set by placing the vat in iced water.

Shredding

The solidified emulsion is then chopped into small 'noodles' and passed through a sieve into the fourth stage of the process.

Washing

This removes from the emulsion the soluble KNO_3 and the excess KBr, which would otherwise degrade its performance. Distilled running water is used, and the process usually takes 1–2 hours.

Chemical ripening

This increases the sensitivity of the emulsion by encouraging the build-up of 'sensitivity centres' within individual AgBr crystals. This increases the speed of the emulsion but does not alter the size and shape of the AgBr crystals.

The shredded, washed emulsion is re-melted and a proportion of gelatine that has been specially produced with high levels of sulphur impurities is mixed in. This mixture is then left at a constant temperature for a certain length of time, at the end of which chemical ripening is complete.

Doctoring

This is the stage at which all necessary additions are made to the emulsion to vary its characteristics:

1. Sensitisers

These extend the spectral sensitivity of the emulsion from monochromatic to orthochromatic, panchromatic or infrared, as required.

2. Hardener

Makes the emulsion resistant to abrasions, etc.

3. Fungicide

Prevents the growth of bacteria and mould.

4. Wetting agent

Reduces surface tension and allows easy penetration of chemicals.

5. Plasticiser

Prevents the emulsion from becoming too brittle.

6. Anti-foggant

Improves the keeping properties of the film.

7. Anti-frothing agent

Prevents bubbles forming during coating.

The emulsion is now ready to be coated on to the base.

Coating

The emulsion is now coated on either side of a base by a mechanical process, giving a thin, even layer. Modern base materials are nearly always polyester for standard X-ray film. This is pre-prepared by adding a thin coating of pure gelatine to act as an adhesive for the emulsion. After coating it is chilled, to set the emulsion, and left to dry. The final stage in the coating process is to add another layer of

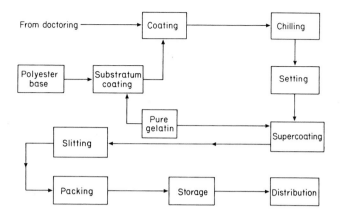

Fig. 1.27 Block diagram of the coating process.

gelatine, called the supercoat, which protects the emulsion. The coating process is summarised in Figure 1.27.

The roll of film is now ready for slitting and packing into suitable containers. After packing, the fresh film is usually allowed to 'stand' for a few weeks to allow the silver bromide to stabilise. It is then ready for normal use.

BIBLIOGRAPHY

Agfa-Gevaert Industrial radiography and holography. 21.7220 (1275). D.I.S. Division, Agfa-Gevaert, N.V. Mortsel, Belgium
Jacobson R E, Ray S F, Atteridge G G, Axford N R 1978 The manual of photography, 7th edn. Focal Press, London
James T H 1979 The theory of the photographic process, 4th edn. Collier Macmillan, London
Ulvarov E B, Chapman D R, Issacs A 1979 Penguin dictionary of science, 5th edn. Penguin, Harmondsworth

2

Sensitometry

Introduction

Sensitometry as a photographic science has been credited to two Americans, Hurter and Driffield, who first proposed a form of evaluation of the performance of photographic material in the late 19th century.

Sensitometry requires that the photographic emulsion be exposed to a specified light source for specified times and then the emulsion is processed under closely controlled conditions. The resultant densities produced on the film are then measured and graphed versus a logarithmic scale of the exposure. Historically the development of the light sources in sensitometry is very interesting indeed. The light sources have been as various as candles with specified burning rates, to lamps which have burnt amyl acetate, acetylene and paraffin. Nowadays the standard illuminant is an incandescent electrical light source of a specified brightness and spectral emission.

The main interest in radiography is how the film will react to (apparently) X-radiation, although usually the real interest is how the film will react to the light produced by the intensifying screens.

The exposure of the photographic emulsion to controlled exposures and controlled processing conditions is a fundamental of all photographic procedures. It is imperative that the student appreciates the relationships which are involved. Sensitometry can be made a very complex subject, but in its basic form it is an extremely easy subject to follow. The only proviso is that the student understands simple logarithmic relationships.

HOW TO DEDUCE DENSITY

Density is the basis of sensitometry, so the sensible way to approach the subject is to consider first of all the derivation of density. Density, of course, can be defined simply as the amount of blackening on the film. As a statement of fact this is correct. Mathematically, however, density is a logarithmic value. It may easily be obtained by deriving two simple ratios from Figure 2.1.

It is safe to say that no light-transmitting material is completely transparent; some light is always absorbed in its passage through the material. In Figure 2.1, the light travelling from the light source (the *incident* light) has been reduced in *intensity* as it passes through the X-ray film to the eye of the viewer (the *transmitted* light).

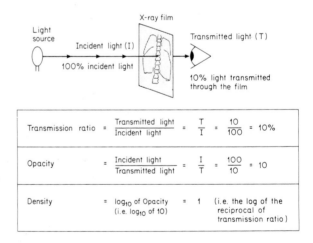

Fig. 2.1 Determining density.

Transmission ratio

The first ratio to obtain is the ratio between incident (I) and transmitted (T) light (expressed as T/I).

Using the figures above we will obtain the following:

T/I = 10/100 = 10%

The figure of 10% is known as the *transmission ratio*.

As can readily be seen, this figure would always be lower than 100%, for the simple fact that it would be impossible to have more light leaving the film than entered it.

The term *transmission ratio* is not used in radiography, but any reader who wears tinted prescription glasses will have heard the optician quote the percentage transmission tint required.

Opacity

The next ratio to consider is the reciprocal of the transmission ratio, i.e. I/T.

$$I/T = 100/10 = 10$$

The value 10 is known as the *opacity*.

This term suffers from drawbacks in its use. It will always be greater than unity and, as will be discovered, can reach quite high values. It is, again, a term which is not used (correctly) in radiography.

It is important to realise that in the examples above, simple integers are used. Both transmission ratio and opacity could be expressed to 2 or 3 significant figures, with the attendant problems of handling the mathematical sums when multiplication is involved. Additionally, both of the figures obtained from these ratios would prove difficult to illustrate graphically.

It is obviously easier to make a graphical representation of numerical values when the numbers are expressed as logarithms. This simple fact leads us to the derivation of density.

Density

Consider the value of 10, obtained for opacity. The log value of 10 is 1.0. This log value, 1.0, is the density of a film when the opacity is 10, or to express it another way:

Density is the log of the reciprocal of the transmission ratio.

There are some important relationships about density which are worth noting. These are shown in Figure 2.2.

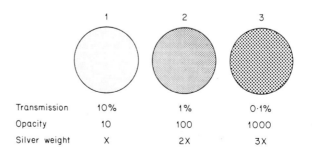

Fig. 2.2 Density: interrelation of silver weight, opacity and transmission.

It can be seen from Figure 2.2 that the silver weight of density on the processed film is related linearly to the blackening on the film, a factor which assumes great importance if films are being sold for silver recovery. Obviously a film with high densities (e.g. an extremity film) will contain significantly larger amounts of silver per unit area than, for example, a chest film.

Figure 2.2 also tells us a great deal about the interrelationships between these. values, pointing to the fact that opacity is going to reach very high numbers when the value of density is 4.

With a density of 4, opacity will be 10 000 and transmission ratio will be down to 0.01%. This demonstrates clearly the mathematical problems concerned. Opacity is increasing to very high numbers whereas transmission ratio is declining to very small numbers.

Perhaps the single most important fact to be gained from the figure is that only 1.0% of the incident light reaches the viewer's eye at density 2. In other words, 99% of the incident light is being absorbed by the film. This fact is worth bearing in mind as it has a great relevance later on.

In addition there are the following important points:

1. Density always increases with exposure (with *one* exception, *solarization*, see p. 72).

2. Density is related directly to silver weight. Bear in mind the relevance to silver recovery.

3. The eye responds to tonal changes logarithmically. This relationship can only be accidental, but it helps.

4. Density, because it is logarithmic, is very easy to manipulate mathematically. Density 1 + density 1 = density 2.

PRODUCTION OF THE CHARACTERISTIC CURVE

In various literature the characteristic curve will be called a D log E curve, an H and D curve (after Hurter and Driffield) or a log It curve. All of these terms refer to the same curve. To draw this curve, the axes are labelled as follows.

Density is represented on the vertical (y) axis of the graph. The horizontal (x) axis carries the (relative or absolute) logarithmic value of the exposure, sometimes called the relative log exposure axis, or the log It (i.e. intensity multiplied by time) axis (Fig. 2.3). Because it is a logarithmic value, it is easy to remember that each increase of log 0.30 represents a doubling of exposure, and each decrease of log 0.30 is equal to halving the exposure.

Having established what is represented by the axes of the graph, the question arises of how to produce the characteristic curve. There are a number of methods, each with their attendant advantages and drawbacks. Each will be considered in turn. It is assumed, for ease, that the initial curves will be produced using the simple relationship of doubling the exposure, usually for 11 steps.

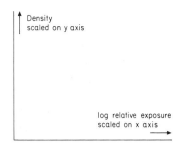

Fig. 2.3 Establishing axes for characteristic curve.

Time scale sensitometry

On the face of it, this is the easiest and the simplest way to produce a characteristic curve. In this case the kV, mA and distance are kept constant and the time of the exposure is varied, always by a factor of 2. This can be done either by simply doubling the time of exposure on the X-ray set, or by covering the cassette with lead rubber and exposing it section by section. In this case the first part exposed will have received the most exposure, the last part, the least. Eleven exposures are sufficient to provide enough points on the characteristic curve to plot a reasonable graph, although 21 would be ideal (this point is considered later in the chapter).

Intensity scale sensitometry

This could be carried out using the same procedure as time scale sensitometry except, in this case, the kV and distance would be constant but the mA values would be altered (i.e. constant time, varying mA).

Intensity scale sensitometry is more usually performed by varying the *height* of the tube in relationship to the film, using the inverse square law to perform the calculations to vary the intensity of the X-ray beam reaching the film. This technique requires great accuracy in the X-ray set and, of course, in the calculations and making of the measurements.

Calibrated step wedge

This method involves the use of an aluminium step wedge which has been calibrated in a specific way. The wedge should have a layer of copper on the base to help create a more homogeneous beam.

It is the calibration of this wedge which is most important; it also requires considerable expertise in the calculations for its construction. It has already been established that to produce a characteristic curve, we have to keep to a doubling of exposures between steps.

Many students feel that making a wedge with regular (i.e. 1, 2, 4, 8 cm increments) steps would give the same exposure increase, i.e.

halving the exposure. Unfortunately, this relationship does not hold because of the differential absorption of the aluminium. The wedge has to be very precisely calibrated so that each step on the wedge produces an exact and regular increase or decrease in exposure. If the wedge is made with these precise calibrations, which demand very high engineering tolerances, it can be a very useful device. Because of the stringent specifications, a large calibrated step wedge can be expensive.

Sensitometer

A sensitometer is simply an exposure device which prints a pre-exposed negative directly onto the film. A sensitometer merely simulates, as nearly as possible, the spectral emission of the intensifying screens in use in the department. Sensitometers exist in many forms, from simple three patch sensitometers to large (and expensive) 21 step negatives for printing.

Whichever one is chosen, care must be taken that the light output of the sensitometer matches the spectral sensitivity of the film. It

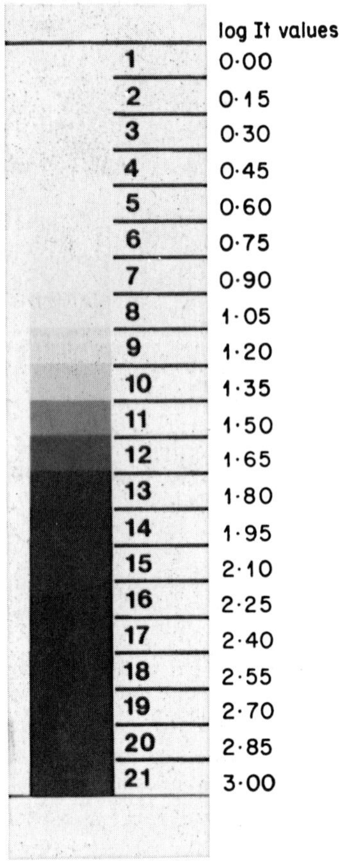

	log It values
1	0·00
2	0·15
3	0·30
4	0·45
5	0·60
6	0·75
7	0·90
8	1·05
9	1·20
10	1·35
11	1·50
12	1·65
13	1·80
14	1·95
15	2·10
16	2·25
17	2·40
18	2·55
19	2·70
20	2·85
21	3·00

Fig. 2.4 Typical sensitometer-produced 21 step wedge.

would be pointless to use a blue-emitting sensitometer with an orthchromatic (green sensitive) film. The result produced would be invalid. The sensitometer allows the users to prepare their own step wedges easily, but it must be checked regularly to make sure that the unit is performing correctly. Figure 2.4 shows the 21 step wedge produced by a typical sensitometer.

Pre-exposed step wedges

These are produced by a number of manufacturers, and are films which have been exposed by the manufacturer in a very accurate sensitometer. Much has been written about the use of these films. Some reports suggest that they are totally unsuitable, some suggest the opposite. It is sufficient to say that films used for this type of work should have stabilised latent image storage and will be usable (after the film has been stored for a while) for a short period of time. This is why this type of film has a very short 'shelf life', usually of the order of 6 months.

The reason that the films are stored before release is that immediately after exposure there can be a number of ways in which the latent image can react. It can begin to fade, or remain the same, or even, over a short period, intensify. To overcome these variations pre-exposed film is stored for a period before it is released. This factor must be taken into account when films are exposed in the department as well (hence the note under 'pros and cons'). It should be noted that some films cannot store a latent image for a long period of time. This is not a film fault, merely a design philosophy of that particular manufacturer.

Pros and cons

All of the methods outlined above have individual 'pros and cons'. Taking time scale sensitometry first, an immediate problem springs to mind.

It has already been established that 11 exposures, doubling exposure in between exposures, will be adequate to produce the curve. If we start with 0.1 s as the first exposure we end up with this series:

0.1, 0.2, 0.4, 0.8, 1.6, 3.2, 6.4, 12.8, 25.6, 51.2, 102.4

It can be seen immediately that the experimenter has to have either a unique timer on the X-ray set, or be an extremely accurate worker with a stopwatch. Of course, there is one other major problem. Using this range of exposures, or even one beginning with 0.01 s, *reciprocity failure* would almost certainly occur. After a timeconsuming and difficult test the result could well produce a curve which, in the higher densities, does not resemble a characteristic curve at all.

Reciprocity failure

This is sometimes referred to as the Swarzschild effect.

As long ago as 1876 two researchers, Bunsen and Roscoe, suggested that a relationship could be placed on E (effective exposure) and I (the light intensity) and t (the time of the exposure.) They expressed the relationship as:

$$E \propto It$$

Swarzschild then modified this formula in the late 1890s to:

$$E \propto Itp$$

where p was a constant for each emulsion, but varied from one emulsion to another.

Basically, these experimenters were discovering that a very long exposure to light does not produce the predicted blackening when related to a very short exposure time. The predicted reciprocity failure for a medical X-ray film would be a film which was stable at short exposure times, with an apparent loss of speed (less blackening) at very long exposure times. The only time a screen film encounters long exposure times to light is in the darkroom. Reciprocity failure at long exposures reduces the effect of long handling times in the darkroom safelight.

As Swarzschild had discovered, this effect can vary enormously between different makes of film, but all manufacturers try to ensure little or no reciprocity failure at normal exposure times in radiography. Modern theory of latent image formation can account for this effect far more readily.

It should be noted that this effect is only apparent where the exposure is due to light from the intensifying screens. With direct exposure to radiation, the X-ray quanta have such high energy, when compared to light, that they produce a latent image immediately in the silver halide grain.

Similar reciprocity problems could arise with intensity scale sensitometry. Also a very unusual X-ray set is required, as well as great accuracy in measurement.

With a calibrated step wedge, the same problems are not encountered. The step wedge can be made with any number of steps, as long as the accuracy has been observed in the specification and manufacture of the wedge, to produce accurate characteristic curves.

The sensitometer, as long as its performance is monitored regularly, has no inherent drawbacks. However, there is a common problem with all three systems.

It is most important that, after exposure, the films are processed at the same time interval after each test, for the test to be valid. Otherwise, due to varying latent image problems (outlined under Preexposed step wedges, p. 53), it is quite possible that very different results may be recorded for different timed 'inputs' into the processor.

One further point could be added here. In laboratory conditions it is always advised to process the films with the low densities entering the processor first. This is to avoid an effect, like bromide drag, causing streaking across the lower densities if high densities are entered first.

In the case of pre-exposed film, the main production drawbacks are overcome. However, one must consider the cost of the films and the fact that, of necessity, they are extremely short dated.

Number of steps

As mentioned before there are three common types of grey scale (or photographic step wedge) produced. They are:

1. The three patch wedge.
2. An 11 step wedge.
3. A 21 step wedge. Usually referred to as a root 2 wedge.

All have a role to play, but the 21 step wedge gives the best results as it gives the user a far better curve. The reason it is referred to as a root 2 wedge is that the difference between each exposure is the previous exposure multiplied by root 2, or 1.414. This fits onto the log It scale very well, as the log value of root 2 is 0.15 (see Fig. 2.5).

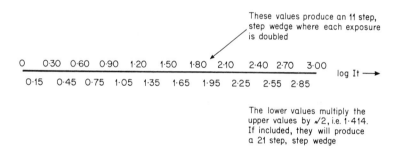

Fig. 2.5 Log It scale, calibrated for both 11 and 21 step wedge.

Calibration of a step wedge

Many X-ray departments have a step wedge, usually made from aluminium, which is used as a routine test tool but which produces totally arbitrary density steps. This step wedge can be calibrated quite easily as long as the department has access to a densitometer, an already calibrated step wedge or a pre-exposed step wedge film of known log It exposures.

The method is quite straightforward. With the calibrated step wedge in position and a piece of lead rubber covering an area on the film equal to the size of the uncalibrated step wedge, an exposure is made.

The uncalibrated step wedge is then placed on what was the

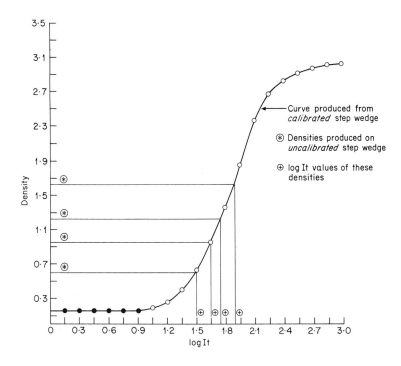

Fig. 2.6 Density values produced by uncalibrated step wedge measured against characteristic curve produced from calibrated step wedge, giving log It values of those densities.

covered area and lead rubber is used to cover all other portions of the same film. Another exposure is now made. The film is then processed.

A characteristic curve is then drawn from the results obtained from the calibrated step wedge. The density values produced by the *uncalibrated* step wedge are now measured. Intercepts are then drawn from each of these density values to the curve and then to the log It axis. These log It values represent the actual values for this step wedge at the kV selected (Fig. 2.6).

INFORMATION FROM THE CHARACTERISTIC CURVE

A great deal of information can be gained from the characteristic curve. The main areas, illustrated in Figure 2.7, are as follows:

1. From 0 to point 1, *Basic fog.*
2. Point A, *Threshold* and from A to B the *Toe.*
3. From point B to C, the *Straight line portion.*
4. The area around D, the *Shoulder.*
5. Point E, *Maximum density.*
6. From F onwards, the *Region of solarisation.*

The best way to evaluate the curve is to look at it section by section.

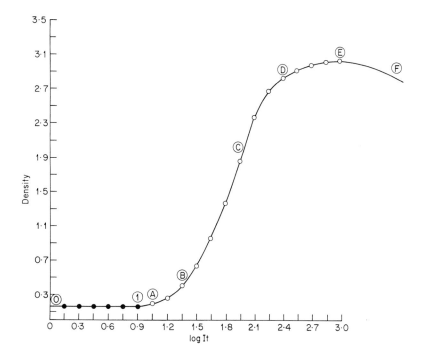

Fig. 2.7 Characteristic curve, illustrating main points of interest.

Basic fog (from 0 to 1)

This section of the curve is often referred to as 'base plus fog' or 'basic fog' (either version is correct). It merely refers to the recorded density of the base, which may be tinted blue for example, plus the recorded density of the chemical fog which may have built up in the emulsion during storage, etc.

An overall increase in basic fog can affect many other measurements on the characteristic curve. How and why basic fog can increase overall is well worth while considering in depth. The following list of causes is fairly comprehensive, but students may like to try and find more. The list has been subdivided into three areas:

1. Faults that can occur in storage.
2. Faults that can occur in the department or darkroom.
3. Faults that can occur in processing.

1. Storage

1. Too long a time in storage

All films have a 'shelf life'. Increased storage time allows chemical fog to build up to sometimes unacceptable levels. Non-screen films fog faster than screen films.

2. Temperature too high

About 10 °C (50 °F) is required for prolonged storage. High temperatures accelerate the aging process.

3. Humidity too high

The relative humidity should be 50%. High humidity, in unprotected boxes, can lead to the film continuing ripening whilst in storage.

4. Films stored horizontally

Films should be stored vertically. If they are stored horizontally then pressure marks are inevitably created on the lowest films.

5. High background radiation

The recommended level of background radiation is 7 $\mu r/h$. The effect of background radiation leads to a linear increase in basic fog.

6. Fumes

A great many fumes can fog film. They are almost too numerous to mention, but a few examples are carbon monoxide, certain paint fumes, formalin, formaldehyde, and mercury vapour.

7. Scattered radiation

It is wise to keep a film store well away from an X-ray room, even if the protection is considered adequate.

2. Darkroom

Many sources of fogging can be found in a darkroom, many of them connected with safelights.

1. Incorrect safelight

If an orange filter is used with orthochromatic film, the film will fog on exposure to the safelight. There is a simple way of remembering safelight colours (see Fig. 2.8). The safest separation should always be two colours away from the maximum sensitivity of the film.

2. Too long handling time

See safelight test, p. 69.

3. Too many Safelights

No explanation is really needed. See Safelight test, p. 61.

4. Safelights too close

About 1 m is the closest that should be considered.

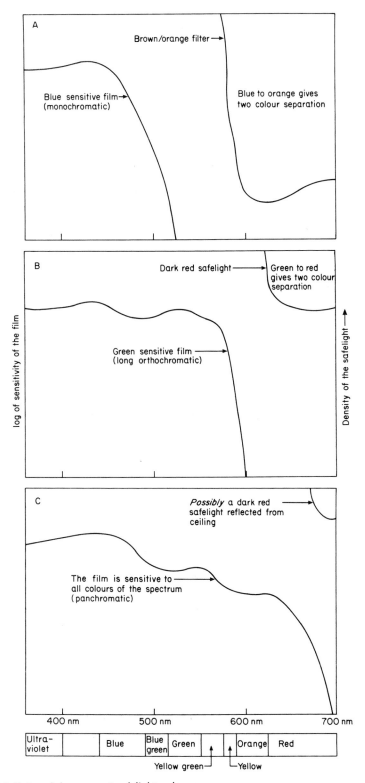

Fig. 2.8 Determining correct safelight colours.

5. Too bright safelights

With a tungsten bulb in the safelight, the maximum wattage should be 25 W.

6. Cracked safelights

A regular check of safelights will obviate this problem.

7. Light leakage

White light of low intensity striking the film in a darkroom can produce an overall fog.

3. Processing

Detailed references to all these faults will be found in Chapter 3, Photochemistry.

1. Over-replenishment

Over-replenishment causes unselectivity.

2. Too high developer temperature

Again, this causes unselectivity.

3. Too long a processing time

Again causes unselectivity. *No* developer is totally selective, all developers will eventually develop every silver halide grain.

3. Contamination

If developer is contaminated by fixer, then basic fog will begin to rise. Eventually, an overall grey film will result, with a density around 1.0. Long before this happens there will be a smell of ammonia. This is the *only* time in the photographic process when ammonia can be smelt.

The only action that can be taken is to drain the developer tank, wash it out thoroughly and start again. Note that fixer contamination of developer can be measured in parts per million.

Fixer

It is also important to remember that fixer can cause an overall increase in basic fog.

1. Temperature

Fixing time is directly related to the temperature of the fixer. If the fixer becomes too cold, perhaps because a heater has broken down in the processor, the film may be only partially fixed. This can result in an overall fog on the film. Of course, the film will not store for a long period and the image will deteriorate rapidly.

2. Time

If a film is in the fixer for too short a time, the result will be exactly as listed under fixer temperature.

3. Under-replensihment

This causes non-fixation of the film. The results are identical to those produced in 1 and 2.

As was said earlier, the above causes are by no means exhaustive. It may be of interest to compile other causes which can produce this result.

It will be seen that increases in basic fog play a very important part in the characteristic curve, as it affects many of the measurements made.

Threshold (point A) and Toe (point A to B)

It is at this point that the film first shows a reaction to exposure; to put it another way, the film could be exposed to an amount of radiation as measured on the log It axis and still show no response. Threshold has a relevance in safelight testing, where the film has to receive a 'flash exposure' to take the film past threshold, before commencing the test. This explains why film is so much more sensitive to mishandling after exposure, i.e. after it has been sensitised. The Toe is an area of rapidly increasing gradient.

Safelight test

In a normal darkroom, the handling time of the film in safelight will be of the order of 45 seconds to a minute. It therefore follows that all safelight tests should at least achieve this sort of time scale.

First of all, the film to be tested should be removed from the hopper in *total darkness*. The film is then given the flash exposure which will take it past threshold, to a density of about 0.6. This action has now sensitised the film and reproduces the normal film use. A degree of practice is needed to achieve this result using white light. If necessary, the film can be loaded into a cassette and an exposure of 5 mAs and 40 kV, with a class 100 system will produce a satisfactory exposure.

The next stage is to place about six coins on the film. The safelights are now switched on and the coins are removed at 10 second intervals.

The safelights are now switched off and the film is processed. As a precaution, another film can be used as a control. This film is removed from the hopper in total darkness and processed along with the test film. When the test film is viewed there may be an image of coins, or only one coin, on the film. If it is the fifth coin, then the safe handling time is 50 seconds.

If this time is considered insufficient, then the safelights should be re-examined and perhaps steps should be taken to remove, or adjust the position of, some of them.

The straight line portion (from B to C)

It is immediately obvious when looking closely at the curve (Fig. 2.7) that there is no 'straight line' portion. The curve on medical X-ray screen film resembles more of an elongated 'S'. However, the name remains, and most students recognise it instantly. It is this section of the characteristic curve which carries a very large amount of information.

Note: The following description of the derivation of Gamma on an X-ray screen film contravenes all the rules of teaching. The description is *wrong*. It should be read very carefully by the student, as it is included to make a very serious point. Gamma does *does not exist* as described below, *on a medical screen film*. It only exists at the point of inflexion. The geometry is correct, it is merely the appliction which is wrong.

Gamma and its other derivatives

At this point it is impossible to deal with the topic until a little geometry is involved. Looking at Figure 2.9, consider the derivation of the tangent of angle A.

$$\left[\frac{\text{Opposite}}{\text{Adjacent}}\right] = \frac{\text{Side } y}{\text{Side } x} = \text{Tangent of angle A}$$

If this triangle is superimposed over the characteristic curve in the region of the straight line portion, it can be seen that a measurement of the slope of the curve can be made.

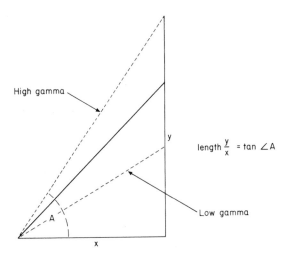

High gamma

length $\frac{y}{x}$ = tan $\angle$A

Low gamma

A

Fig. 2.9 Determining Gamma.

It is important to appreciate that the angle of this slope, when expressed as a tangent, is exactly equal in numerical terms to the Gamma. It also follows that the larger the angle, i.e. the steeper the slope, the higher the Gamma. This means, in photographic terms, that the film will have a higher contrast. The exact opposite is also true; the smaller the angle, the less steep the slope, the lower the overall contrast.

If there had been a true straight line section, the triangle could have been superimposed exactly. Unfortunately, on medical X-ray screen film there is no straight line. In fact the curve represents more of a flattened 'S'. Therefore, an estimate has to be made of where the straight line portion is, and this will vary from individual to individual. An estimate is clearly unsatisfactory, therefore a better method has to be used.

True Gamma

It is usually said that Gamma (identified by the Greek letter γ), is not found on medical X-ray screen film. To be strictly accurate, it can be found at the point of inflexion of the curves and, as can easily be seen, will be the highest contrast available on the curve (Fig. 2.10).

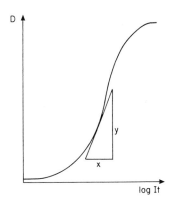

Fig. 2.10 Gamma is recognised as the maximum gradient exhibited by a characteristic curve and is equal to the slope of the straight line portion of the characteristic curve. However, a modern X-ray emulsion does not have a straight line portion to the curve and we cannot adopt the measurement. To be pedantically accurate, the Gamma for a curve without a straight line portion is measured at the point of inflexion of the curve, i.e. at the intersection of the increasing and decreasing point of the slope.

Average gradient (or average Gamma)

Usually denoted by $\bar{G}$. Again, a triangle has to be constructed using the same principles as in Gamma but now two defined points, *net density* 0.25 and *net density* 2.0, are used to construct the triangle (Fig. 2.11).

With this measurement of the slope we gain the true value of the

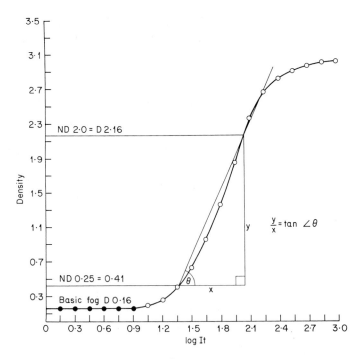

Fig. 2.11 Determining average gradient ($\bar{G}$).

average contrast available in the straight line portion of the characteristic curve.

Net density is simply defined as 'the density required plus basic fog'. It is a means of equalising the results on varying types and standards of films by asking, for example, 'what amount of energy is required to raise this film to net density 1?'. If one film has a basic fog of 0.6 and another film has one of 0.18, unless net density were used the first film would appear to be much faster (Fig. 2.12).

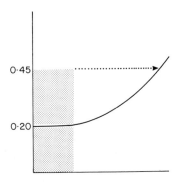

Fig. 2.12 Net density is that density which the film achieves solely by actinic radiation. Therefore, when determining a net density the amount of basic fog present on the film must be taken into account.

The basic fog present is 0.20; the net density required is 0.25. The basic fog and the net density are added (0.20 + 0.25) and the measurement is made at 0.45.

But why are 0.25 and 2.0 chosen as the points on the curve to establish average gradient? Consider the derivation of transmission ratio for a moment. Only 1.0% of the incident light reaches the viewer's eye at density 2. On the average viewing box (if such a thing exists!) there is simply not enough light emitted to penetrate through density 2. Hence the choice of density 2.

But why 0.25? The higher the slope of the curve the higher the contrast, the lower the slope the lower the contrast. If an average value is taken of the contrast available in the toe of curve it will be extremely low indeed. As the eye can only discern differences in contrast of about 10% it becomes obvious that there is simply insufficient contrast available much below net density 0.25. Hence the choice of 0.25. These are also the values of the maximum and minimum useful densities.

Variants

The two points used to measure average gradient mentioned will vary with the type of material used, as the curves will vary considerably according to film type. The following film types require the different values shown, to measure average gradient.

Cinefluorography	0.25 and 1.25 + basic fog
Image intensifier	0.25 and 1.75 + basic fog
Monitor photography	0.25 and 1.75 + basic fog
Photofluorography	0.25 and 2.0 + basic fog
Film/screen techniques	0.25 and 2.0 + basic fog

It is worthwhile to stop here and make a brief résumé of what has been said so far.

1. The tangent of the angle the slope makes is numerically equal to the average gradient.
2. The value of this tangent tells us the average value of contrast available with in the straight line portion.
3. The steeper the slope, the higher the contrast and vice versa.
4. Two points are used to construct the triangle, net density 0.25 and net density 2.0 for screen films.

But what practical use is there in knowing the value of the average gradient? One simple formula is all that is needed to put this question into perspective.

Image contrast = subject contrast × average gradient

The above formula spells out the fact that the final contrast seen on the film is a result of the initial subject contrast multiplied by the average gradient. Consider the two films in Figure 2.13. With an average gradient of 2.5 for film A (a good average value), there is an amplification of the subject contrast by a factor of 2.5.

Subject contrast is very difficult to arrive at absolutely and some explanation may be necessary. It means that a curve has to be drawn and then the maximum and minimum values of mAs (as log It values)

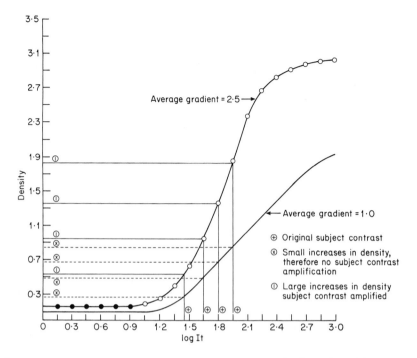

Fig. 2.13 Average gradient for two films, showing potential effect of amplification of subject contrast.

passing through the body areas are assessed. The intercepts are then drawn from these points to the curve and then to the density axis. With an average gradient of 2.5, large increases of density are produced, *in the region of useful exposure*, for relatively low increases in exposure.

With a very low average gradient of 1.0 with film B (which incidentally is an unusable value in medical radiography), the image contrast is equal to the subject contrast, no amplification of contrast is possible. Now, only small increases in density are produced for the same increases in exposure as were used with film A.

The value of the average gradient is not the only information which can be gained from this section of the curve. Information on the useful exposure range, speed and latitude is readily available.

Useful exposure and density range

This is the ideal way to consider exposure latitude. If the full characteristic curve is constructed and then two vertical lines drawn from the intercepts of the two net densities, the useful exposure range for the film can then be determined.

In the case of Figure 2.14, the log It axis of the curve is intercepted at 1.36 and 2.05. If this axis is considered as a log relative exposure axis, the figures will seem to be fairly arbitrary. It becomes clearer if the log It axis is considered to be the *absolute* value of mAs at a certain kV and that these values have been used to plot the curve.

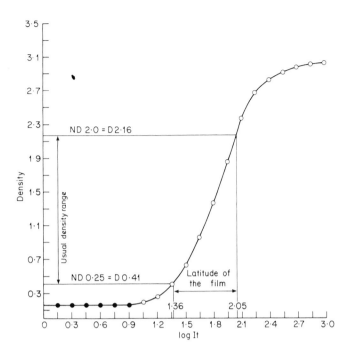

Fig. 2.14 Usual exposure and density range

Incidentally, the mAs values were obtained by taking the antilogs of each log It value on the scale.

Absolute values as an example

log It 0 = 1 mAs
log It 0.30 = 2 mAs
log It 0.60 = 4 mAs
log It 0.90 = 8 mAs
log It 1.20 = 16 mAs
log It 1.50 = 32 mAs
log It 1.80 = 64 mAs
log It 2.10 = 128 mAs
log It 2.40 = 256 mAs
log It 2.70 = 512 mAs
log It 3.00 = 1024 mAs

Note that these values have been taken as actual mAs values of log It. However, the relationship between exposures for these log It values always remain the same.

As these values are now assumed to be the *actual* mAs values at a certain kV, the useful range of exposures would be between 23–112 mAs at that particular kV.

These figures were obtained by finding the antilog of 1.36 and 2.05 respectively. On the scale showing actual mAs values as an example, 1.36 will equal 23 mAs and 2.5 will equal 112 mAs.

Below an exposure of 23 mAs actually reaching the film, a very low density film would be obtained. Above 112 mAs reaching the film, a very black film would be obtained. Both of these exposures would not utilise the film correctly. In the first example, exposures will have been made in the toe area of the curve, whereas in the second example, exposures were made in the shoulder. In both cases, the exposures would have been made outside the straight line portion of the curve. It might therefore be better to consider that the straight line portion is more correctly named 'the region of useful exposure'. This exposure latitude is irrevocably linked to the average gradient of the film. The higher the average gradient, the lower the latitude of the film. The lower the average gradient, the higher the latitude.

This knowledge is of particular use when setting up automatic exposure devices, so that they can be triggered to stop when the exposure has reached the mid-point of the curve. Usually, however, the log It axis is used merely to refer to the relationship between the exposures. For example, starting with 6 mAs as log It 0, then log It 1.20 will be 96 mAs, etc. This figure is obtained as follows:

log It 0   =   6 mAs
log It 0.3 = 12 mAs
log It 0.6 = 24 mAs
log It 0.9 = 48 mAs
log It 1.2 = 96 mAs

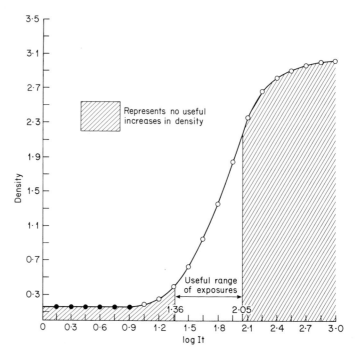

Fig. 2.15 Small increases in exposure in the useful exposure range will increase density appreciably; above net density 2.0 and below net density 0.25, only small or non-existent gains in density are made for the same increases.

Similar relationships exist across the log It scale. It only means remembering that log It 0.3 is equal to doubling (or halving) the exposure.

It can be seen from the above explanations that only in the region of useful exposure are almost linear gains made in density increase. Below the intercept from net density 0.25, there are small or non-existent gains in density. Above the intercept of net density 2.0, similar small gains are made for the same increase in exposure. It is only in the useful range of exposures that large density gains are made *for the same increases in exposure* (see Fig. 2.15).

Latitude of the film

The region of useful exposure can be used to define the latitude of the film. Looking at Figure 2.14 we can see the useful exposure range which will also tell us the amount of under-or overexposure the film will tolerate. In other words it defines the 'getawayability' of the film.

Speed

If a 35 mm film is purchased for a camera, it is easy to determine the speed of the film by the ISO number: the higher the number, the faster the film. This is not so easy with X-ray film.

To define the speed of an X-ray film can sometimes be difficult. Consider the curves illustrated in Figure 2.16. Note that two of these

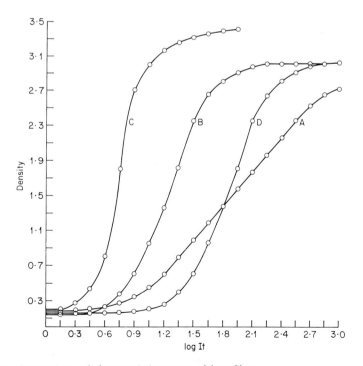

Fig. 2.16 Comparison of characteristic curves of four films.

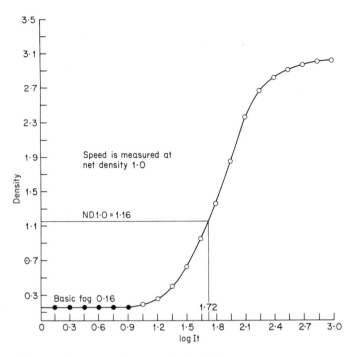

Fig. 2.17 Film speed is measured at net density 1.0.

films (C and A) are unusable in an X-ray department as screen films. Film C has an unusable latitude and film A has an average gradient of 1.0 (see under Variants, p. 65). Films B and D are almost identical, apart from speed differences.

One film must be faster than another, if it reaches a certain density with a lower exposure than the other film. Considering films B and C, film C is obviously the fastest film because it reached density 1 well before film B. However, films A and D create a different problem. A is faster than D below density 1.35, and slower than D above density 1.35.

It is usual to say simply that the further over to the left the curve lies, the faster the film. This is, of course, absolutely true, but the statement remains a simple statement. In the case of films A and D it has to be qualified, by adding 'above or below a certain density'.

In the ANSI (American National Standards Institute) specifications, X-ray film speed is defined as the exposure required for the film to reach net density 1 (see Fig. 2.17).

If this fact is now transferred to Figure 2.16, it can be seen that:

Film A has a speed of log It 1.67
Film B has a speed of log It 1.14
Film C has a speed of log It 0.68
Film D has a speed of log It 1.73.

This fact can be extremely useful when films are being compared using an accurate exposure device. It provides a very accurate figure

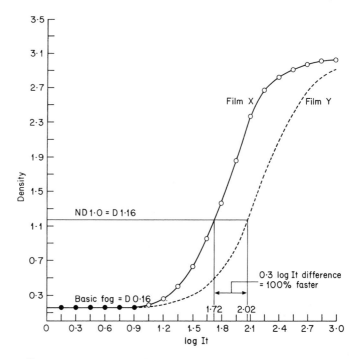

Fig. 2.18 Full sensitometric curves of two films, allowing speed to be compared.

which can be expressed in percentage terms (e.g. 25% faster) or in log It exposure differences. For example, if full sensitometric curves are produced, the speed of both films may be measured and compared, as shown in Figure 2.18.

In this case the films are separated by a log It difference of log It 0.3. This means that film X is 100% faster than film Y, i.e. film Y requires twice the exposure of film X, or within the range 50–80 kV, there is a 10 kV difference in speed. Thus, absolute values can be found for differences in film speed.

It might be instructive for the reader to discover for him-or herself why 0.10 log It difference in speed does not represent a 33% increase or decrease in exposure. Remember that log values are being dealt with.

When speed comparisons are made in the X-ray department, the measurements are usually comparative. In this case the two films to be tested are placed in the same cassette and an exposure is made through a step wedge. (Incidentally, it is not necessary for this wedge to be calibrated.) It is then easy to see which film produces the higher densities for the same exposure through the wedge. In which case, the film producing the highest density at the same step is the fastest.

A similar type of test can also be used to compare screens. In this case the step wedge exposure would be made on the two cassettes to be tested, ideally with the wedge covering the two cassettes so that only the one exposure is required. The films may then be compared in the way described above for density differences. Of course, complete sensitometry can be undertaken and very accurate figures obtained by measuring the actual log It differences.

Shoulder (area around point D)

It is at this point that the film's reaction to exposure begins to fall off. In the straight line portion of the curve, large increases in density were achieved by relatively small increases in exposure.

In the shoulder of the curve, the density increases are very small indeed for the same increases in exposure. Eventually, the curve begins to flatten completely and it is at this point that D max, or maximum density, is reached.

Maximum density (point E)

This name speaks for itself. It is the maximum density which can be reached on the film, under this set of exposure and processing conditions. Very often it is referred to as Max D, or D max.

Region of solarisation (point F onwards)

At this point on the characteristic curve, the density on the film begins to *decrease* for increases in exposure, i.e. a reversal image can be obtained.

To reach this area on the film a large amount of overexposure is required, usually of the order of several thousands of times.

It is caused by the silver halide grain not being able to absorb any more energy and the grain beginning to re-associate into the silver bromide, instead of breaking down into silver and bromine ions.

Solarisation is sometimes observed on X-ray films in the department. It is safe to say it is never caused by direct overexposure, but may be the result of prolonged exposure to safelight after exposure in the X-ray room.

The phenomenon of solarisation is used in the manufacture of copying films. In this case the desired effect is that the film should react so that any light areas are produced as light areas and dark areas as dark. If ordinary X-ray film was used to make a copy, the light areas would be reproduced as dark areas. When the film is manufactured as a solarised film, pre-solarisation is produced, usually, by chemical means.

SPEED vs DEFINITION

This section of the text should be read in conjunction with Chapter 7, Image Quality, as the information in that chapter is apposite to the area under discussion. In Chapter 7, reference is made to the way in which the image quality can be affected by a change in the speed of the film. The illustrations of the arrowhead (Fig. 7.12) explain in detail how the resolution, and hence the image quality, can be altered. The essential conclusion arrived at is that the faster the film, the worse the definition (this, of course, implies the use of similar emulsions).

Quantum mottle

Much has been written about quantum mottle, which is really a phenomenon which interferes with diagnosis and appears as marked 'graininess' on the film. It is directly related to the dose (mAs) reaching the film, i.e. the lower the dose the higher the quantum mottle and vice versa.

It should be said that the illustrations for quantum mottle were produced using a random number generator to position the 'quanta'. On a macroscopic scale it could be said that they fairly represent actuality.

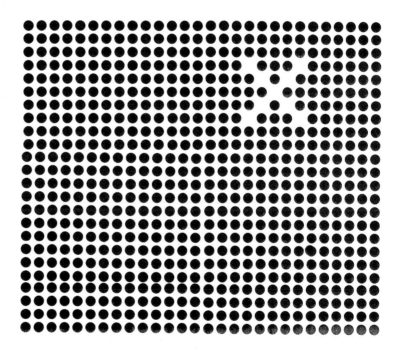

Fig. 2.19 X-ray quanta striking film (theoretical representation).

In Figure 2.19, the dots represent X-ray quanta arriving at the film. The figure also illustrates the perfect world, which does not exist. X-ray quanta do not arrive evenly at the film, but vary randomly over the film surface. Nevertheless, the shape of an 'X' can be clearly seen.

Figure 2.20 represents reality. Exactly the same number of quanta are present, but they are now striking the film randomly. Statistically, with high levels of irradiation the quanta are scattered fairly evenly over the film surface. Because of this high level of irradiation, the image can still be clearly seen.

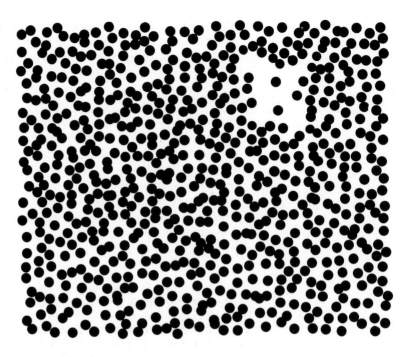

Fig. 2.20 X-ray quanta striking film (representation of reality, with quanta striking film randomly).

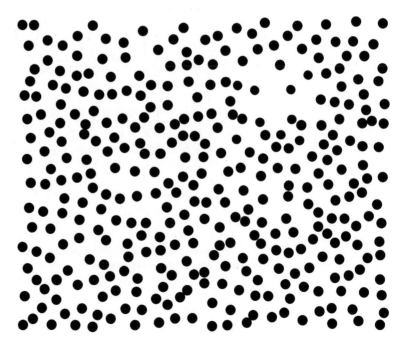

Fig. 2.21 X-ray quanta striking film, half exposure of Fig. 2.20.

With half the exposure, only half the quanta are available (Fig. 2.21). Now the image is not clearly rendered, as the randomness of the quanta landings produces marked variations of density over the film. The dose is now so low that the film now begins to record individual quanta and the apparent 'grain' (the record of the single quanta) begins to appear.

It does not take much imagination to realise that exposures can be so low that only individual quanta will be recorded, insufficient even to record an image. It has been suggested by many sources that quantum mottle is the factor which limits the ultimate speed of any film/screen system.

Quantum mottle, therefore, has an effect similar to an increase of film speed, in that it reduces the ultimate definition of the system by increased graininess. The effects of both the speed of the film and quantum mottle are similar, but the causes are very different.

CONCLUSIONS

Sensitometry is a part of photography which, if well understood, can give the user a great deal of information about the behaviour of film, screens and the automatic processor within the department. It also plays a major part in a quality assurance programme (see Ch. 6).

Anyone using a video imager (see p. 271) is well advised to be familiar with sensitometry so as to gain the best quality images from the imager.

The principal uses of sensitometry are:

1. To compare different types of film.
2. To compare different types of screens.
3. Useful tool for setting up exposure devices.
4. To determine average gradient, and therefore subject contrast amplification.
5. To find film and exposure latitude.
6. To find the absolute value of the speed of films.
7. To monitor the performance of an automatic processor.

There is, finally, one extremely important point to remember:

The characterisic curve is only valid under a certain set of processing conditions.

Any alteration of processing conditions in terms of speed of throughput, changes in temperature, changes in chemistry, etc., can drastically alter any results.

3
Photochemistry

Introduction

Photochemistry is a complex topic requiring a vast amount of specialist knowledge and experience. However, an empirical appreciation does not have to draw on complex formulae or physical principles and can be gained with logical reference to a few simple chemical ideas.

The topic in its widest sense covers everything from the chemistry used in holographic films and processing to that used in the production of holiday colour slides. It is not generally appreciated that advances in these fields and associated camera topics led us to the mass production of the silicon chip. Historically, photochemistry was a somewhat haphazard affair, with many discoveries made completely by accident and many hazardous processes, including the use of mercury vapour as a developer, as common practice.

As far as we are concerned, photochemistry can conveniently be divided into five sections:

1. The latent image and its formation
2. Development process
3. Fixation process
4. Washing
5. Silver conservation.

Obviously all these topics are highly interrelated, not only with themselves but also with the chemistry of the film emulsion, the required sensitometric characteristics of the film and the automatic processor.

THE FORMATION OF THE LATENT IMAGE

Introduction

The production of the latent image is the first stage of the photochemical process. It is here that all the information eventually seen is recorded as minute changes in the silver bromide crystal. These changes are so small that even an electron microscope reveals no difference between an exposed crystal and an unexposed crystal, and only development will show which is which. Even with modern computer techniques of image manipulation, if the information is not in the latent image no further 'processing' will increase or reveal more detail, although it may improve certain areas of particular interest.

Definition

The dictionary definition of latent is literally 'hidden'. However, this literal 'hidden image' translation is inadequate; it is more formally defined as 'the image produced on the film after exposure but prior to development'. The exposure need not be useful exposure, as in the production of a radiograph; it may be from any source that is sufficient to produce the minute changes within the silver bromide crystal necessary to render the crystal developable.

An understanding of latent image formation is important as it allows:

- A full understanding of the development and fixation process.
- A better appreciation of the factors governing quality, e.g. resolution, basic fog, etc.
- An increased appreciation of the effects of X-radiation and light in relation to exposure and the final result.

Emulsion and silver bromide

The emulsion is a suspension of silver bromide and certain impurities in gelatine. The nature of the silver bromide is, however, somewhat unusual, as will be appreciated later. In the laboratory silver bromide is made in the following reaction:

$$AgNO_3 + KBr \rightarrow AgBr + KNO_3$$

i.e., Silver nitrate + potassium bromide gives silver bromide + potassium nitrate.

The silver bromide produced in this way is what is known as a univalent ionic cubical lattice (Fig. 3.1). It has a structure similar to that of common salt, and after the initial formation of the cube shape grows simply by the addition of further ions of silver and bromine (i.e. Ag^+ ions and Br^- ions).

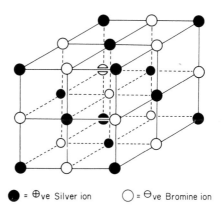

$\bullet$ = $\oplus$ve Silver ion $\bigcirc$ = $\ominus$ve Bromine ion

Fig. 3.1 Cubical silver bromide crystal lattice.

Unfortunately, if this reaction is carried out in light the silver bromide immediately dissociates, turning the solution black (the silver bromide has effectively been exposed). There is another problem associated with this reaction; the perfect crystal formed in this process is of no use photographically, as it exhibits none of the properties necessary for the formation of the latent image. In practice, therefore, the reaction is carried out in the gelatine suspension medium with excess amounts of potassium bromide.
In practice:

$$AgNO_3 + KBr(excess) \rightarrow AgBr + KNO_3$$
In gelatine   Suspended in gelatine
(Reaction carried out in total darkness)

Effects of gelatine

Gelatine is obtained from the skins of dead animals, and occasionally from ligaments and bones, by the hydrolysis of the collagen fibres that are present in such skins. Fortunately, from the photographic point of view, these fibres possess four principal features that are important in the formation of the latent image.

1. Chemical impurities

Photographic quality gelatine has had all the impurities removed from it before it reaches the production stage. However, this purification removes not only useless substances but also very useful ones. These useful substances are compounds of sulphur which form silver sulphides (AgS) and produce 'active' areas within the silver bromide crystals. It is therefore necessary to carefully add controlled amounts of sulphur to give the film its required latent image characteristics.

2. Physical defects in the crystal lattice structure

These are very significant in the production of the latent image, as they establish so-called electron traps within the lattice structure (see below).

3. Provides suitable growth medium

The reaction for the production of silver bromide is carried out in gelatine. Gelatine has the property of being able to keep forming and growing nuclei of silver bromide apart, thus allowing crystals to grow without impinging on each other. This allows fine control of emulsion grain size.

4. Suspension and binder agent

Gelatine also acts as a suspension and binding agent for silver bromide when it is coated onto the film base and, fortunately, is totally inert even with prolonged storage. It is also thought that it prevents re-association of the silver and bromide ions released by exposure.

Electron traps

These are the main factors involved in latent image production, and they consist of areas of 'low energy' within the crystal lattice. Initially they are termed 'shallow', but they can be 'deepened' by various means and this deepening can be significant in the later stages of the latent image process.

'Shallow' traps are of two kinds:

1. Neutral colloids from impurities

These have two effects:

- Deepen electron traps, thus increasing stability in the early stages of image formation
- Consume certain photo by-products.

2. Defects in crystal lattice

These defects are called kinks and jogs, and are areas of crystal lattice fracture where the full bonding potential between two ions is not used but stored between two or more points (as in Fig. 3.2). They are mainly formed by growing crystals coming into contact with each other. This produces forces within the crystal lattice causing the crystals to break up and produce 'free' lattice chains. These free chains possess ions that are not completely neutralised by their opposite ion and attempt to share their charge with adjacent points on the structure (point 'b' in Fig. 3.2). At this point the electrical potential of the crystal differs and an area of 'low energy' is produced. There are many such areas in a single crystal and these are the most significant factor in electron trap production.

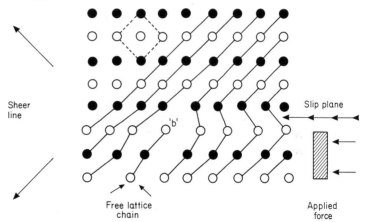

Fig. 3.2 Production of crystal lattice defects.

Effects of excess potassium bromide

The reaction to produce silver bromide is carried out in excess potassium bromide. This produces two main beneficial effects:

1. Alters crystal shapes

This has the advantage of producing more crystal defects and consequently more electron traps.

2. Increases surface barrier of individual crystals

This surface potential barrier is produced to protect individual crystals against unselective developers and certain other by-products of exposure and processing. It consists of a barrier of bromine ions (Br$^-$) that collect at the surface of the crystal. Excessive potassium bromide ensures an adequate supply of these ions as the crystal is formed.

Free interstitial silver ions

These are positively charged silver ions that are trapped within the crystal during its formation. The presence of these ions is not obvious from the simple equation, however their presence is vital for two main reasons:

1. They provide the free silver that is necessary during the early stages of latent image formation.
2. They assist the balancing of the negatively charged bromine ion barrier, thereby ensuring the silver bromide crystal is electrically neutral.

They are also free to migrate around the crystal, and this ability to travel assists in the formation of the latent sub-image centre (see next section).

MECHANISMS OF LATENT IMAGE FORMATION

The actual way in which the latent image forms falls into the all-too-frequent category of 'no one really knows what happens but we do know how altering various components alters the end result'. Bearing this in mind, there are two main theories of formation:

1. The Gurney Mott (classical) theory.
2. The Mitchell (modern) theory.

All other theories, of which there are many, broadly fall into one of these catagories.

Both the Gurney Mott and Mitchell theories are based on the partial reduction of silver bromide crystals during exposure. This partial reduction is achieved by the free interstitial silver ions (Ag$^+$) gaining an electron from some source (usually exposure to light, X-rays or both).

Effects of exposure

The desired result of exposure as far as the latent image is concerned is the release of an electron within the silver bromide crystal lattice. It is well known that exposure of any substance to a source containing the correct wavelengths and energy produces three effects:

1. Compton effect
2. Photoelectric effect
3. Pair production.

In the X-ray to blue range (1 nm to 430 nm) used to expose conventional unsensitised (monochromatic) film, only the first two effects occur in the silver bromide crystal: the Compton effect and the photoelectric effect. Of these two, the photoelectric effect predominates, as silver bromide is an ionic compound and has very few of the unbound electrons that are necessary for the Compton effect to occur. Approximately 96% of the electrons produced are from the photo electric effect. In any case, both effects release a high kinetic energy electron that can be used in latent image formation. Unfortunately, not all these electrons remain useful.

Energy of the released electrons

The energy of the electrons released by exposure is very important, as to be useful in image formation they must be able to enter the conduction band of the silver bromide crystal.

This band is one of the three energy bands that exist in metallic crystalline solids. The three bands are:

1. Valency band
2. Forbidden gap
3. Conduction band.

These bands can be represented as an energy level diagram (as in Fig. 3.3).

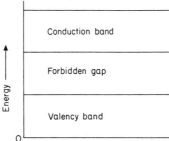

Fig. 3.3 Energy level diagram.

Actual values in terms of energy levels are not shown, as real values are unnecessary for our discussion. In any case they vary from substance to substance and also in range and 'depth'.

1. Valency band

Simply, this is the range of energies that may occur in the outer electrons of an atom. These allow the electron to take part in ionic or covalent bonding. In other words, if the electrons in the outer shells are within this energy band they may be useful in forming bonds with other atoms and forming, perhaps, a new compound.

2. Forbidden gap

In order to enter the conduction band, electrons must traverse the forbidden gap. This is a range of energies that are not allowable according to the theories of wave mechanics. Those with enough energy pass through and become 'free electrons' within the crystal and are available to form the latent image. Those with insufficient energy eventually fall back into an orbit.

3. Conduction band

If an electron has a certain range of energies it can exist within this band and may be available to form the latent image. This does not alter the electronic configuration of the atom but, providing it retains the range of allowed energies, moves as a free electron within the crystal.

An electron that is successful in entering the conduction band leaves a 'gap' in a higher orbit of the atom concerned in the initial interaction. This gap is called a 'hole' and is effectively a unit of positive charge. The hole would make the structure of the crystal 'unstable', but the migration of a colloidal sulphur particle to the site renders the hole ineffective.

Theory of latent image formation

As stated previously, there are two principal theories of latent image formation:

- Gurney Mott
- Mitchell.

Both of these suggest that it is a two stage process involving *nucleation* and *growth*, and whilst both have general agreement on the growth process they differ on the mechanism of the nucleation process.

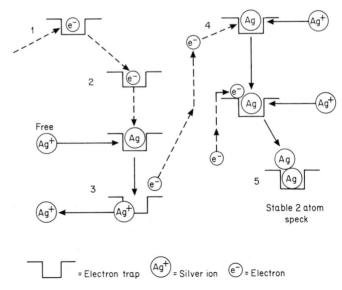

Fig. 3.4 Diagrammatic representation of the Gurney Mott theory.

Gurney Mott theory

Nucleation

This is best described by a diagram (see Fig. 3.4) showing the various stages involved.

Stage one

An electron that has been released by exposure is captured by a trapping centre and temporarily localised. A mobile, positively charged silver ion may migrate to this centre and form a silver atom, but. . .

Stage two

Before the arrival of this silver ion, the electron may escape from the trap due to its vibrational energy and again become free in the conduction band. Eventually it remains captured long enough to be joined by a silver ion giving a silver atom. . .

Stage three

Unfortunately, a single silver atom is unstable, separation occurs and stages one and two happen again.

Stage four

Fortunately, during its short life the single silver atom can act as a trap for another electron, and if another silver ion is attracted to this site. . .

Stage five

A stable two-atom silver speck is formed and is called a latent sub-image centre. This then grows as detailed later.

Mitchell theory

Nucleation

As previously, this is best described by the use of a diagram (Fig. 3.5).

Stages one and two

A free silver ion comes near to a shallow electron trap and deepens it. Whilst this trap is deepened a free electron, released by exposure, and another free silver ion approach the trap together and immediately form a silver atom. This is called a pre-image centre.

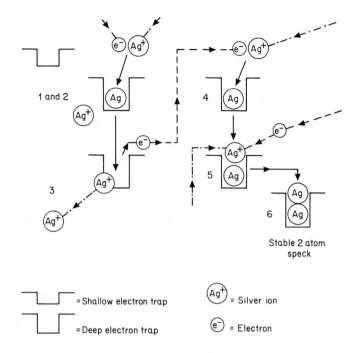

Fig. 3.5 Diagrammatic representation of the Mitchell theory.

Stage three

Unfortunately, as in the Gurney Mott theory, the single silver atom is unstable and it dissociates into a silver ion and an electron.

Stages four and five

Stages one and two re-occur. During its life the single silver atom does not act as a trap for a further electron (as in the Gurney Mott theory) but must aquire a second silver ion. If it is successful and an electron arrives before the escape of this second silver ion, a stable latent sub-image centre forms.

Growth

There is, fortunately, general agreement on the growth process. Both the Gurney Mott and Mitchell theories support that this is due to the deepening of the electron traps, because of the presence of the latent sub-image centre, increasing the attraction of that site compared to the shallow trap.

The increasing electrical attraction of these points in the crystal attracts the electrons from exposure and the silver ions from the crystal lattice, or from the supply of free interstitial ions, causing a build-up of silver atoms.

Many sub-image centres are formed throughout the crystal on one single exposure, but growth does proceed in a preferential way as the

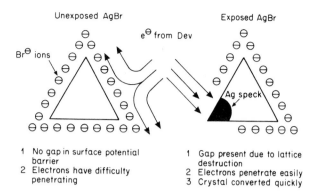

Unexposed AgBr

e⊖ from Dev

Exposed AgBr

Br⊖ ions

Ag speck

1 No gap in surface potential barrier
2 Electrons have difficulty penetrating

1 Gap present due to lattice destruction
2 Electrons penetrate easily
3 Crystal converted quickly

Fig. 3.6 Effect of the bromine ion barrier.

first formed sub-image centres tend to exhibit greater electrical attraction. During their growth, the ever-enlarging silver specks start to invade the surface of the crystal. This reduces the surface potential barrier (Fig. 3.6) by destroying the crystal lattice in that area, therefore rendering the crystal more susceptible to development.

When growth is complete the sub-image centres are commonly called development centres.

Action of developer on silver bromide crystals

The function of developer is to reduce the exposed silver bromide crystals to metallic silver. This function is performed by the donation of electrons in a selective fashion (see Selectivity, p. 92). No developer is completely selective and therefore the developing agent that reduces exposed crystals more quickly is used. The exposed crystals have a gap in the surface potential barrier, therefore allowing electrons from the developer easier access (see Fig. 3.6) to perform this reduction.

It is interesting to note that the use of excess potassium bromide in the production of the crystal increases the surface potential barrier, thereby assisting the process of selectivity.

SUMMARY

1. The production of the latent image is the first stage of the photochemical process. It is defined as the image produced on the film after exposure but prior to development. Changes produced after exposure in the silver bromide crystals of the emulsion are so small that even an electron microscope cannot reveal them.

2. Film emulsion is a suspension of silver bromide in gelatine; pure silver bromide is a cube-shaped crystal lattice (see Fig. 3.1). However, this crystal is of no use photographically, as it has none of the properties required to obtain a latent image.

3. Gelatine is vital to the production of the latent image because it provides:

a. Chemical impurities

These consist mainly of sulphur and produce 'active' areas in the silver bromide crystal.

b. Physical defects in crystal lattice structure

These are most probably the most important factors in the latent image production, as they introduce electron traps (see 4, below).

c. Growth medium

Allows silver bromide crystals to grow during the chemical reaction.

d. Suspension and binding agent

It is used to coat the emulsion onto the film base.

4. Electron traps within the crystal are areas of low energy that are caused by lattice defects and impurities from the gelatine. They are significant because it is in these areas that, after exposure, the latent image starts to form (see Fig. 3.2). Also it will be noticed that there is an excess of potassium bromide used in the emulsion production. This has two beneficial effects:

- Alters crystal shapes giving more electron traps
- Increases the surface potential barrier of the crystal, thus improving selectivity (see Fig. 3.6).

5. During the production of the emulsion, free interstitial silver ions are contained within the silver bromide crystal and provide the free silver that is necessary during the early stages of latent image formation.

6. There are two main theories of latent image formation:

- Gurney Mott
- Mitchell.

Details of these theories can be found in the main text. However, both make use of the electrons that are released in the crystal due to exposure, and the fact that these electrons may become free in the conduction band of the crystal. Once the electrons released by exposure become free electrons, they eventually combine with a silver ion to produce a silver atom at an electron trap and eventually a latent sub-image centre, which grows by attracting more silver atoms until it becomes a development centre.

The process of combination of silver ions and electrons is called nucleation; the enlargement of the sub-image centre is known as growth. There are many nucleation and growth centres produced in one crystal by one exposure, but the first formed latent sub-image centre tends to become the largest because of its greater electrical attraction. Growth also causes the breakdown of the crystal lattice structure which allows entry of the developer electrons. This entry is easier than in the unexposed crystal (see Fig. 3.6) and helps with the selectivity of the developer, i.e. its ability to distinguish between exposed and unexposed crystals.

7. It is interesting that the mechanics of latent image formation are still only theory; the actual process is still not fully understood.

DEVELOPERS AND FIXERS

Introduction

Next to film, developers and fixers are probably the most consumed photographic products used in the X-ray department, yet their use is often taken for granted and little consideration given to the complex chemical systems that have been designed to give high image quality, solution stability and easy practical use. Although obviously complex in nature, a basic appreciation is not beyond the capability of the reader with little formal knowledge of chemistry, but some understanding is an obvious advantage.

Developer and fixer chemistry depend a great deal on the ability to understand and apply the concept of pH. This subject is the starting point of our consideration of the second and third parts of photochemistry.

The concept of pH

In simple terms, pH is a quantitative method of measuring the degree of acidity or alkalinity of a solution. It is based on the fact that concentrations of ions that co-exist in solution may be described by a number called the equilibrium constant.

Equilibrium constant = concentration of products in a chemical reaction/concentration of reactants.

Pure water is chosen as the basis of the pH scale. Under normal conditions this is very slightly ionised into H^+ ions and OH^- ions and has a specially-named equilibrium constant called the ion product of water. This is written Kw; it is equal to the product of $[H^+][OH^-]$ and has the value 10^{-14} mol^2/l^2 at 25°C, i.e.

$$Kw = [H^+] [OH^-] = 10^{-14} \text{ mol}^2/\text{l}^2$$

The square brackets are used to indicate that concentrations are being considered and the mol/l is a method of measuring these concentrations.

It is well known that the acid 'portion' of a substance in solution is the H^+ ion content, whilst the alkaline portion is the OH^- ion content. Water is neither acid nor alkaline, therefore these ions are present in equal concentrations. From the above equation it can be seen that the total concentration of both the H^+ and OH^- is 10^{-14} mol^2/l^2; as they are present in equal proportions there must be 10^{-7} mol/l of H^+ ions and 10^{-7} mol/l of OH^- ions.

Table 3.1 Hydrogen ion concentrations and related pH values

	[H$^+$] (mole/litre)	pH
	1 or 10^0	0
	0.1 or 10^{-1}	1
	0.01 or 10^{-2}	2
Increasing acidity	0.001 or 10^{-3}	3
	0.0 001 or 10^{-4}	4
	0.00 001 or 10^{-5}	5
	0.000 001 or 10^{-6}	6
Pure water	0.0 000 001 or 10^{-7}	7
	0.00 000 001 or 10^{-8}	8
	0.000 000 001 or 10^{-9}	9
Increasing alkalinity	0.0 000 000 001 or 10^{-10}	10
	0.00 000 000 001 or 10^{-11}	11
	0.000 000 000 001 or 10^{-12}	12
	0.0 000 000 000 001 or 10^{-13}	13
	0.00 000 000 000 001 or 10^{-14}	14

This shows that only one in every thousand million water molecules is ionised.

Acid solutions are those with H$^+$ ion concentrations greater than 10^{-7} mol/l, whilst alkaline solutions have a H$^+$ ion concentration of less than 10^{-7} mol/l. This is demonstrated in Table 3.1.

As the manipulation of such figures proved to be inconvenient, a simpler method was devised by stating that 'pH is the log of the reciprocal of the hydrogen ion concentration'. This removes the large number of zeros in the values and the negative value of the power:

$$pH = \log_{10} \frac{1}{[H^+]}$$

Developers

Most developers for automatic processing have a pH range of 9.6–10.6, and to work to optimum efficiency must be maintained within ±0.2 of the manufacturer's recommended value, otherwise detrimental effects may occur to the final image quality, thus reducing diagnostic information (Fig. 3.7).

Fixers

Fixers for automatic processing have a pH range of 4.2–4.9, and again must be maintained at the recommended value to work efficiently. If allowed to rise above 4.9 they will still perform fixation, but problems will arise with the hardener present in modern fixers, causing

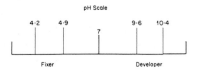

Fig. 3.7 The pH scale and its range for developers and fixers.

transportation difficulties in the processor and eventually destroying the solution (Fig. 3.7).

Summary

1. pH is a measure of the degree of acidity or alkalinity of a solution.

2. Its value is the log of the reciprocal of the hydrogen ion concentration of a solution (see equation, above).

3. A pH value of 7 is neutral.

4. Higher than 7 is alkali.

5. Lower than 7 is acid.

6. As pH is a log scale, small changes in value are large changes in ion concentration.

DEVELOPER

The features of a developer for use in automatic processing are not easy to define. However, it is possible to generalise:

1. All conventional radiographic emulsions are subject contrast amplifiers when correctly processed. They have an average gradient that is greater than 1, usually between 1.8 and 3.5. The chemistry of the emulsion and the developer are arranged so that these limits are available over a wide range of different conditions. Many people are of the opinion that X-ray developers are 'high contrast'. This is a vague term, as the comparison used to detemine 'high' is often not specified.

2. X-ray developers are considered to be high speed, and have the ability to produce an image in approximately twenty seconds, thereby enabling 90 second processing. This speed is mainly due to working at high temperatures, but unfortunately this tends to increase the base + fog level of the film. In an attempt to reduce this, a move to two and three minute processing would have to be made.

3. A base + fog level of less than 0.2 is desirable, but this is problematic due to the reasons outlined above.

4. Developer must produce a maximum density of between 3.0–4.0.

5. Must contain additives that allow the emulsion to be transported through high speed, high temperature roller processing.

6. Must contain additives that absorb detrimental by-products of the developer action as well as guarding against auto-oxidation and the non-uniform nature of water supplies. This allows solutions to be used for long periods without excessive maintenance or replenishment.

7. Concentrated solutions must store for long periods in a wide range of conditions without undesirable effects.

8. Chemicals must be as non-hazardous as possible, to conform with Health and Safety regulations, and be simple to use.

Functions

For a chemical to be a developer it must possess two main properties, conversion and selectivity.

Conversion

The chemical must be able to precipitate metallic silver from the silver salts of bromide, chloride and iodide or combinations of these salts (Fig. 3.8).

The most common silver halide in X-ray emulsions is silver bromide (AgBr). This is normally mixed with a small proportion of silver iodide (AgI) to produce an emulsion with the desired characteristics. The ratio is of the order of 96% AgBr to 4% AgI. Figure 3.8 shows the reaction that occurs when AgBr is placed in a developing agent.

The developer reduces the AgBr to metallic silver and itself becomes oxidised, therefore developers are reducing agents. It can be seen that the desirable reaction has occurred. However, two by-products have also been formed, both of which adversely affect further development and must be combatted by other agents (see Developer constituents, below). Interested readers should note that the developing agent donates electrons to the AgBr crystal during the reduction process.

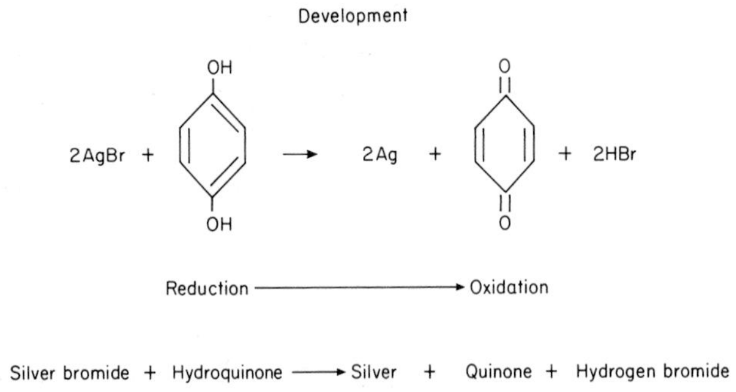

Development

$$2\,AgBr + \text{(hydroquinone)} \longrightarrow 2\,Ag + \text{(quinone)} + 2\,HBr$$

Reduction ⟶ Oxidation

Silver bromide + Hydroquinone ⟶ Silver + Quinone + Hydrogen bromide

Fig. 3.8 The chemical action of developer on silver bromide (simplified).

Selectivity

This is the ability of a developing agent to differentiate between exposed silver halide and unexposed silver halide, changing only the exposed crystals to metallic silver.

Many chemicals are able to reduce AgBr to metallic silver but few have the property of selectivity. It is an unfortunate fact that even those used as developing agents are not completely selective. In practice, therefore, developers reduce exposed AgBr quicker than unexposed AgBr. This differential ability can be evaluated and is called the selectivity ratio. It is the difference in the rate between the development of exposed and unexposed grains of silver bromide. The ratio is high in selective developers and low in unselective developers.

Again, there are additions which may be made to developer solutions to try and improve this ratio. Examination of published data reveals that in general terms, highly selective developers are slow acting whereas unselective developers are fast. In practice, a trade-off exists between speed and selectivity (see also Latent image, p. 87).

Amplification gain

It is this feature of the film, latent image and developer system that makes photography, as we know it, a viable proposition. Amplification gain is a measure of the extent to which the developer amplifies the initial effect of exposure on the silver halide grains. Many experiments have been carried out to assess the numerical value of this gain, giving results ranging from 10^6 to 10^{12}. However, the most widely accepted figure seems to be 10^9:

Ag + development = Amplification gain of 10^9

The photographic process is the only process known at this time which gives gains of this order. A close rival is a heat transfer process (Diazo), having a gain factor of about 10^3. To put this value in perspective, a hi-fi system giving amplification of 10^9 would produce approximately 200 000 W. An average domestic system gives about 20–30 W.

Due to the relatively high cost of silver-based recording systems, many millions of pounds have been spent trying to find alternatives that approach this enormous gain factor, with little success to date.

DEVELOPING SOLUTIONS IN THE AUTOMATIC PROCESSOR

Introduction

Automatic processing developers have special features that make them quite different from manual processing solutions. It is important therefore not to infer similar properties, and to realise that, due to advancements in technology, certain substances are given traditional names that are not strictly accurate in chemical definition.

Table 3.2 The constituents of developer

Developer replenisher	Machine tank

1. Developing agent(s)
2. Preservative
3. Accelerator
4. Restrainer
5. Buffer
6. Sequestering agent
7. Solvent
8. Other additions:
    Hardening agent
    Wetting agent
    Anti-frothant
    Fungicide
	+ 9. Starter solution

In the following sections, reference will be made to machine tank developer (MT) and developer replenisher (RT). These should be considered as separate entities, and care should be taken to state which is being considered.

The major differences between the two are shown in Table 3.2. In general, most have a pH in the range 9.6–10.6.

Constituents

The constituents of developer replenisher and machine tank developer are shown in Table 3.2. It is important to remember that:

Developer replenisher + starter = machine tank developer.

The need for replenishment

As previously stated, certain by-products of development affect its activity, and as development proceeds the developing agent is used up, its concentration falls, and the developer becomes less active (exhausted). In a practical situation this would necessitate frequent changing of the developer to maintain consistent results, both from the image and the machine/mechanical point of view. In order to obviate this, a certain amount of replenisher is added to the machine tank every time a film is fed into the machine. The replenisher replaces the exhausted developer and maintains the concentration of the other active components at the correct levels. It also maintains the physical quantity of the solution in the tank.

The principal factors affecting developer replenishment are:

1. Area of film processed
2. Average density of the film
3. Silver content of the film
4. Maximum density required
5. Thickness of the emulsion
6. Single or duplitised coating
7. Processor work load
8. Amount of aerial oxidation.

Note: Many of the factors listed above are related to each other and decided by the film chemistry. However, knowledge of this data is essential to correctly replenish solutions, even though the manufacturer freely provides this information in the form of recommended replenishment rates.

Replenishment in most processors is usually governed by an average rate per length of film (for developer, the average rate is 40–60 ml for every 35 cm). This means that large films are actually receiving slight under-replenishment, whereas small film sizes receive over-replenishment, the net effect being that over an average working day, replenishment is correct. However, most modern machines are capable of assessing actual film size and replenishing accordingly. Some advanced processors also calculate average density as well as size, giving even more accurate replenishment. This is achieved by a suitably programmed microprocessor (i.e. computer) which will also monitor all other automatic processor functions (see Ch. 4, Automatic processing).

Starter solution

In theory, once correctly set, replenishment could continue indefinitely; but emulsion flaking and dirt accumulation in the developer tank necessitate regular cleaning.

After draining and cleaning the main tank, fresh developer replenisher is added to fill the tank to the recommended level. If the rollers were replaced and a film developed, it would exhibit all the features shown in Figure 3.9

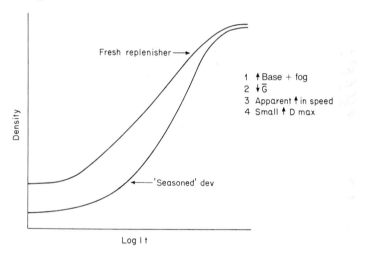

Fig. 3.9 The effect of processing a film in replenisher as compared to 'seasoned developer'.

The change in the characteristic curve is due to the high activity of replenisher. If films are still processed through this solution, its activity will eventually fall and balance at the correct level. This is due to the increase in bromine ion (Br⁻) concentration and depression of the pH value, both of which are caused by development (Fig. 3.8). To enable immediate use of the processor, starter solution is added to the machine tank. This is a restrainer solution which adds weak acid and Br⁻ ions, therefore depressing activity to the required level before films are processed.

Starter solution is usually supplied separately, a certain quantity being added for every mixed litre of solution in the machine tank. However, some manufacturers supply the whole MT developer, which just requires mixing with water, whilst RT developer is available separately.

Developing agents

There are two principal agents used in automatic processor developers:

- phenidone (P) and
- hydroquinone (Q).

P and Q are not used separately but in combination to produce a Phenidone hydroquinone (PQ)-type developer. Using two agents in combination produces considerable advantages, which will become apparent (see Fig. 3.10).

Early developers used metol in place of phenidone in this combination, but phenidone is used exclusively today in X-ray developers because of its many advantages (see Table 3.3 and Superadditivity and Regeneration, below).

Combining agents this way enables the manufacturer to control

Table 3.3 Characteristics of different developing agents

Developing agent	Characteristics

Common name:
  Phenidone (P)
Chemical name:
  1–phenyl 3–pyrazolidone
Discovered by:
  Ilford Labs, 1940
Main modern use:
  General use
	1. High speed
	2. Low selectivity
	3. Low contrast
	4. Only 10–15% compared with Q to give similar activity
	5. Activity not so dependent on Br^- concentration
	6. Liquid concentrate

Common name:
  Metol (M)
Chemical name:
  monomethyl-paraminophenol-sulphate
Discovered by:
  Hauff, 1891
Main modern use:
  In MQ powder developers
	Characteristics of no interest, as use as a radiographic developer largely obsolete (included for interest only)

Common name:
  Hydroquinone (Q)
Chemical name:
  para-dihydroxybenzene
Discovered by:
  Sir W de W Abney, 1880
Main modern use:
  Graphic arts
	1. High contrast
	2. Slow speed
	3. High selectivity
	4. Susceptible to auto-oxidation
	5. Activity very dependent on temperature and pH

Phenidone hydroquinone (PQ)	1. High speed 2. Higher contrast than MQ 3. Low auto-oxidation rate 4. Not excessively Br^- ion dependent 5. Susceptible to pH variations 6. Temperature dependent 7. Greater superadditivity than MQ 8. Liquid concentrate 9. Less likely to cause dermatitis than MQ 10. Causes less staining than MQ 11. Long shelf life

base + fog, contrast, speed, etc., as well as making full use of the superadditive effect. Correct replenishment removes most of the problems experienced with a PQ combination.

Superadditivity and regeneration

This is another almost unique effect of the photographic process. It is an advantage that arises when using agents in combination. Superadditivity may be described as 'the combined activities of two developing agents in the same solution which is greater than the sum of their separate activities'. This is illustrated in Figure 3.10.

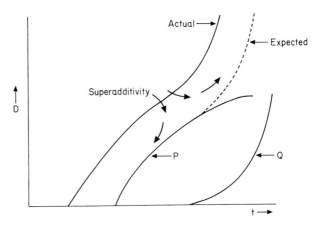

Fig. 3.10 Diagrammatic representation of superadditivity.

It is still not completely clear how this mechanism functions, although it is believed to be due to:

1. The relative size of the ionised form of the developing agents in the early stages of their effect on the sensitised AgBr crystal.

2. Hydroquinone developers that contain sulphite (of which radiographic developers are a good example) form a first oxidation product of hydroquinone called hydroquinone monosulphonate. In the presence of phenidone this forms a superadditive system of great power.

3. Regeneration — in this reaction the first oxidation product of phenidone reacts with hydroquinone to yield ordinary phenidone. This means that the concentration of the most active ingredient is kept high, thus assisting the left shift shown in Figure 3.10.

Advantages of phenidone hydroquinone (PQ) developers

PQ developers have certain advantages over their MQ counterparts, so much so that only PQ developers are now used for radiographic developers. This is because:

- PQ developers have a more efficient superadditive system and greater regeneration effect

- PQ is cheaper than its MQ equivalent
- Easier to make liquid concentrates
- Longer shelf life
- Longer working life
- Greater activity at equivalent pH values
- Easier control of replenishment
- Less susceptible to Br^- concentration
- Easier to handle, as PQ developers are less likely to cause contact dermatitis and/or staining of hands and clothing, and do not have an unacceptable odour after prolonged use.

Preservative

Developer activity is reduced by oxidation. This oxidation takes place in two ways:

1. Normal development action (Fig. 3.8)
2. Aerial or auto-oxidation.

Developing agents + oxygen $\rightarrow$ Oxidised dev. agents + OH^- ions.

The problem is aerial oxidation; if not reduced to a minimum, it soon produces coloured insoluble products which depress, and would eventually destroy, the activity of the developer. To reduce this aerial oxidation to an acceptable level, various forms of sulphite can be added to the developer solution.

Agent

The most common agent used in automatic processing developers is potassium metabisulphite. This is used, especially in liquid concentrate developers, because of its high solubility and greater preserving efficiency compared to other preserving agents (such as sodium sulphite).

Function

The active 'ingredient' is the sulphite ion. This forms sulphonates with early oxidation products. These sulphonates are colourless and inert and have two properties:

- They slow down formation of discoloured products
- They discourage oxidation.

A highly simplified view of how this works is to imagine that the sulphite combines with dissolved oxygen, in the developer solution and at the surface of the developer, to produce the sulphonates in solution. However, in practice it is not as simple as this, as it is not a case of preferential absorption of oxygen by the preserving agent.

Any reader with some chemical knowledge may have spotted that potassium metabisulphite is acidic. This is peculiar, as it was stated earlier that developers were alkaline and very pH dependent. However, this acidity is more than compensated for by the addition of sufficient alkali to counteract its effect.

Aerial oxidation is kept to a minimum in automatic processing by four methods:

1. High preservative level in the developer;
2. Floating lid in the developer replenisher tank to reduce the surface area of the developer in contact with the air;
3. Closely fitting rollers, again to reduce surface area in contact with the air;
4. Deep narrow tanks in the processor so that the surface area to volume is kept as small as possible.

All these four methods, or a combination, may be used in practice to keep oxidation to an acceptable level.

Accelerator

As established previously, developers are very pH dependent and must be alkaline to work effectively and produce the desired result. Unfortunately, neither hydroquinone nor phenidone are particularly alkaline, and if simply dissolved in water do not produce a working developer. Both agents require an activator to stimulate their developing properties. This activator is called the accelerator; it is alkali, which is added to the developer solution. By varying the amount of accelerator present, the activity of the developer is closely controlled.

Agent

Automatic processing developers are considered to be highly active and therefore have a high amount of accelerator present. The agent used is either sodium or potassium hydroxide. Both these agents are strongly alkaline and are particularly useful in high contrast developers containing hydroquinone, as their high solubility makes them ideal for production as liquid concentrates.

Function

The accelerator controls developer activity by assuring correct pH value. It affects contrast and speed so that, in balance with other agents in the developer, the desired image quality is produced.

Restrainer (Anti-foggant)

As stated previously, restrainer is added to replenisher to produce machine tank developer when starting the machine from 'dry'. In this case it is known as starter solution (see Starter solutions, p. 95).

However, restrainer is also present in normally prepared developer replenisher where it may be called an anti-foggant. It is therefore good practice to consider starter solution as additional restrainer.

Agent

There are two principal types of restraining agent in use:

- Inorganic restrainers, e.g. potassium bromide;
- Organic restrainers e.g. benzotriazole.

Developer replenisher uses an organic benzotriazole-type restrainer. This is principally because of two main factors:

1. Organic restrainers appear to be capable of restraining base + fog with little or no effect on film speed. This is not true of inorganic restrainers, which are occasionally deliberately used to control film speed during processing.
2. With high speed developers, the amount of inorganic restrainer required to keep 'fog' within acceptable limits would be such that image staining may occur, as potassium bromide in large quantities is a silver bromide solvent.

Because of these features it is common to find organic benzotriazole used in developer replenisher, and potassium bromide plus acetic acid used in starter solution (see also High and low temperature chemistry, p. 107).

Function

The function of the restrainer is to improve the selectivity of the developer, ensuring low fog and high image contrast. Its action is to increase the effective bromine ion barrier that exists around silver bromide crystals (see Latent image, p. 87). The barrier is increased around both exposed and unexposed crystals. However, exposed crystals have some crystal lattice destruction where the protection is useless (Fig. 3.11).

The amount of restrainer provided in developer is sufficient to give adequate protection of the crystals when the replenisher is used in the conventional manner. When starter is added (it will be recalled that there is some acetic acid present in this solution, as well as potassium bromide) this depresses the pH of the replenisher, thereby giving the correct activity. The potassium bromide provides the small additional amount of restrainer to give correct selectivity.

Buffer

If Figure 3.8 is studied, it will be noticed that the development process releases bromine ions from the silver bromide complexes within the emulsion and hydrogen ions from the developing agent, due to the donation of electrons from, in this case, the hydroxyl

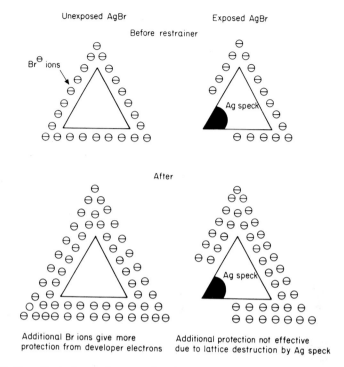

Fig. 3.11 The effect of restrainer on silver bromide crystals.

groups in hydroquinone. These combine to form hydrogen bromide, but as this occurs in an aqueous solution it becomes hydrobromic acid. This by-product will depress the pH value of the developer solution and take it away from its ideal level. As previously discussed, this would affect the activity of the developer and if allowed to persist would render the developer useless.

Agent

A buffer is normally a solution of weak acid and alkali compounds, and in the automatic processor is usually something like boric acid and sodium hydroxide.

Function

The Penguin Dictionary of Science defines a buffer as 'a solution the hydrogen ion concentration of which, and hence its acidity or alkalinity, is practically unchanged by dilution, and which resists a change in pH on the addition of acid or alkali'. In simple terms, in the case of developers, it can be considered that this is achieved by the absorption of the hydrogen ions before they combine with the bromine ions. In fact the actual effect of the hydrobromic acid is limited by the equilibrium concentrations that are allowed by the equilibrium equation. This limits the number of free hydrogen and bromine ions available and therefore the amount of acid produced. It is interesting to note at this stage that a buffer helps maintain pH and therefore activity by absorbing harmful by-products of development action, whilst the preservative maintains activity by absorbing products of auto-oxidation.

Sequestering agent

This addition is used to counter the problems that may occur if hard water is used to make up developer solutions. It prevents the precipitation of calcium sludge which would otherwise show up as chalky deposits on the dry film or cause scaling of the developer tank. The scaling would be somewhat similar to lime scale found in domestic kettles.

The calcium sludge is caused by a reaction that takes place between the calcium and magnesium salts present in the water supply and the sodium sulphite compounds in the developer. Under normal conditions this does not present a problem as caustic alkali developers (i.e. X-ray developers) do not suffer from calcium precipitation. However, extremes do occur and sufficient sequestering agent is added to cope with even the hardest water supplies.

Agent

1. Sodium salt of ethylene diamine tetra-acetic acid (EDTA Sodium salt).
2. Sodium hexametaphosphate (not now in general use, commercially known as Calgon).

Function

The function of this agent is to soften hard water supplies, thus preventing precipitation of the calcium and magnesium salts onto the surface of the film. This is achieved by transforming the calcium and magnesium salts into soluble complexes. These complexes are inert to the sulphite components of the solution and, as a result, do not precipitate out.

Solvent

The solvent used in the photographic process is almost always water, and although ideally distilled water is the solvent of choice (because of its purity) it does not produce significantly better results as far as we are concerned. However, it does have its use in highly specialised scientific applications such as holography, for example.

Normal tap water is more than adequate for use with conventional X-ray developers and has two often quoted advantages, relatively low cost and availability.

There is also an advantage that arises because of a very useful coincidence. It is a fact that all the salts produced in the photographic process, with only one exception, are soluble in water. This removes the need for any intermediate steps to remove deleterious by-products that beguile many other processes. Unfortunately, there is one problem with using available water supplies.

Disadvantage

The water supply is not constant in character.

There are various problems associated with the non-constant nature of domestic and industrial water supplies. Table 3.4 itemises the major problem areas.

The most significant practical precaution that can be taken is the use of filtered water in the preparation of solutions. It can be quite alarming to see the amount of foreign material present in a filter that has been in use for even a short time.

Table 3.4 Problems associated with water supplies

Problem	Indication	Solution
Hard water	Excessive calcium + magnesium salts Chalky deposits on film	Sequestering agent: sufficient included for hardest water supplies
Excessive iron + copper content	Can cause fogging + oxidise developer (usually from copper pipes used to supply water to processor)	All specifications for installation of automatic processors now include the use of plastic pipes
Suspended solid matter	Particles of grit, dirt, etc., scratching of film in processor	Use of filtered water supply for mixing chemicals, usually from output side of water panel
Fluoride and chlorides	Added at water treatment works to control bacteria content	No photographic effects in concentrations usually present

Other additions

It is the so-called other additions that principally distinguish developers for automatic processing and those for manual processing. However, commercially available solutions differ very little whether for manual or automatic processing, and as these additional chemicals provide significant improvements to both manual and automatic processing situations, examination of actual formulae will probably reveal little difference between the two. There are four principal other additions:

1. Hardening agent
2. Wetting agent
3. Anti-frothant
4. Fungicide.

Hardening agent

Probably the worst situation in which to place the photographic emulsion (especially the gelatine used as the suspension agent for the silver bromide) is a warm aqueous alkaline solution. Developer is an excellent example of such a solution. The high temperatures in use can cause excessive swelling and softening of the emulsion, by encouraging water absorption. By controlling this effect the hardener reduces to a minimum the following problems:

- Chances of mechanical damage (e.g. scratching) due to roller transport
- Non-transportation, due to the film being too 'thick' to pass through the rollers
- Sticking of films in the crossover assembly due to the soft gelatine adhering to dry crossover rollers
- Sticking of the film in the fixer and/or wash racks
- Chances of frilling, i.e. the separation of the emulsion from the base (this is of no practical significance)
- Chance of reticulation, i.e. a network of cracks on the processed film (this is of no practical significance).

Various hardening agents are in common use, e.g. certain aldehydes and sulphates. However, all modern emulsions are pre-hardened as part of the manufacturing process and this greatly assists in the protection of the film in high temperature roller transportation.

Wetting agent

This is added to stimulate uniform development by reducing the surface tension between the developing solution and the film emulsion. It allows easy penetration of the developer into the emulsion, which would otherwise prove difficult (in the short period spent in the developer tank in automatic processing), due to the presence of hardener.

Some developer formulations may not contain this agent, as emulsions do contain a proportion of wetting agent added during manufacture. Most agents are detergent-based derivatives and because of this an additional inclusion is needed to combat problems that may arise due to the agent's basic property of foaming (see Anti-frothant, below).

Anti-frothant

The automatic processor relies, for replenishment and recirculation, on the use of pumps. These pumps deliver developer under some pressure to the main tank. This pressured delivery, and the action of the rollers, provides a very important feature of the automatic processor, that of constant agitation. However, this raises the problem of foaming and frothing, mainly due to the presence of the wetting agent. Therefore an anti-foaming agent is included to reduce foaming, which if allowed to occur would contaminate the inside of the processor.

Fungicide

The developer tank of the automatic processor provides ideal conditions for the growth and multiplication of certain strains of fungi. It provides a continous and uniformly warm moist area within which is a good deal of suitable food, in the form of gelatine which is stripped off the surface of the film during transportation through the rollers. This removal of the emulsion is unfortunate but is taken into account in film and processor design.

Fungi growth can also take place within the various lines transporting fluids in the processor (especially in the wash tank and pipes), causing blockage and incorrect flow. It usually has the appearance of a slightly opaque strand-like slime.

The addition of fungicide usually controls this growth, but in extreme cases it may persist. This necessitates the complete drainage and cleaning of tanks and lines with a powerful fungicide, to remove this growth and any spores that may be present.

The advent of the first generation of cold water processors exacerbated this situation, as the low water throughput (about 1.5 l/min, compared to about 14 l/min in tempered water processors) caused great problems; many processors had to be converted back to mixed water machines. Second generation (so-called total cold water processors) solved this problem by recirculating the water at higher pressures but still using only about 1.5 l/min from the main supply.

Starter solution

As stated previously, this is added to developer replenisher to produce machine tank developer, when starting the processor from 'dry'. It has two main functions:

1. It depresses the pH of the developer, therefore reducing the activity of the solution.
2. It adds bromine ions to the solution, thereby restraining the action of the developing agents on the unexposed $AgBr$ grains (i.e. increases selectivity).

The amount to add is critical, as under- or over-addition greatly affects the developer's characteristics and therefore affects final image quality. It is usually supplied in a separate bottle, with instructions to add so many millilitres per mixed litre of developer in the machine tank.

Agents

Usually potassium bromide plus acetic acid.

Commercial preparations

Developer chemical available from manufacturers is normally supplied as a liquid concentrate to make up so many mixed litres, and sometimes packed containing three parts, A, B and C. Each of the three parts comprises various items of the final developer that, for chemical reasons, need to be kept apart until working developer is required. It is not possible to be specific about the constituents of each part (as exact formulations are normally trade secrets). However, generalisations can be made to illustrate actual solutions. Table 3.5 is an indication of the contents of developer solutions, if packed as three separate parts.

Never bring part B into direct contact with water; always dilute the solution with part A. This is important, as phenidone is insoluble in water and is kept in solution by the fact that it is mixed with ethylene glycol. Direct mixing with water that does not contain part A will cause the phenidone to precipitate out. Unfortunately this process is irreversible.

Table 3.5 Developer constituents in commercial preparations

Part	Danger	Content
A	Causes burns	Developing agent (hydroquinone) Preservative (sulphite) Buffer + Accelerator (alkali — hydroxide)
B	Causes burns	Developing agent (phenidone) Solvent for phenidone (ethylene glycol) Restrainer (acetic acid + benzotriazole) Restrainer (potassium bromide)
C	Irritant	Hardener (gluteraldehyde) Acetic acid

Mixing

Developer should be mixed carefully, with due regard to the fact that both parts A and B can cause burns and part C is an irritant. Suitable protective clothing should be worn in the form of gloves, aprons, etc. This is particularly relevant not only for reasons of personal safety, but also because of the Health and Safety at Work Act.

Before mixing the replenisher, check the volume remaining in the replenisher tank and ensure that there is sufficient space to accept the additional solution. Then:

1. Add the volume of water stated in the instructions.
2. Add slowly the whole of parts A, B and C in order, with continuous stirring.
3. Continue stirring for at least 2 minutes to give a uniform mixture.

Stirring is very important, as it prevents the formation of insoluble precipitates. It is also a wise precaution to use separate stirring rods for developer and fixer, as even small amounts of contamination may be detrimental.

High and low temperature chemistry

The normal range of temperatures within which developers operate can conveniently be divided into two sections. These are so-called high and low temperature, and their ranges are only relevant when considering radiographic processing (Table 3.6).

Table 3.6 Temperature ranges

Division	Temperature	Normal pH
High temp. chemistry	31°C–39°C	9.6*
Low temp. chemistry	26°C–33°C	10.00*

* Actual values depend on manufacturer

The advent of the demand for low temperature chemistry posed many problems for the designers of chemical systems, as it was still necessary to retain the same total processing cycles (i.e. 90 seconds, 2 minutes, etc.) which meant staying with short developing times and also retaining the same image quality.

The main problem was that of processing the film at lower temperatures for the same time, but still producing the same maximum density, contrast, speed and base + fog levels. In order to achieve this, three principal alterations have been made in the production of low temperature chemistry. These are:

1. Higher concentration of hydroquinone
2. Different restrainer
3. Higher concentration of preservative.

The increase in the hydroquinone level provides the higher activity needed at lower temperatures to give the required densities. Unfortunately hydroquinone is more susceptible to aerial oxidation and therefore requires a higher concentration of preservative. The higher pH, caused again by the large amount of hydroquinone, also has an adverse effect on the usual restrainers, requiring a change in this agent as well.

It is debatable whether the use of low temperature produces a better or worse image. However, it is true that there is a limit as to how much temperature decrease can be compensated for by altering other constituents. The advantages of low temperature are rather vague, but a definite *disadvantage* is that they are less stable than their high temperature counterparts.

Practical tests

These are the subject of Chapter 6 on Quality assurance, but are included here for completeness:

- pH of the machine tank developer
- pH of the replenisher tank developer (these can be plotted on a graph and any variations studied)
- Measure replenishment rates
- Specific gravity of the machine and replenisher solutions
- Sensitometric evaluation, i.e. full sensitometry; fog, speed and contrast index; visual comparisons.

Summary

1. For a chemical to be useful as a developer it must possess two main properties: conversion and selectivity. It must be able to convert exposed silver bromide to metallic silver whilst leaving unexposed silver bromide relatively unchanged (Fig. 3.8).

2. The amplification gain of the silver + developer system is of the order of 10^9.

3. Developers for automatic processing have special features that distinguish them from their manual counterparts, and although it is possible to use auto-process developers in a manual situation it is usually not possible to do the reverse. The developer used in the machine tank and the developer used in the replenisher tank have different properties and pH values, e.g. pH machine tank 10.00, pH replenisher tank 10.30. But they are related by the fact that:

Developer replenisher + starter = machine tank developer

4. Developer replenisher is a very important solution, mainly because it is used to maintain constant solution activity and quantity. There are many factors affecting the degree of replenishment required.

5. Starter solution must be added to developer replenisher when chemicalising the processor from 'dry'. This is because it has two important effects. Firstly, it increases the bromine ion concentration; secondly, it depresses the pH to the correct value, enabling immediate use of the processor to give correct film quality.

6. A typical developer comprises many agents. Table 3.7 shows the general names of these agents, their probable chemical composition and their functions.

7. Commercial developer preparations may be supplied in three parts. These can be hazardous if handled incorrectly and must be kept apart for complex chemical reasons (see Table 3.5). For use, these should be mixed carefully, with suitable precautions, according to the manufacturer's instructions and always with continous stirring.

8. 'Low' temperature chemistry differs from 'high' temperature chemistry in that it has a higher hydroquinone concentration, a different restrainer and a higher preservative concentration.

9. Practical tests, given as a list (above), are also the subject of Chapter 6, Quality assurance.

10. The constituents of developer can easily be remembered by using the mnemonic 'SOAPRADS':

Table 3.7 Developer constituents: probable composition and function

General name	Chemical used	Function
1. Developing agents	Phenidone plus hydroquinone	Selective conversion, AgBr (exposed) to metallic silver Also possesses the feature of superadditivity
2. Preservative	Potassium metabisulphite	Reduces aerial oxidation to a minimum
3. Accelerator	Sodium or potassium hydroxide	Gives the developer its pH value, therefore ensuring correct activity
4. Restrainer (anti-foggant)	Organic: benzotriazole, potassium bromide	Improves developer selectivity, therefore reduces fog level Also found in starter solution
5. Buffer	Boric acid + sodium hydroxide	Maintains pH within defined limits and therefore activity of developer constant
6. Sequestering agent	EDTA sodium salt	Softens hard water
7. Solvent	Water	Acts as solvent for all chemicals and by-products of developer action
8. Other additions Hardening agent Wetting agent Anti-frothant Fungicide		Reduces emulsion swelling and softening Reduces surface tension Prevents foaming due to reduced surface tension Reduces growth of fungi

S — Solvent
O — Other additions
A — Alkali buffer
P — Preservative
R — Restrainer
A — Accelerator
D — Developing agents
S — Sequestering agent.

Fixers

The fixer bath is in most cases the least understood solution used in processing. It is not generally appreciated that while it is possible to produce an adequate image in a development time of, say, ten seconds, it is not possible to completely fix the image in such a short period without the use of expensive and perhaps potentially hazardous solutions, both of which features are undesirable in a hospital situation.

In the early days of automatic processing, most of the problems associated with the chemical side of the processor were eventually traced to the fixer, so much so that the modern processor is designed primarily around the fixer solution. This in no way decreases the importance of the developer or the other processing systems, but indicates the importance attached to ensuring that the film is correctly fixed.

Previously it was stated that very rapid fixation was not possible using conventional agents; however, these agents can be used to provide, in certain situations, a 'quick look' facility. In these cases, the film must be returned for completion of the process if any degree of archival permanence is to be achieved.

Function

For a chemical to be a fixer it must possess two properties: conversion and selectivity.

1. Conversion

It must be able to convert unexposed, undeveloped silver halide into a form that can be removed from the emulsion layer by the water present in the fixing bath, thus rendering the image permanent. To this end the agent present must therefore be a silver halide solvent that produces salts that are soluble in water. This can be briefly described by the following equation:

Silver halide + fixing agent →
  Water soluble silver complexes + inert by-products

2. Selectivity

In this sense, 'selectivity' means that the agent must have no effect on either the metallic silver in the developed image or the gelatine in which it is suspended. Again, however, as with developer it is far from a perfect world, and unfortunately all fixing agents are to some extent mild silver solvents. It is therefore just as detrimental to image quality to leave a film in fixer for too long a period as too short a period, and although only relevant in practical terms to manual processing, a film left overnight in an X-ray fixer will have little or no image on it when viewed in the morning.

There are many agents that possess the above required features, although only two are in common use:

- Ammonium thiosulphate $(NH_4)_2S_2O_3$
- Sodium thiosulphate $Na_2S_2O_3$.

Only one of these — ammonium thiosulphate — is used in radiographic processing. Other fixing agents that are found in use in other fields, but not in medical X-ray departments, are the alkali cyanates and thiocyanates. Even though they are very much more rapid in action, unfortunately they may have a detrimental effect on the silver image and gelatine.

The conversion process occurs in three stages when a thiosulphate is used, the middle step producing the only salt in the photographic process that is not soluble in water. This apparent disadvantage has an interesting use, as it provides a useful test to see if the film is correctly fixed (this is discussed further in the next section).

Fixing solutions

All automatic processing fixers used in X-ray departments are of the ammonium thiosulphate acid hardening type. This is significant because ammonium thiosulphate is the most rapid, easily prepared and easy to use fixing agent in terms of mixing and safety (although it still needs to be prepared and used with some care). The acid present in these fixers negates the need for a rinse or stop bath process between development and fixation, and also allows the use of very efficient hardening agents which are essential when rapid drying at high temperatures is required (as in an automatic processor).

These factors mean that maintenance of the fixer pH value within fine limits is essential, and to this end all fixers commercially available have a pH range of 4.2–4.9 (approx.), depending on the manufacturer, and a tolerance of $\pm$ 0.2 pH (approx.) about the recommended value.

Constituents

The constituents of fixer replenisher and machine fixer are shown in the list below. It is interesting and important to note that unlike developer, there is no difference, between replenisher and machine tank fixer in terms of the actual agents employed or their pH.

1. Fixing agent
2. Acid
3. Buffer
4. Preservative
5. Hardener
6. Solvent.

Need for replenishment

It is obvious that as the fixing process progresses, there is going to be a decrease in the level of the active ingredients of the fixer solution and also an increase in the level of by-products. The fixing agent is used up as it converts the silver bromide into soluble silver complexes; this leads to an increase in the silver concentration of the fixer, and if allowed to climb above 7–8 g/l results in insufficient fixation because the rate of diffusion of the soluble silver complexes out of the film falls below a minimum safe level. This cannot be compensated for by increasing the fixing time, as in automatic processing this cannot be changed.

Similarly, the pH of the fixer will alter due to carry-over of alkali developer in the emulsion of the film, and although the squeegee rollers of the automatic processor reduce this to a minimum, it cannot be completely eliminated. An increase in the pH value of the solution away from its ideal eventually affects the hardener, which becomes less efficient, resulting in problems with transportation of the film through the rollers as well as scratching and inadequate drying.

In practice these problems would necessitate constant changing of the fixer solution to maintain consistant results, this change being necessary approximately twice as often, in a given solution, as with developer in a similar situation (although this comparison is very much simplified and leaves out relevant data such as development auto-oxidation rates, etc., which would complicate the comparison).

To obviate this, a certain amount of replenisher is added to the machine tank every time a film is fed into the processor. When added in the correct proportions this ensures that the level of the active ingredients is maintained at the correct concentration by adding fresh solution. It also results in removal, usually to a silver recovery unit, of the same amount of used fixer. This keeps the volume constant and also, if correctly replenished, the silver level constant (usually 5–7 g/l); this final fact ensures that the soluble silver complexes are completely removed from the film, providing pH and fixing time remain constant. It also ensures that the physical amount of fixer used is not excessive (see Chapter 6, Quality assurance). The factors affecting fixer replenishment are:

- Area of film processed
- Average density of the film, i.e. amount of unexposed, undeveloped silver bromide to be removed
- Thickness of emulsion and silver coating weight
- Single or duplitised emulsion
- Type of fixing agent (in theory only, as the agent is always ammonium thiosulphate).
- Silver level required
- pH level required.

Many of the factors listed are closely related to each other and are decided by the manufacturer in the film and chemical manufacturing process (e.g. type of fixing agent, thickness of the emulsion, silver coating weight, etc.).

Replenishment in a normal situation is usually governed by an average rate per length of film processed, and for fixer this is approximately 80–100 ml for every 35 cm. A useful rule-of-thumb guide is that fixer replenishment should be twice that of developer in any given situation, but again this depends on other factors and really an objective evaluation is the most desirable course to take. Again, as with developer, the average rate for the 35 cm length of film means that large films actually receive under-replenishment whereas small films receive over-replenishment, the net effect over a typical working day resulting in, on average, correct replenishment. 'Chips with everything' applies here too, as a microprocessor can be programmed to scan the film via a series of detectors, and to replenish correctly according to all the pertinent variables.

Fixing agent

There is only one agent used in automatic processing fixers. This is ammonium thiosulphate. This is used exclusively because of its ability to fully fix the image in a considerably reduced time compared to its sodium thiosulphate counterpart. The decrease in time is entirely due to quicker diffusion of the ammonium thiosulphate into the emulsion layers and associated quicker removal of by-products.

Traditionally, fixing times have been quoted as multiples of a factor known as clearing time.

Clearing time

The clearing time is defined as the time taken for the 'milky' appearance of a film that is receiving fixation, to just disappear, leaving the expected 'transparent' image.

The clearing times and associated fixing times for the two common agents are:

Ammonium thiosulphate
Fixing time = 1.3 × clearing time
Clearing time = 8–10 seconds (approx.)
Sodium thiosulphate
Fixing time = 2 × clearing time
Clearing time = 4–5 minutes.

All the above figures are quoted for the same film type at temperatures typically found in automatic processing. Again, this indicates the superiority of ammonium-based products in terms of speed of action. Finally, one other advantage is the fact that ammonium thiosulphate fixers are always provided in liquid concentrate form. This enables easy storage and preparation of working solutions.

Sodium thiosulphate fixers, as stated previously, are not generally in use in X-ray departments of the so-called 'developed countries'. However, it is incorrect to think that these fixers are totally unused, as in many circumstances where speed of action is not important their use is still widespread. They are also extensively used in 'third world' and developing nations, where they are sold in powder form.

Function

The function of the fixing agent is to convert unexposed, undeveloped silver bromide into water soluble silver complexes that can be removed from the film by the solvent present in the fixing bath.

When correctly carried out this renders the image permanent, as it removes any remaining silver bromide that would otherwise begin to break down under the action of light and cause the image to fog.

It also produces the 'transparent' appearance of the film, as the areas of the film that have received no exposure, if viewed directly after development, have an opalescent 'green' appearance. This is the undeveloped silver bromide that must be removed if the image is to become stable and useful on storage.

The removal of the unwanted silver bromide is a three-stage process, involving the initial neutralisation of developer carried over within the emulsion layer. Stage two of this process produces the only salt in photographic process that is insoluble in water.

Initial stage (Fig. 3.12)

The film transported from the developer into the fixer still contains alkali developer within the emulsion layers. Most of the surface developer has been removed by the action of the squeegee rollers as it passes out of the developer tank (see Automatic processing). However the remainder must be neutralised as quickly as possible before the fixing agent can get to work. This is achieved by the acid in the fixing bath working in the 'neutralisation zone' (Fig. 3.12).

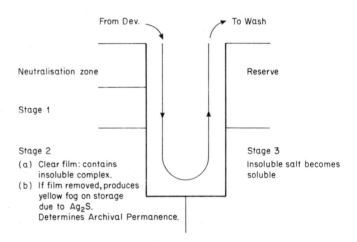

Fig. 3.12 The stages of the fixation process.

Stage one (Fig. 3.12)

When the film has passed through the neutralisation zone the fixing agent plus other active ingredients, e.g. the hardener, diffuse into the emulsion. This rate of diffusion depends on the type of fixing agent, the steepness of the diffusion gradient and the temperature of the solution. It is this rate that determines, primarily, the speed at which fixing occurs. Once within the emulsion, the ammonium thiosulphate reacts with the silver bromide to produce silver sulphate and certain by-products.

Stage two (Fig. 3.12)

The silver sulphate is further acted on by more ammonium thiosulphate to produce a simple salt of silver ammonium thiosulphate. This salt is insoluble in water. When all of the silver sulphate has been converted into this intermediate salt, the image will appear clear but is still not fully fixed. The time taken for the silver sulphate (green in appearance) to be converted into the simple salt (which is clear in appearance) is called the clearing time.

Stage three (Fig. 3.12)

The third stage is the conversion of the simple salt, by the further action of ammonium thiosulphate, into a complex salt of silver ammonium dithiosulphate which is soluble in water and is washed out of the film. When all of this complex salt has been removed from the film it is considered to be fully fixed.

Reserve capacity (Fig. 3.12)

Fixation, as can be seen from studying the previous stages, is a complex process involving many chemical reactions. As time is both limited and constant in automatic processing, it is prudent to have available a reserve capacity to ensure that correct fixation occurs. This allows for variations in, for example, temperature and replenishment that may result in prolongation of one or more of the stages just described.

If all of the intermediate salt, i.e. the silver ammonium thiosulphate, is not converted into its soluble version, fixation remains incomplete and degradation of the image, on storage, will occur even though the film may have been adequately washed (poor washing being the most important factor in image deterioration on storage). An interesting feature of the intermediate salt is that it has a bittersweet 'saccharine' taste. This can be put to good practical use, for if fixation is suspect it can easily be tested by tasting the corner of a completely processed film (i.e. one that has been developed, fixed, washed and dried). If it tastes bittersweet then it is not correctly fixed; the stronger the taste, the worse the fixation. This, of course, should only be carried out on a film with no diagnostic value, in addition to other quality assurance procedures, and with due regard to good hygiene practice.

Acid

As the film is transported from the developer section of the processor to the fixer it passes through a pair of squeegee rollers that remove surplus developer from the surface of the film. However, the developer remaining within the emulsion still continues to develop the image. If allowed to continue this would lead to degraded image quality. This is prevented by the acid component neutralising the alkali developer, thus stopping development as soon as the film enters the fixing tank. The process is carried out in the neutralisation zone (Fig. 3.12).

A fortuitous additional advantage is that the hardeners used in fixers are very pH dependent and need an acid environment in order to work at their most efficient.

Dichroic fog is a problem quoted in association with the fixing solution. It is caused by the continuation of development in the presence of the fixing agent and appears pink when viewed by transmitted light and green/silvery when viewed by reflected light. Dichroic fog does not occur in practice in automatic processors, as the pH value of the fixer would have to rise to such a level (certainly greater than 5.0) that the hardening action would be impaired to the extent that the film would not be transported through the processor (see Hardeners, p. 120; Buffers (below)).

Agent

The agent chosen to provide the acid content depends on which hardener is to be used. In radiographic fixers these are normally:

- Acetic acid with aluminium chloride as hardener
- Sulphuric acid with aluminium sulphate as hardener.

The association of a particular acid with a particular hardener should not be taken as definitive, as it is quite possible to have an acetic acid fixer with an aluminium sulphate hardener or a sulphuric acid fixer with an aluminium chloride hardener.

The choice of an acid paired with a certain hardener is made to ensure that sufficient active ions are available to produce a stable solution over a range of both storage and usage conditions.

Function

From the previous discussion it can be deduced that the main functions of the acid are to stop development by neutralising the alkali developer, and to provide the correct pH level for the hardening agent.

Buffers

As previously stated, even though the processor is designed to keep the carry-over of developer into fixer to a minimum, it cannot completely prevent it. The continual addition of even small amounts of alkali would eventually result in an increase in the pH value away from its desired level, eventually leading to problems with the hardening activities of the fixer and, if allowed to progress, would result in reduced hardening, non-drying and eventually non-transportation of the film through the processor. The classic definition of a buffer is 'a solution whose acidity or alkalinity is practically unchanged by dilution and which resists a change in pH on the addition of acid or alkali'. In the case of fixer, this solution is a mixture of two different agents, both of which have significant properties apart from their combined action as a buffer.

Agent

In nearly all cases, this is a mixture of acetic acid and one of a number of sulphite-based compounds, such as sodium sulphite or potassium sulphite to name but two. These sulphites also possess the property of exerting a preserving action on the thiosulphate complex of the fixing agent (see Preservatives (below)). To this end, a fixer buffer can be considered as:

Fixer buffer = acetic acid + preservative.

Acetic acid is nearly always the acid of choice, even when sulphuric acid is used for the acid component in aluminium sulphate-hardened fixers, as it has a very large buffer capacity. When acetic acid is used for the main acid content, obviously it can also act as part of the buffer combination.

Function

The single purpose of the buffer agent is to maintain the pH of the fixing solution within fine tolerances. This ensures correct neutralisation of developer contained within the emulsion as it enters the fixing tank (Fig. 3.12), and correct hardening of the emulsion by maintaining the pH level for optimum hardening action (see Hardeners, p. 120).

Preservatives

The many advantages of maintaining fixing solutions at a constant acid pH value have been established in the previous sections. Unfortunately, there is one disadvantage that cannot be conveniently ignored. If ammonium thiosulphate is placed in even a mild acid solution, it has a tendency to break down to form sulphur particles: this is known as sulphurisation. If allowed to progress, this would eventually render the fixer useless, producing a colloidal suspension of sulphur with a yellow/green 'particulate' appearance.

When the fixer is at the correct pH value, the production of sulphur particles is prevented by the preservative's active ions combining with any sulphur that may have formed, to produce a soluble complex that leads to the sulphur being re-dissolved. This effectively cancels out any effect that the sulphur would have had on the fixing bath.

Maintenance of correct pH values is very important, as this can have serious effects on the preservative's action:

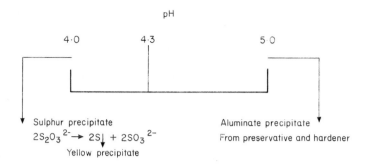

Fig. 3.13 The effect of pH on the preservative.

1. If the pH is allowed to rise above 5.0, a white crystalline deposit forms. This is a precipitate of sodium aluminate due to the action of the preservative and the hardener. Unfortunately, this is almost totally insoluble and is very difficult to remove. In practice it is probably true to say that the problems associated with decreased hardening action would be noticed before any white precipitate is formed (Fig. 3.13).

2. If the pH is allowed to fall below approximately 4.0, massive sulphurisation occurs due to the increased acidity. In practice the reduction of the pH to below 4.0 should not occur, providing certain simple precautions are taken during the mixing of fixer replenisher. Normally fixer hardener is added last to the combination of fixing agents and water. The hardener solution has a very low pH value (i.e. high acidity) of approximately 1.0–1.5. If this is added without sufficient agitation, it may cause localised depression of the pH to below 4.0, resulting in the production of sulphur. This can easily be seen during the mixing process. If precipitation does occur it can, apparently, be dispersed by further vigorous agitation. This does not cause the sulphur to re-dissolve; it simply mixes it throughout the replenisher tank, and when left to stand (say, over night) precipitates to the bottom of the tank where it can be seen as a light yellow crystalline deposit (Fig. 3.13).

Again, vigorous agitation will disperse this deposit, but it will reappear on leaving the solution to stand. The quantity of this deposit poses no particular problem unless present in excessive amounts, when it may cause partial filter blockage within the automatic processor or replenisher tank, resulting in reduced flow rate.

3. The third problem with the preservative, whilst not directly associated with the pH level of the fixer, is nevertheless significant and is not generally recognised.

It is easily appreciated that it is very important to reduce to a minimum aerial oxidation of the developer (see Developer preservative, p. 98). However, it is often erroneously stated that fixers do not suffer from oxidation due to the air. The facts are that whilst the *fixing agent* (i.e. ammonium thiosulphate) is not affected by the oxygen in the air, the *preservative* is significantly affected, its

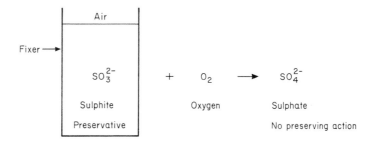

Fig. 3.14 The effects of oxygen on the fixer preservative.

efficiency decreasing according to the length of time of exposure. This decreasing efficiency is due to the sulphite ions combining with the oxygen to produce a sulphate which has no preserving action (Fig. 3.14)

Reduction of the sulphite preservative level in this way renders the fixing agent more susceptible to sulphurisation even at correct pH values, due to the decrease in the available sulphite causing a reduction in the efficiency of the conversion of any free sulphur into soluble inert (as far as the fixer is concerned) complexes.

In order to combat this problem it is useful to remember two precautions:

1. If possible, fit the fixer replenisher tank with a floating lid, similar to that in use in the developer replenisher tank; this reduces the surface area of the fixer in contact with the air. To be fair, this is only required when fixer use is very low, e.g. a theatre processor.

2. When preparing a solution for use in an area of very low film through-put, i.e. where there is very low fixer usage, do not make up more solution than is necessary to do the amount of work required.

In the majority of situations, auto-oxidation of the sulphite does not present any particular problem due to the high usage of fixer found in most departmental automatic processors. However it is not unusual to find the yellow precipitate (even if only a small amount) associated with sulphurisation due to poor mixing.

Agent

In all cases this is one of a number of sulphite-based compounds, the important criterion being the number of free sulphite ions liberated when the agent is in solution. It is the sulphite ion that has the preserving action on the ammonium thiosulphate. As there are a number of suitable agents, just two will be quoted as examples: sodium sulphite (Na_2SO_3) and potassium sulphite (K_2SO_3).

Function

The function of the preservative is to prevent or reduce to a minimum the breakdown of the fixing agent into sulphur particles. This breakdown is due to the action of the acid components of the fixing solution on the thiosulphate complex, and is called sulphurisation. Any free sulphur particles produced within the solution are converted by the sulphite ions present into a soluble complex that can be re-absorbed.

Hardeners

One of the major problems associated with rapid film processing is the necessity of using high processing temperatures and high pH values to reduce processing times. This has undesirable effects on the emulsion, causing excessive absorption of the processing solution; this leads to swelling and softening of the gelatine, leaving the film in a very delicate condition. In order that the film may be processed in a roller-type processor, the emulsion must be hardened to control the moisture absorption and, therefore, swelling and softening. If the film were not hardened, even a human hair on the surface of the emulsion would cause significant scratching. Hardening is so important that it is carried out during:

- Film manufacture
- Development and
- Fixing.

Film manufacture

The film is hardened at this stage to enable it to resist the abrasions caused by packing, unpacking, loading/unloading into the cassette, etc. It is not possible to completely protect the film from the effects of careless handling, as this would be practically impossible. To this end there is sufficent hardening to afford reasonable protection, but the film is still able to absorb the developer quickly enough to develop the image in about 22 seconds in a 90 second processor.

Development

Here the film is further hardened, as part of the development process, to resist the swelling and softening caused by the high temperatures and pH values of the developing solutions. However, it is important not to over-harden at this stage, as this would make fixation more difficult by slowing down the rate of absorption of fixing solution into the emulsion.

Fixing

The hardening is continued as part of the fixing process, where it prepares the film for the wash tank. It is here that the film is brought to its final degree of hardness, so that it does not absorb too much water during the washing process. If too much is absorbed the film would not become completely dry in the limited time available in the automatic processor dryer. Therefore, the amount or degree of hardening of the film in the fixer determines how efficiently the film will dry. Other factors are also significant, for example temperature, humidity, etc., but still one of the most common causes of the film coming out of the processor wet or damp is inadequate hardening, usually due either to failure to add sufficient hardening solution or to under-replenishment of the fixer.

Over-addition of the hardener can also cause problems as this leads to inadequate washing, due to reduction in the rate at which the wash water diffuses into and out of the emulsion, and consequently inadequate drying. A further problem that may not be immediately apparent concerns the archival permanence of the image. The film may be just dry enough to be handled, but may still contain thiosulphate complexes that have not been removed by washing. These decompose on storage and cause image staining to such a degree as to render the film useless.

The fixing bath is the only place where, in practice, the concentration of the hardener can be affected to any significant extent. This is due to the fact that during emulsion coating it is controlled by the manufacturer, and because hardening variations in development are not normally associated with immediate processing problems. For some reason it is all too common to discover that either no hardener or insufficient hardener has been added to the fixer replenisher. The problems associated with this occur quickly, starting with damp films and leading eventually to the film sticking in the processor, usually just at the entrance to the dryer where the wet sticky emulsion meets the hot dryer rollers.

Figure 3.15 shows the approximate moisture absorption caused by the addition of too much and too little hardener to the fixer replenisher.

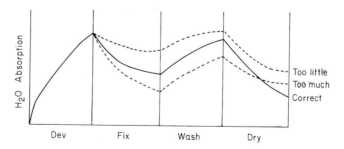

Fig. 3.15 The effects of hardening on emulsion water absorption.

Hardener and pH values

In the section on acid it was stated that one of its functions was to provide the correct pH value for the hardener to work. The efficiency

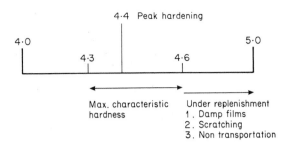

Fig. 3.16 The effect of pH on the hardening characteristics of fixer.

of the hardening action is very pH dependant, even small variations giving considerable changes in emulsion moisture absorption. Most conventional aluminium-based agents have their maximum characteristic hardening between a pH of 4.3–4.6, with a peak at 4.4 (Fig. 3.16). Consistant pH values above and below these limits soon manifest themselves as damp films coming out of the processor, and while it is difficult to produce low pH values (unless due to very poor mixing), high values (i.e. above 4.6) are easily produced by under-replenishment (Fig. 3.16).

Agent

The agent used as hardener varies according to which manufacturer produces the fixer. It is paired with a particular acid. This pairing increases the stability of the particular hardening agent in use. There are two principal aluminium-based compounds to be found in modern fixing solutions:

1. Aluminium chloride (Al Cl$_3$) with acetic acid
2. Aluminium sulphate (Al$_2$ (SO$_4$)$_3$) with sulphuric acid.

Both agents have advantages and disadvantages; the choice of which to use depends on the manufacturing process to be followed and the particular school of thought favoured by the chemical research team. However, there is no doubt about the active ingredient of the combination as this is always the aluminium ion.

Function

The function of the hardening agent is to control the swelling and softening of the emulsion, i.e. moisture uptake, thereby allowing roller processing, high processing temperatures and rapid drying times. It also protects the film from moderate forms of mechanical damage that may occur during processing.

The control of moisture uptake is achieved by the aluminium ions causing cross-linking of the gelatine polymer within the emulsion, thus keeping the chain-like molecule 'tightly packed', even though its spiral structure tends to unwind when placed in water.

Solvent

Again, as with developer this is almost always water. Normal tap water is more than adequate but the use of a filtered supply from the output side of the water mixing panel has the added advantage of reducing to a minimum the presence of particles of grit, dirt, etc., that may scratch the emulsion if allowed into the machine tank of the processor.

Tap water has all the advantages and disadvantages stated in the section on developers, but in this case there is the additional problem associated with the presence, in the film emulsion, of the only non-water soluble salt in the photographic process.

Commercial preparations

Fixer replenisher available from manufacturers is normally supplied as a liquid concentrate to make up so many mixed litres, typically containing two parts. These parts are either marked 'A' and 'B' or Replenisher and Hardener (part 'A' corresponding to the replenisher and part 'B' to the hardener). Unlike developer, some manufacturers provide replenisher and hardener as separate items and require a separate order for each (rather than combining them in one complete pack). The exact contents of each part are normally trade secrets, but in general are as summarised in Table 3.8.

Table 3.8 Fixer contents in commercial preparations

Part	Danger	Content
A Replenisher	Causes burns	Fixing agent Acid Buffer Preservative Solvent
B Hardener	Causes burns pH 1.0–1.5	Hardener Acid

It is very important never to add concentrate part 'B' (i.e. hardener) to concentrate part 'A' (i.e. replenisher), as an instant precipitate of aluminium forms, 'plates' onto any metallic components and is extremely difficult to remove. This precipitate can form even when there are relatively low concentrations of part 'A', so it is good practice to add only hardener to correctly diluted part 'A' (see below, Mixing).

Mixing

Fixer should be mixed carefully with due regard to the fact that both parts can cause burns. Suitable protective clothing should be worn in the form of gloves, apron, glasses, etc. These basic precautions are often ignored, and whilst it is considered tedious by some people to put on protective aprons, etc., it does prevent fixer splashes burning holes in clothing and prevents dermatitis from splashes on the skin.

Before mixing the replenisher, check the volume remaining in the tank and ensure that there is sufficient space to accept the additional solution. Then:

1. Add the volume of water stated in the instructions.

2. Add slowly the whole of part 'A' (or the part marked 'replenisher') with continuous stirring.

3. Add the whole of part 'B' or, if the hardener is supplied separately, the correct amount according to the instructions. This is usually so much hardener per mixed litre of solution; typical volumes are 25 ml per litre. Thorough stirring at this stage is vital to prevent localised production of insoluble sulphur particles.

4. Continue stirring for at least two minutes to ensure a uniform solution mixture.

Some manufacturers offer the option of diluting the replenisher either 3:1 or 4:1 (i.e. three parts water to one part fixer), the choice depending on the particular application the fixer will be used for. This also alters the amount of hardener required. There is no advantage in under-diluting fixer in an attempt to obtain more rapid fixing; in fact the amount of water present is vital as this is the solvent for the final product of the fixation process. An easy proof of this is trying to fix a film in a dish of concentrated fixer; no matter how long the film is left it will not clear. However, if this concentrate is slowly diluted with increasing amounts of water, the film will clear rapidly.

Temperature ranges

The temperature of the fixer is vital if correct fixation is to be assured. Simply: the higher the temperature the shorter the fixing time. Within certain limits, there is an almost linear relationship between increasing temperature and decreasing fixing times. In most cases it is not possible to alter fixing times during automatic processing, therefore accurate temperature is essential.

Fixer temperatures are closely related to developer temperatures, and in an ideal situation both solutions should be identical (e.g. 32°C). However, in practice it is quite common to find slight variations between the two and, in general, the maximum variation allowable is that the fixer should not be more than 2°C lower in temperature than the developer.

All commercially available solutions are designed to work in the ranges 26–39°C, allowing alterations in fixing times away from the approximate 22 seconds found in 90 second automatic processing. This means that these are suitable for use with both high and low temperature developer chemistry. Problems may occur at the lower end of this temperature range, but these probably would not be visible until after a period of storage. Increasing to a two minute processing cycle may prove to be the cure for this situation if this is convenient from a departmental point of view.

Practical tests

These are the subject of Chapter 6 (Quality Assurance), but are included here for completeness.

- pH of the machine tank fixer
- pH of the fixer replenisher
- Measure replenishment rates
- Measure silver concentration levels
- Specific gravity of the machine and replenisher solutions
- Sensitometric evaluation.

Summary

1. For a chemical to be a fixer it must possess two main properties, conversion and selectivity. It must be able to convert unexposed, undeveloped silver halide into a form that can be washed from the emulsion, but it must not degrade the newly-developed image or affect the gelatine in which it is suspended.

2. All fixers used in automatic processers are of the acid hardening type, using ammonium thiosulphate as the fixing agent. This agent produces the most rapid fixers without having to resort to the cyanates (although these have a more rapid action).

3. The pH of the fixer must be maintained within fine limits to ensure rapid neutralisation of the alkali developer and to provide the correct environment for the hardener to work. Automatic processor fixer has a pH range between 4.2–4.9, and should be maintained within 0.2 of its recommended value.

4. Fixer replenisher is important as it is used to maintain solution activity and quantity. There are many factors affecting the degree of replenishment required and these are listed in the main text.

5. A typical fixer comprises many agents; Table 3.9 shows the general names of these agents, their probable chemical composition and their function.

Table 3.9 Fixer constituents: probable composition and function

General name	Chemical used	Function
Fixing agent	Ammonium thiosulphate	Conversion of undeveloped AgBr into soluble silver complexes
Acid	Acetic or sulphuric acid	Stops development Provides correct pH for hardener
Buffer	Acetic acid + preservative	Maintains pH of solution
Preservative	Sodium or potassium sulphite	Reduces sulphurisation to a minimum
Hardener	Aluminium chloride + acetic acid Aluminium sulphate + sulphuric acid	Controls emulsion water absorption
Solvent	Water	Acts as solvent for fixer chemicals and by-products of fixation

6. Commercially available fixer may come in two parts, marked 'A' and 'B' or Replenisher and Hardener, respectively. These concentrates should never be mixed without the correct amount of water being added first.

7. When mixing chemicals, follow carefully the manufacturer's instructions, wear protective clothing and use continuous stirring.

8. Fixer temperature is closely related to developer temperature and should be no more than $2°C$ cooler than the developer.

9. Practical tests, given as a list above, are the subject of Chapter 6, Quality assurance.

WASHING

Compared with the previous sections the consideration given to the washing process will probably seem trite. This is not because the washing process is unimportant; on the contrary, all the effort given to maintaining correct replenishment rates, pH values and other factors connected with the 'chemical' balance of the processor and production of the final image can be severely damaged by neglecting the simple process of adequately washing the film. In automatic processing it is not usually possible to significantly alter wash rates, other than to forget to turn on the water supply to the processor; and in any case the water flow to the processor is normally set by the engineer on installation, according to the manufacturer's recommendations. It must also be remembered that the water supply can be responsible for assisting in the control of other important processor functions, for example developer temperature control, etc. (see Automatic processing, p. 151); therefore altering water flow to increase the efficiency of the wash process may affect other systems whose immediate importance outweighs the necessity for better washing.

In general, however, when operating correctly the processor is designed to more than adequately wash the films for conventional purposes.

Function

The function of the washing process is to remove from the film emulsion, fixer that has not been used in the conversion of unexposed, undeveloped silver bromide into soluble complexes, and also to remove the remainder of the soluble silver complex salts that have not been removed by the water present in the fixing solution.

The removal of the substances is of vital importance, as it is the level of these salts in the film after washing that determines its archival permanence.

Archival permanence

Archival permanence is defined as the length of time a film will store without significant deterioration in its image quality. In practice the tests carried out in most X-ray departments are quite inaccurate and only give a vague idea of safe storage times. The normal bands considered are: less than 5 years; 10–20 years; 20–25 years, and greater than 25 years. These bands are then measured using a colour comparison chart. More accurate methods of determining archival permanence are available but require some knowledge of chemistry and access to chemical analysis equipment, e.g. BS 1153/1955. It is traditional to test for residual thiosulphate to measure archival permanence, as this proves to be most convenient. (See Chapter 6 Quality Assurance.)

The salts responsible for image degradation are silver complex salts and residual thiosulphates.

Silver complex salts

These consist of the intermediate insoluble silver salts that remain in the emulsion due to inadequate fixing (i.e. not all have been converted to the soluble silver complex salt for some reason), and the soluble silver complex salt that has not yet been dissolved by water. Obviously, washing the film is not going to remove the insoluble salt, as this is a problem of poor fixing, but it will remove the soluble complex. This soluble complex deteriorates with time to form a silver sulphide which produces an overall yellow/brown 'fog', therefore its reduction to a low level is important.

Residual thiosulphate

This is the remaining ammonium thiosulphate that is present in the emulsion. If not completely removed it decomposes to produce a very mild acid which attacks the silver image and converts it to a silver sulphide. This results in a yellow/brown staining and image fade, due to the reduction in the amount of silver forming the image.

As previously stated, it is traditional to test for archival permanence by estimating or actually measuring the amount of residual thiosulphate present in the emulsion after it has been dried. This test is chosen because ammonium thiosulphate is present in the largest quantities, it is easier to detect by chemical test, and both the soluble silver complexes and the thiosulphate are removed from the emulsion at the same rate.

Residual thiosulphate test

This assesses the archival permanence of the processed film. It can be carried out using a commercially available preparation, or failing this by using a 1% solution of silver iodide in a weak acid solution. To carry out the test, place a small drop of the solution on the emulsion surface in a clear area of the film to be tested. If the film is duplitised, this should be in the same place on both emulsions. Blot off the excess using a paper towel and wait the period of time recommended in the instructions (usually about 30 seconds, in subdued lighting). Compare the colour on the film with the comparator chart and assess the archival permanence range. This should be carried out in daylight to obtain the most accurate results. Do not place the film on a viewing box after the solution has been applied, as this accelerates the reaction that is occurring and gives a false indication of the archival permanence; also, do not attempt to compare the film with the colour chart after about 30 seconds beyond the recommended waiting time as this also gives false indications.

If thiosulphate is present it is indicated by a yellow colouration that gets progressively darker the worse the archival permanence.

Stages of washing

Washing is essentially a diffusion process that occurs in three stages:

1. Due to the concentration gradient that exists between the high salt concentrations within the emulsion as compared to the water in the wash tank, the residual salts diffuse out of the emulsion.

2. The dissolved salts within the water around the film are removed by the constant circulation of water within the automatic processor wash tank.

3. The contaminated water within the wash tank is replaced by fresh incoming water, thus helping to maintain the high concentration gradient required to wash the films to the correct degree.

Diffusion of the salts out of the emulsion occurs until an equilibrium situation exists between the concentration in the emulsion and the concentration in the wash water around the film. In theory, the decrease in the thiosulphate content of the film follows an exponential curve with the result that no matter how long the film is washed there is never a zero thiosulphate count. However, this is of no practical significance as the lowest thiosulphate count possible depends on the proportion of other dissolved salts in the wash water. To carry this argument further, it seems logical to use demineralised water to wash the film to its ultimate extent, but if this is done, excessive swelling of the gelatine occurs; this destroys the capillaries within the emulsion and causes sludging in the wash tank.

In practice even the most efficient washing systems do not approach the level of the emulsion salt content equalling that of the water supply. This is mainly due to the short washing times found in automatic processors and the fact that there is no need to wash to such high standards. Most modern processors will comfortably wash to 175 mg of thiosulphate per square metre, which in average storage conditions gives greater than 25 years archival permanence.

Factors affecting wash rate

Most of the factors affecting a film's wash rate are beyond practical control, as they are a function either of processor design or of the chemical composition of the water supply. However, for the sake of completeness the following list gives the most significant factors (and a brief explanation where necessary).

1. *Steepness of the concentration gradient*

This is the difference in the concentration between the salts within the emulsion and those in the wash water. The steeper the gradient, the more rapid the washing.

2. *Rate of water flow*

The more rapid the water change the more rapid the washing, as this keeps the concentration gradient high and provides agitation.

3. *Degree of agitation*

High agitation levels provide high levels of fresh water to the surface of the film, helping the factors above.

4. *Temperature*

In theory, an increase in water temperature provides quicker washing. However, in practice there is little choice that can be made, as wash temperature is a function of individual processor systems.

5. *Degree of hardening*

This is a function of fixation, and in a correctly operating processor is constant at a pre-determined level. Over-hardening of the emulsion results in poor washing, due to salts in the emulsion having difficulty in diffusing out. Under-hardening results in over-absorption of water giving transportation problems.

6. *Time in the wash tank*

This is of little practical significance, as this is constant in an automatic processor and depends on the time cycle as a whole.

7. *pH of the wash water*

This is of no practical significance.

Many of these points are interrelated and dependant on factors such as processor design, chemical design, and the degree of archival permanence required from the stored image. Conventionally it is unusual to store films for periods much in excess of seven years, however, recent EEC recommendations suggest that archival storage up to and in excess of 21 years may be introduced; this would certainly require a much closer look at present standards of washing. Microfilm archiving systems are designed to provide this level of permanence but still require careful monitoring of residual thiosulphate contents.

Summary

As this is only a short section, a lengthy summary is unnecessary; however, a few points are significant.

1. The wash process is carried out to remove soluble silver complex salts and residual fixing agent from the film emulsion.

2. The degree to which a film is washed, in most cases, determines its archival permanence.

3. There are both objective and subjective tests to determine archival permanence, the most common one in X-ray departments being the residual thiosulphate test.

4. Washing is a continuous three-stage diffusion process, the rate of which depends on a number of closely related factors.

5. The testing for residual thiosulphate is especially significant for microfilm archival systems.

SILVER CONSERVATION

Silver conservation has always been desirable. It has assumed greater significance in recent years due to the increased financial constraints placed on the X-ray department and the widely varying price of silver. Fortunately the last factor, at the time of writing, seems to have stabilised following the 'silver crisis' of the late 1970s. Figure 3.17 shows how the silver price varied between July 1984 and July 1985. It has been estimated that the photographic industry consumes about 40% of the total silver used, and that approximatly 66% of this is recoverable. The cost benefits are obvious. The main reasons for carrying out silver recovery are:

- The high price of silver can bring profitable returns
- Silver is a diminishing natural resource that requires conservation
- Effluent that contains high silver concentrations can cause ecological damage.

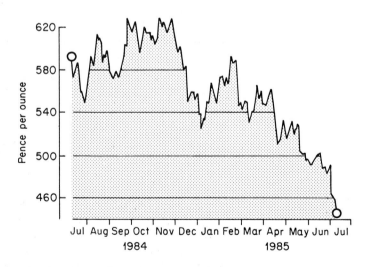

Fig. 3.17 Variation of silver price July 1984–July 1985, showing downward trend. Since July 1985 a further 100p has been lost, leaving the price at 350p/Troy oz (March 87); this is still not cheap. Source: The Times 16/7/85 and Datastream.

As a basic guide, 1000 35 × 43 cm films contain approximately 32 Troy oz of silver. Assuming silver at £5/oz, this gives £160 of totally recoverable silver. After 1000 average-sized films have been processed, there are approximately 13 Troy oz available for immediate recovery. Again assuming £5/oz, this gives a return of £65.

Methods of silver recovery

A number of methods of silver recovery are available. For the sake of completeness the main methods are listed below; some are easier to utilise than others and the choice of method will depend on local circumstances, amount of fixer used, financial return expected, staff available, etc.

- Collection of fixer
- Metal (ion) exchange
- Electrolytic recovery
- Precipitation
- Collection of old films.

Collection of used fixer

This is perhaps the easiest and most straightforward of the methods listed. A number of specialist companies will collect the used fixer in containers and the silver is recovered and refined elsewhere. Credit can be given either for an estimated silver concentration at the time of collection, or for the assayed quantity after refining. Most reputable collectors will provide an estimate on collection and an assayed valuation as a check of the true silver content.

Metal exchange

When a silver salt solution is brought into contact with a base metal (i.e. steel wool, zinc, etc.) the base metal is replaced by the silver, and the base metal ions are released into solution. The sludge produced can be collected and dried, and the silver refined. In a steel wool silver recovery unit this principle can readily be exploited. A steel wool cartridge of 5 kg can, theoretically, recover 20 kg of silver; in practice, an amount between 5 and 15 kg should easily be obtained. Figure 3.18 is a simplified diagram of such a unit.

The steel wool is held in a plastic container and the processor fixer overflow is connected directly to the unit via a bypass valve. This prevents the overflow of fixer should the unit become blocked. As the fixer passes over the steel wool in the cartridge, metal exchange takes place and the silver is deposited as a sludge. A secure lid is essential to prevent the escape of fumes. The unit should be kept in a well-ventilated place away from the general working environment.

To ensure maximum efficiency, particular attention should be paid to the following points:

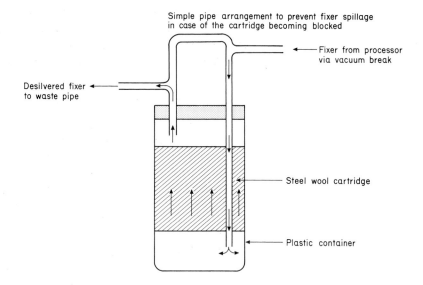

Fig. 3.18 Diagrammatic cross-section of metal (ion) exchange in the silver recovery unit.

1. Ensure that the steel wool remains below the fixer solution level. This reduces oxidation of the wool and ensures that any build-up of heat caused by that oxidation is kept to a minimum.

2. Ensure that solution flow through the cartridge is at the correct speed. Too high a flow will reduce the efficiency of recovery.

3. Monitor the outflow for the presence of residual silver. This can be done with silver estimating papers, but these can be unreliable.

4. The fitting of a similar unit in tandem may improve the efficiency of the whole system.

5. Remove exhausted cartridges as soon as possible.

Although this method is cheap and easy to run, some significant problems exist, such as the danger of clogging the cartridge and discharging iron ions into the drains. The variable workload experienced in most departments could mean that the automatic processor, working under peak load, would flood the cartridge and silver would go to waste.

Theoretical efficiency is of the order of 95%, but in practice 70% is a more realistic target.

DHSS document DA(83) 23 recommends metal exchange as the recovery method of choice when fixer use is below 20 litres per day.

Metal replacement with zinc dust

This is NOT recommended for use in an X-ray department. Zinc dust is scattered over the surface of used fixer; because the dust offers a very large surface area to the fixer solution this method can be extremely efficient, more so if the solution is agitated. The fixer should be acidified with glacial acetic acid for the best results and the solution should be regularly checked for silver concentration to ensure that all the silver is being converted. When the silver level is sufficiently low the sludge can be removed, collected and refined.

Electrolytic recovery

This is the most popular method of silver recovery. Providing the unit is working correctly very pure silver is produced (of the order of 95–98% purity), very little further refining is required and the possibility of re-using the fixer exists. It is based on the principle that when two electrodes (usually a carbon anode and a stainless steel cathode) are placed in a used fixer solution and a direct current is passed between them, positively charged silver ions ($Ag+$) are attracted to the cathode, where their charge is neutralised and they plate out as metallic silver (Ag). If the current is increased the silver is deposited faster. However, if the current is too high or the silver concentration too low, the ions cannot get to the cathode fast enough and 'sulphiding' occurs. This is a black layer of silver sulphide which can eventually stop the plating process altogether. These factors influence the construction of the two types of electrolytic units.

Low current density

Usually found in situ in manual processing units. They use large electrodes with a very low current in order to reduce the risk of sulphiding. However, the current must not be too low, as no transfer of the silver ions will occur at very low current densities. They are of little significance in the modern department.

High current density

In high current density units the fixer solution is under constant agitation. This allows operation at a higher current and the use of a smaller surface area cathode without the same danger of sulphiding. Agitation is achieved by rotation of the cathode and/or the anode, a separate stirring device or by bubbling air through the solution. This has the advantage of bringing fresh silver ions close to the surface of the cathode and speeding up the rate of deposition of metalic silver.

The output of these units can range from 10–400 g per hour.

Regular checking of the silver levels and adjustment of the current density is required to avoid sulphiding and thus ensure maximum silver returns. However, in most departments this would be too time-consuming and units are set to a current value that corresponds to an 'average' silver concentration of the fixer.

Modern units have solved this problem by incorporating a micro-processor that monitors silver concentration and adjusts the current supplied to give maximum returns.

No diagram has been included to describe these units. This is deliberate, as so many different units are available and a specific example would only confuse. The reader is referred to the one in use in his/her department for complete details.

Precipitation

This method is included for the sake of completeness, but it is *not* recommended for use as it is difficult to carry out and can produce poisonous fumes which can also fog films.

When sodium sulphide (20%) is added to waste fixer, a silver sulphide sludge is produced in the bottom of the container. This sludge requires collection, drying and refining. Alternatively, ferrous hydroxide or sodium hydrosulphate can be added to waste fixer. If the latter is used a particularly pure form of silver is produced. If ferrous hydroxide is used the solution must first be made alkaline. The resultant precipitate must be skimmed and dried.

Collection of old films

It should not be forgotten that old films have a considerable amount of silver content. A number of specialist companies operate collection services for quantities of used film. The company will normally offer a price for each kilogram of film to be collected; this will depend on an estimate of the recoverable silver available and whether the films are in envelopes or not. Credit is normally given against the assayed value of the recovered silver, minus an amount for the service provided by the company.

Estimation of silver yield

This is fraught with many problems and no firm indication can be given, as numerous variables are involved, for example: the average density of the films after processing, the average silver content of the fixer before recovery, the average silver content of the fixer after recovery, the silver content of all the different types of emulsion being used in the department, the exact efficiency of the recovery methods in use, etc., etc.

It has been suggested that there are, on average, approximately 4 g of recoverable silver per square metre of film used. Whilst this may be a reasonable guide, it does not take into account advances in emulsion technology resulting in lower silver coating weights or local variations in the factors mentioned above. It seems reasonable to suggest that an estimate for the potential amount of recoverable silver is made over, say, a six month period and that this is compared to actual returns.

The amount recoverable can be estimated by multiplying the amount of fixer used in the period by the average silver content of that fixer, less an amount for fixer that has been wasted. This of course is only very approximate but may serve as a rough guide. It has also been suggested that the fixer leaving the recovery unit be regularly monitored: providing that this is somewhat below 1 g/l, this is an acceptable indication of an adequate standard of recovery. Readers are left to make their own decisions.

Ecological considerations

When the degree of pollution caused by the waste water from X-ray film processing is examined it is found that, when compared to other industries, very few problems exist.

It is important that both the fixer and developer are emptied into the same sealed drain, as this will mean that the pH value of the waste water will lie between the permitted tolerance of 6–9 pH value. There are no solids, oils or fats, the temperature is not excessive, and there is a total absence of chromium or ferricyanide ions. The main problems arise due to the probable presence of silver and the Biochemical Oxygen Demand (BOD).

Adequate silver recovery procedures should ensure that pollution from this source is minimal.

> The BOD is a measure of the content of organic matter in water and wastes. It is the amount of oxygen when a sample containing a known mass of oxygen in solution is kept at 20°C for five days. The oxygen is consumed by microorganisms that feed on the organic matter in the sample. *Penguin Dictionary of Science 1979*

Processing 15 m^2 of film per day requires a BOD of approximatly 600 g oxygen per 24 hours. This is similar to that of domestic waste water. It is accepted that the pollution caused by one person in an industrialised country requires a BOD of 54 g oxygen per 24 hours. Calculations reveal that processing 1–1.5 m^2 of X-ray film gives approximately the same pollution as one person in one day.

In addition to the BOD per day, the BOD per litre of waste water is also important. A typical value for processor effluent would be 650 mg oxygen/l. This is about twice the average value of domestic waste water, but considerably less than other industries, e.g. the food industry (2000–5000 mg oxygen/l) or intensive stock-breeding (30 000–50 000 mg oxygen/l).

Other factors that may be considered are the Chemical Oxygen Demand (COD) and the Total Dissolved Solids (TDS).

It is important to get these values into perspective. The effluent discharge from the processor is diluted many thousands of times before it leaves the hospital, continues to be diluted in the main sewage system and by the time it reaches the treatment plant should pose no problems to purification. However, this is no excuse for complacency, and regular monitoring of the efficiency of silver recovery is essential.

Special precautions may be necessary if the processor is not connected to a mains sewage system or if discharge is directly into surface water drains. Consultation with the local water authority will always be required.

REFERENCES

Christensen E, Curry T, Dowdey J 1978 An introduction to the physics of diagnostic
   radiology, 2nd edn. Lea & Febiger, Philadelphia
Jacobson R E, Ray S F, Attridge G G, Axford N R 1978 The manual of photography,
   7th edn. Focal Press, London
James T H 1979 The theory of the photographic process, 4th edn. Collier Macmillan,
   London
Uvarov E B, Chapman D R, Issacs A 1979 Penguin dictionary of science, 5th edn.
   Penguin Books, Harmondsworth

4

Automatic processing

Introduction

The final link in the production of the X-ray image is processing, manual or automatic. This final process is as vital as any other procedure in the imaging chain. No matter how good the radiographer, the film or the screens, the final result is made or marred in processing.

The purpose of this chapter is to look at the advantages of automatic processing. The history of its development is also considered. The inside of an automatic processor is usually a mystery to those who use it: to this end a processor is constructed from 'scratch'. The modern developments of automatic processors are also considered.

Modern automatic processing produces few film faults and these are almost always the same. These faults are listed, as are general film faults.

MANUAL PROCESSING VERSUS AUTOMATIC PROCESSING

Before automatic processing is discussed, it is worthwhile to look closely at manual processing and then to examine the reasons why automatic processing was an inevitable and invaluable progression.

Time

Table 4.1, below, illustrates the relative differences in time required by manual and automatic processing. The times illustrated are average values.

Table 4.1 Time requirements of manual and automatic processors.

Process	Manual	Automatic
Development	3–5 min	22 s
Stop bath or rinse	10–20 s	Nil
Fixing	10 min	22 s
Wash	15 min	22 s
Drying	20 min	24 s
Total	(approx.) 50 min	90 s

Convenience

In manual processing there are nine distinct steps:

1. Unloading the film
2. Loading the film onto a hanger
3. Development
4. Stop bath or rinsing
5. Fixing
6. Washing
7. Immersion in a wetting agent
8. Drying
9. Reloading the cassette, possibly with wet hands.

These steps give nine opportunities for damage to the film or screens. In automatic processing, the list comes down to three:

1. Unloading the film
2. Inserting into processor
3. Reloading the cassette.

It may be interesting for the student to consider daylight handling systems at this point.

1. Insert the cassette into the system.

In a centralised daylight system, one single operation is all that is required!

Economics

Very often, justification has to be made for the purchase of an item such as an automatic processor. Listed below are the various considerations of manual versus automatic processing.

1. Automatic processing eliminates all hangers and their replacements.

2. There is little or no difference in the electrical consumption of the two systems, assuming there is thermostatic control on the manual system and there is an electrical dryer. Indeed, with modern processors the current drain could be typically 6 A.

3. Water consumption is significantly lower in automatic processors than in manual processors. Water in a manual system has to run continuously in the wash tank. Typically, this can be about 12–15 l/min. With modern energy-saving devices, automatic processors use about 1.5 l/min, and that only whilst there is film in the processor.

4. Film wastage can be reduced, simply because of standardising the development process.

5. Chemical costs for both manual and automatic systems will be approximately the same, as long as correct replenishment procedures are applied.

6. An average darkroom technician can process about 5 m^2/h manually. With an automatic processor, this increases to 15 m^2/h.

7. There is a considerable saving in space using automatic processing.

As a very rough guide, if film consumption of the department reaches 10 m^2 a day (about 138 24×30 films), then automatic processing is the cheaper of the two systems, bearing all the above in mind. This saving can be as much as two thirds of the cost of manual processing.

Advantages of automatic processing

All the factors which can influence the photographic quality of the radiographs are kept within very fine limits. Automatic processing therefore provides consistent, uniform results.

1. Time in the developer, fixer, wash and dryer is constant, due to a controlled drive system.

2. In normal conditions the temperature of all the solutions is unaffected by outside conditions.

3. The quality and the quantity of the solutions are maintained to a high standard, due to automatic replenishment.

4. Pump-driven circulation of the processing solutions along with continuous movement of the rollers ensures constant agitation,

giving uniform penetration of the chemicals into the emulsion layer of the film.

5. Constant dryer temperatures along with even distribution of the drying air ensure even drying and a uniform surface quality of the film.

6. Because of all these factors, coupled with the exposure latitude of modern X-ray film, satisfactory results can be obtained with exposure discrepancies as great as ± 25%.

7. Very short exposure times are to a large extent made possible by absolute uniformity of these factors, which is almost impossible to achieve with manual processing.

In short, the modern automatic processor may be considered as its own compact environmental control unit.

HISTORY OF AUTOMATIC PROCESSING

It is always interesting to look at the historical developments which have led to a finished product. The evolution of automatic processing almost demands that the history should be studied, to lead to a clearer understanding of why and how things are as they are.

The development of the processor starts at the beginning of the 20th century, but at that early stage it was not concerned with X-ray film. A number of attempts were made in the early 1900s to mechanise the development process, with little or no success. Then in 1910, Glen Dye, the founder of the Pako Corporation in the United States, introduced the first motor driven printer to process photographic paper. In 1918, he automated the drying process for photographic prints. In the 1920s he produced the first washing process for prints.

All of these early developments were concerned with the 'paper' side of photography. Then in 1929, Pako introduced the Senior Filmachine, which made it possible to automatically process amateur roll film in large quantities, with the consequential substantial savings in labour costs. This was the nearest stage at this time to dealing with a sensitive emulsion coated on a clear base.

Anyone who has watched a Walt Disney cartoon cannot fail to appreciate the skill and ability of the animators who draw the characters. However, not many people appreciate that for a single character in a 2-hour cartoon film, there would be approximately 180 000 separate drawings. That number only includes the one figure; backgrounds and any other characters inserted in the cartoon would make the figure astronomical. In the mid-30s, Walt Disney was looking for a process which would help minimise the handwork in the production of animated cartoons. Pako, at this stage, were contemplating the construction of an X-ray processor. Disney approached the Pako Corporation and a processor was devised to handle the (then) oversized negatives used in cartoon work. This experience was a major stepping stone in the later development of the X-ray film processor we know today.

Just before the start of World War Two, Pako had worked in the Mayo Clinic to try and perfect a 'dip and dunk' processor. The technical know-how gained from the Disney experience proved vital during the war, as these processors were used to process industrial X-ray film in many military applications.

In 1946 the first of the commercial Pako 'dip and dunk' machines was installed in a New York hospital. The analysis of operation of this machine is staggering by today's standards. To start with, the machine was about 2′6″ (76 cm) wide by about 15′ (457 cm) long. The description of operation (from a fact sheet c. 1949) makes interesting reading:

> The film is initially loaded on to a hangette which can accomodate 2 17×14 inch films, or 4 8×10 inch films. The hangette is then placed on a bar at the loading end of the machine. A lever is operated which then drops the hangette into an automatic conveyor. The film is then immersed in the developer for half a minute. It is then removed, automatically, and transferred one step forward in the developer for one minute. There were three more one-minute stops and a one-half minute stops that completed the five minute cycle of development. There is then a one and a half minute stop in an acetic acid stop bath to neutralise the alkali of the developer and to protect the acidity of the fixer. This also has the benefit of stopping development almost immediately. There is a total of 15 minutes in the two separate fixer tanks; 22 minutes are then taken up in the two wash tanks. A further one-minute immersion in a wetting agent to complete the wet processing cycle. The film then enters the infrared dryer. The dryer takes 35 minutes to dry the film.

The total dry-to-dry time was 1 h 19½ min. There was, however, provision to view emergency films one minute after their immersion in the fixer.

It can be seen from this description of the machine that the appoach was to make an 'automatic' darkroom technician with 'automatic' arms. There was obviously no saving in time but a trend to *consistent quality* had evolved.

Although only the Pako Corporation developments have been looked at above, this should not be taken to imply that other companies and individuals have not contributed to the evolution of automatic processing machines.

For example, around the time of the original Pako 'dip and dunk' machine, Dr Hills of Guys Hospital was developing another 'dip and dunk', without a dryer. This had a 35 min cycle; 5 min development, 3 min fixing, 25 min wash. The later model of the Hills-Russell machine had a dryer added, which took another 15 min to dry the film.

Also, at the end of World War Two some considerable expertise had built up in the roller processing of dental film. This work was not to materialise until some 10–15 years later.

The magic words in the above paragraph are 'roller processing'. During the early 1950s the attitude of manufacturers began to polarise as some parts of the industry publicly stated that X-ray film would be unable to stand the rigours of roller processing.

At this stage, parallel developments took place, on the one hand the 'dip and dunk' processor, on the other the roller processor.

Roller processor

Three companies — Gevaert, Kodak and Pako — were looking closely at the development of roller processors. Kodak introduced the first roller processor with stepped roller film drive, whereby the film was carried in and out of deep tanks.

Pako had also settled for a deep tank, with a sun and planetary roller drive system (Fig. 4.1).

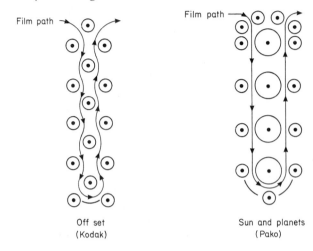

Off set
(Kodak)

Sun and planets
(Pako)

Fig. 4.1 Transport systems: off set and 'sun and planets'.

Gevaert had developed the Curixmatic processor. This had shallow tanks and an opposed roller drive system. The processor, because of this drive system, was significantly longer than its contemporaries (Fig. 4.2).

It says a great deal for these manufacturers' research teams that these drive systems are still in use today, in varying forms.

All the above processors had a time cycle of about $7\frac{1}{2}$ min, which was revolutionary at the time. It is important to note that the processors were capable of dealing with the film *in use at the time*, i.e. a manual process film coated on an acetate base.

It became very apparent at this stage that special processing chemistry had to be developed. Both the fixer and developer needed hardeners. Then the film emulsion was scrutinised and optimised so that, in the relatively short time the film was in the processing

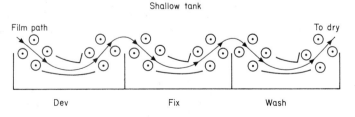

Shallow tank

Film path

To dry

Dev   Fix   Wash

Fig. 4.2 Transport systems: shallow tank.

solutions, it was capable of being processed to its fullest extent. In fact, the link between processor/film/chemistry was being inexorably forged.

The trend to words faster processing cycles then appeared. The half cycle ($5\frac{1}{2}$ min) arrived on the scene along with smaller processing machines, but still faster machines were demanded by the X-ray departments. Then in 1965, polyester base was introduced by Dupont.

Other companies followed with similar-type bases for films, and this finally established the processor/film/chemistry link. The manual film had been acetate-based, difficult to transport at the best of times. It was thicker than polyester and less optically clear. Polyester had a major advantage in its chemical 'memory'. It always 'remembered' it had been made flat. It was firm and rigid and yet was flexible enough to transport easily through an automatic processor. In addition (and this was to become very important in 15 years' time) the film had less silver in the emulsion. The film was also suitable for manual processing. This was quite a feat, as the film was now capable of being processed in the range 65°–105°F, an operating range of 40°F.

Machine speeds came down to $3\frac{1}{2}$ min and then 90 s. The machines also got significantly smaller. The Dupont T3, the Gevaert Gevamatic 110, the Kodak M6 and the Pako XU were all examples of this genre. This was followed by the 'table top' processor, a compact automatic processor, usually running at about a 2 min cycle. The Pako 14X and the Kodak M100 were good examples of this. Currently the Agfa-Gevaert Gevamatic 60 offers almost the ultimate in table top processing, including self-contained replenishment for developer, fixer and wash.

For roller processors, evolution is still carrying on. The introduction of microprocessors has again revolutionised the automatic processor. This development is looked at more closely later in the chapter.

Dip and dunk processors

The parallel development of this type of processor never equalled the technical achievements of the roller processor.

In the early 1950s, Elema Schonander introduced a very large machine which required a big room to house it. Ilford marketed the Pixamatic, which was superseded by the Kenex and then the Merlin.

It is almost certain that the demise of the dip and dunk machines was due to their lack of technical sophistication. They were simply darkroom technicians with automatic arms; big, noisy and cumbersome. In short, the dip and dunk machines were incapable of taking advantage of the huge technical advances made in films and chemistry in recent years.

Specialised processors

These can only be briefly touched upon, as many came and went very quickly. The market seemed to require specialised dental processors and dedicated cine processors, such as the Gevamatic R10 and Scopix 12. Almost without exception, the specialised processors settled for roller processing.

In a topic as wide ranging as the history of automatic processing, it is inevitable that the subject can only be briefly touched upon. It is impossible to mention every individual or every manufacturer who has made an incursion into automatic processing. To those who have been missed, apologies are due.

THE AUTOMATIC PROCESSOR

The long historical introduction to this chapter is necessary to help the student understand the evolution of the automatic processor. Evolution is still continuing, albeit with help of the ubiquitous computer. There are now many and various types of processors, all with idiosyncracies that would be impossible to describe. Therefore, it would seem best to start with a description of a typical automatic processor and look at some ways, in mechanical and engineering terms, that the sometimes complex problems have been tackled. It should be stressed that no processor exactly like this exists. Students should familiarise themselves with the automatic processor in their own department. Ample literature exists which describes particular makes and types of processors.

A TYPICAL AUTOMATIC PROCESSOR

A typical automatic processor consists of a number of separate but interrelated systems. These can be listed as follows:

- Film entry system
- Transport system
- Chemical and re-circulation system
- Replenishment system
- Water system
- Dryer system
- Electrical system.

Each of these will considered in turn and a processor will be 'constructed' using the equipment suggested.

Film entry system

Every processor must have some apparatus which will take the film into the processor. Usually this is linked to the Replenishment system so that the act of feeding the film into the processor activates the replenishment pumps for a period of time. An ideal film entry system would consist of:

- A pair of rollers

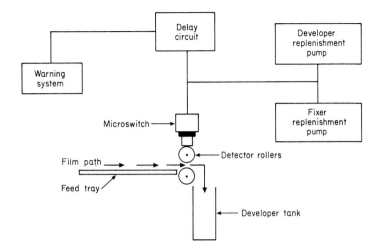

Fig. 4.3 Film entry system.

- A microswitch, above the rollers.

These would be combined to make a system as illustrated in Figure 4.3.

There are many versions of the microswitch: examples include infrared light beam which is stopped by entry of the film; trip wire, which in turn operates a microswitch; even a steady stream of air, which again is interrupted by the film's entry.

In this 'ideal' processor, the lower roller is fixed and the top roller, which is of significant weight, has a small movement allowed. When a film leaves the feed tray, the top roller is forced upwards. If the microswitch has been set correctly this movement will trip the switch and activate a number of electrical systems.

Subsystems

The feed system is usually interrelated to:

- The replenishment system
- Some warning system.

In basic automatic processors, the action of inserting the film activates a relay which switches on the replenisher pumps. It becomes obvious that if a simple switch is used the processor is only capable of recognising the *length* of the film being inserted. The pumps are therefore only working when the film is going through the film entry system.

The warning system is used in many different ways, but it is usually used to tell when the next film is to be inserted, i.e. when the first film is clear of the entry rollers. This warning could be a bell, a buzzer or a warning light. Many departments have a safelight over the feed tray which is switched off as the film goes into the processor.

Transport system

In modern processors the transport system consists of a series of rollers which are used to move the film through the processing tanks (see Fig. 4.4). This system also relies on an electric motor driving all the racks at a constant speed. The constant speed is very important, so the drive system will be a common one to ensure that there is no possibility that, for example, the developer rack will move faster than the fixer rack.

The rollers can be arranged in many and varied formations, but essentially they will be arranged in either deep tanks or shallow tanks.

Within the racks will be found guide plates. These plates are used to keep the film within the transport path. They are stainless steel or plastic. They have to be kept meticulously clean, particularly if they are above solution level. If lengthwise scratches occur on the film, it is almost 100% certain that guide plates are the cause.

Rollers fall into various types. They can usually be described as hard or soft.

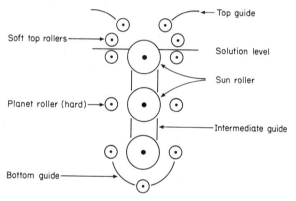

Fig. 4.4 Rack arrangement.

Hard rollers

These can be made of stainless steel or (nowadays more usually) paper wound on a stainless steel core and impregnated with an epoxy resin. This explains why great care must be taken when cleaning this type of roller. Coarse cleaning materials can seriously damage the surface of the 'paper' rollers, causing permanent damage. This will cause marks to be printed on films.

Soft rollers

Usually found in crossovers in the machines. They can be used as 'squeegees' to squeeze the excess chemicals off the films and thereby reduce carry over of chemicals. They are usually constructed of a neoprene-type substance (certainly not rubber, which is not inert as far as processing chemicals are concerned).

There are advantages and disadvantages to both of these systems, but essentially they relate to cost. A shallow tank system will be simpler and cheaper to make and run, as far fewer rollers are used. Usually the capacity (i.e. the number of films per hour) is lower than a deep rack system.

The deep rack system can be of very high capacity, but will usually be more costly because of the large numbers of rollers involved.

In terms of processing quality it is almost impossible to decide. It really boils down to 'horses for courses' in each department.

Chemical system

This system comprises the tanks for developer and fixer and the allied subsystems.

The tanks themselves must be constructed of some inert material such as stainless steel or plastic. They merely act as containers for the developer, fixer and wash water.

Once developer and fixer have been made up in the processor and the processor started, the chemicals have to be circulated constantly and maintained at the correct temperature.

It can be seen from Figure 4.5 that the chemical system is closely interrelated to the other systems, i.e. the replenishment, water and heating systems. In any processor, no matter what type or make, this interrelationship must exist.

Circulation of developer

In the recirculation system, the developer is constantly passed through the following (Fig. 4.5):

- Thermostat
- Temperature gauge

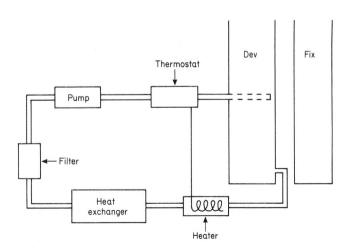

Fig. 4.5 Recirculation of developer.

- Heat exchanger (water system)
- Circulation pump
- Heater
- Filter.

Thermostat

Note that *thermostat* and *thermometer* are not synonyms. The thermostat *controls* the temperature; the thermometer merely *measures* the temperature.

The thermostat is the device which senses the temperature of the solutions. Once the operating temperature is set, the thermostat will automatically switch the developer (or fixer, if fitted) heater off and on at the appropriate temperature.

Thermometer

It is extremely important to have a constant display of developer temperature wherever possible. In some machines, the thermometer may be replaced by a simple light which will constantly cycle between off and on, indicating that the correct set temperature is being maintained.

Heat exchanger

This is also part of the water system. The developer and water circulate (separately) through this device. The operation of the heat exchanger is fully described under the water system, p. 151.

Circulation pump

This pump forces circulation of the developer through the various devices listed above. Note that ideally the developer would be taken from the bottom of the tank, circulated through the system, and then be brought back to the middle of the tank. It can then be forced through a 'spreader' which will ensure adequate spread of the solution throughout the tank.

Heater

The developer is passed over this small, relatively low consumption in-line heater. The heater, in turn, is linked to the thermostat.

Filter

Certainly not obligatory, but the use of an in-line filter helps to keep the developer cleaner. The filter could be as simple as a stainless steel or plastic mesh, or as complex as sophisticated renewable device filtering down to about 25 μ.

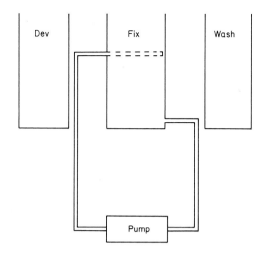

Fig. 4.6 Fixer recirculation.

Fixer circulation system

The fixer circulation system is constructed in almost exactly the same way as the developer. If the processor is a so-called 'cold water' processor there will certainly be an in-line heater and thermostat. If it is a 'tempered water' processor, i.e. it uses both hot and cold water, a heat exchanger would certainly be used in the fixer circulation system to utilise waste heat from the developer, via the water system, to maintain the fixer temperature (Fig. 4.6)

A filter is sometimes found in a fixer circulation system.

Replenishment system

The replenishment system preserves both the *quality* and *quantity* of the chemicals in the processor. The basic system consists of:

- Replenisher tanks
- Filters
- Replenishment pumps (linked to the film entry system; see Fig. 4.7).

Replenishment tanks

These must be constructed of an inert material such as stainless steel or plastic. Whilst the developer and fixer tanks perform exactly the same function, i.e. to hold the replenisher, they differ in their construction.

The developer tank has a floating lid on top of the developer replenisher. This is used to reduce the auto-oxidation of developer replenisher solution. Remembering that developer is a reducing agent and has an affinity for oxygen, care must be taken to reduce auto-oxidation at every opportunity.

It is a sensible practice to make up only enough developer replenisher to last for about a fortnight. It is also necessary to keep the floating lid clean and not to allow any oxidation products to build up on the surface.

In addition to the floating lid, there is usually a cover. This cover is there merely to prevent easy access for dust or dirt.

Filters

Filters are usually found in the line from the tanks to the processor. These can be a simple stainless steel mesh, to catch large particles which may block the pump or the line to the processor.

The fixer tank will exactly duplicate the developer tank, apart from the floating lid.

Replenisher pumps

These pumps are operated from the microswitch in the film entry system. The pump can be a single electric motor which drives two impellers, forcing the solutions up to tank level. There is always a device either in the pump itself or in the replenisher line which allows individual adjustment of the developer and fixer replenishment rates.

It is very important that there should be no flow back into the replenisher tanks from the main processor tanks. This can be prevented in two ways; either by creating a break in the line so that the replenisher is fed over the top of the tank via a 'hook', or by having a one way valve in each line.

In shallow tank processors a simple 'chicken feed' system can be used. This consists of a bottle containing the replenisher, inverted over the processing solution. When the level of the solution drops,

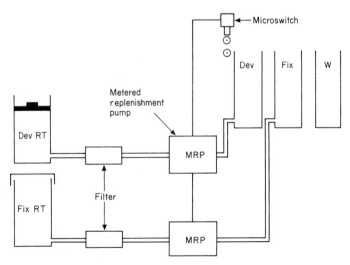

Fig. 4.7 Replenishment system.

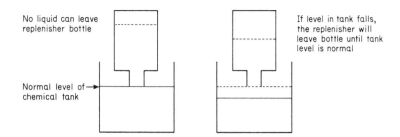

No liquid can leave
replenisher bottle

If level in tank falls,
the replenisher will
leave bottle until tank
level is normal

Normal level of→
chemical tank

Fig. 4.8 Replenishment system in shallow tank processor.

the solution from the bottle automatically refills the solution back to the preset level. Replenishment then stops (Fig. 4.8).

Water system

This is sometimes considered to be the simplest of the systems within the processor. This is certainly not the case.

The water system is influenced by the type of processor, i.e. whether it is a 'cold water' processor or a 'tempered water' system.

Tempered water processor

This will consist of the following components (see Fig. 4.9).

1. Cold and hot water supply
2. Filters
3. Mixing valve
4. Flow gauge
5. Temperature gauge
6. Heat exchanger (developer)
7. Heat exchanger (fixer).

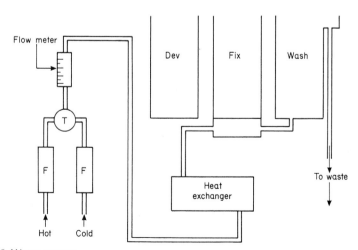

Fig. 4.9 Water system.

Cold and hot water supplies

Ideally these should be of equal pressures, about 5 psi being the minimum pressure which is acceptable. The ideal solution would be to have two water header tanks of the same height. Unfortunately this is not always possible and pumps (to increase the pressure) or valves (to reduce the pressure) may have to be considered.

Filters

Ideally, both hot and cold water supplies should be filtered, to avoid contaminants in the water and to avoid clogging the mixing valve.

Mixing valve

This item is not as simple as a shower valve; it is a sophisticated water/temperature control valve operated by a thermostatic motor. This valve is capable of controlling water flow and temperature to a very high degree, typically ±0.5°C.

When the valve is set for temperature it will maintain a constant flow of water. Most valves have a cut-off device which will not allow only hot or only cold water to flow into the processor.

Flow gauge

This is a gauge utilising a stainless steel float. The scale is calibrated to indicate the flow rate of water into the processor.

Temperature gauge

Not obligatory, but certainly it is very useful to see at a glance the operating temperature of the water in the processor.

Heat exchanger

This is basically a box containing a series of tubes through which water and developer (or fixer) run. The tubes are, of course, totally separate (Fig. 4.10).

The purpose of the heat exchanger(s) is to absorb any waste heat from the developer and to finely control the developer temperature. If the heat exchanger is used in the fixer, the reverse operates. The waste heat from the developer is passed to the water and then re-absorbed by the fixer.

To consider the operation in the developer circulation system we must look at what happens when the heater is switched on.

The developer reaches its correct temperature and the thermostat recognises that the correct temperature has been achieved (for example 36°C). Anyone who has ever boiled milk on an electric stove will know what happens with electric heaters. There is a considerable

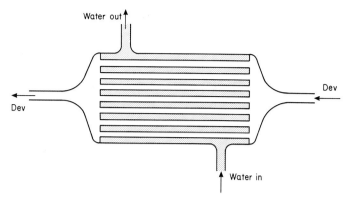

Fig. 4.10 Heat exchanger.

amount of residual heat left in the heater and this will continue to (over) heat the developer.

At this stage the heat exchanger comes into play. Wash water should always be at least 3°C below the developer temperature. The excess heat from the developer is now absorbed by the cold water in the heat exchanger and the overswing in developer temperature is brought down. When the developer temperature reaches the correct temperature the thermostat recognises this and switches the heater on. However, there is a slight delay in heating, and the developer temperature goes below the correct temperature until the heater takes full effect.

If a graph is drawn of this response it will be seen as a sinusoidal curve, keeping the swing of temperature under very fine control (Fig. 4.11).

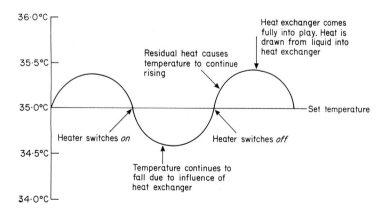

Fig. 4.11 Graph of thermostat response.

6. Dryer system

This is almost a totally self-contained unit. It is comprised of the following:

- Roller transport system

- Blower
- Heater
- Thermostat
- Filter
- 'Air knives'.

Roller transport system

This is driven from the main drive shaft to ensure that the speed of the film through the dryer is the same throughout the processor.

Blower

This unit generates the air flow used in drying the film.

Heater

The blown air is driven over the heater.

Thermostat

Used to set the temperature of the drying air. This is usually about 120°F. It should be noted that there is also a safety thermostat incorporated in the dryer. This cannot be adjusted, and it will switch the dryer heater off if the temperture exceeds 140°F.

Filters

On some processors, the air coming in to the blower is filtered as well as the outgoing air to the heater.

Filters are obviously fairly essential in the dryer area, as any dirt blown into the air system will be virtually blasted into the film surface.

'Air knives'

These are used to increase the velocity of the air as it strikes the film surface.

They use the principle of the Venturi effect. This simply means that air at low velocity forced through a large diameter bore will increase in velocity if it is forced through a smaller diameter bore.

It should be noted that the dryer transport section is constructed such that the first third of the section is used to heat the water carried in the film and make it vapourise. The second third is used to blow the water vapour away from the film surface very rapidly. The last third is there for spare capacity.

If a film leaves the dryer wet, it is very rarely due to the dryer temperature. It is nearly always due to poor fixation, perhaps because

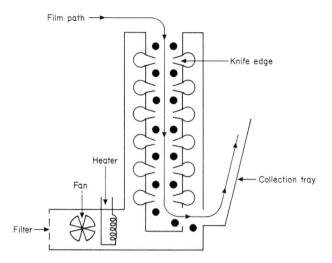

Fig. 4.12 Drying system.

of under-replenishment or lack of hardener. Film should dry, if all the parameters in the processor are correct, at fairly low temperatures.

Electrical system

The combination of water and chemicals with electricity could be fatal. To this end, great care must be taken in the installation of an automatic processor. Various standards are applied in different countries, but they all specify precautions to be taken at installation in terms of electrical safety, any pollution effects (i.e. discharge of developer and fixer) and connections to water supplies.

Standby system

There is also a requirement for processors to have a standby system to reduce running costs.

The standby system will automatically shut down some operations of the processor as listed below, if a film has not entered the processor for a predetermined interval. In a 90 s processor, a typical interval would be two minutes.

Water supply

This will be reduced to an absolute minimum, typically 5 l/min. This will be just sufficient to maintain the correct developer temperature via the heat exchangers.

Circulation system

The developer circulation system must be left on, to maintain the correct temperature. Sometimes, fixer circulation is shut down.

Transport system

The processor transport system will stop completely until the next film is inserted or the standby system is re-cycled.

Dryer

This again is shut off until the next film is inserted, or until the standby system has re-cycled.

Re-cycling is not always fitted to a standby system, but it is a useful addition. The system switches the machine on if a film has not entered the processor for a predetermined interval, usually about half an hour. This action prevents the drying out of the crossover rollers (which can create 'pie' lines; see p. 162), prevents the dryer and perhaps fixer getting too cold, thus ensuring that the processor is always ready for use.

Processors may run on 3 phase or single phase electricity supplies. It is essential that before installation, close contact is maintained between the company representative and service engineer to ensure that the correct electrical supply is installed, along with the other installation requirements.

The final processor 'built' from the descriptions contained in the chapter is merely a composite of all the parts outlined.

Cold water processor

The description of the cold water processor is almost identical to that of the tempered water processor, apart from some minor details. The water system will differ in that only cold water is used. This can simplify and reduce the installation costs for the automatic processor. A mixing valve is not required. Because of this, the description is based mainly on the tempered water system.

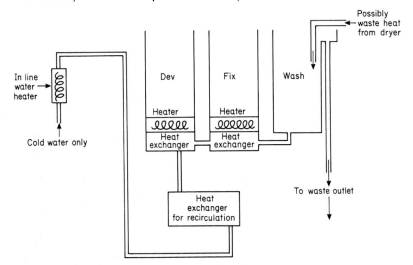

Fig. 4.13 A typical cold water processor.

The cold water processor (Fig. 4.13) uses in-line heaters to heat both the developer and fixer. Any waste heat from the water, developer and fixer is utilised by heat exchangers. Some processors even use waste heat from the dryer to heat the water. In other words, the cold water processor is a large energy saving device!

As outlined in the beginning of the chapter, as far as the authors are aware, no processor available on the market looks and operates exactly as the above processors.

Features from many different types and makes of machines have been incorporated, to give a *general* description. It is up to the individual student to study the machine in his or her own department and to become familiar with it.

MICROPROCESSOR CONTROL

In recent years, microprocessors have been fitted to automatic processors.

If Chapter 10 (Computing) is consulted, it will be seen that the price of computer memory has plummeted over the years and is still continuing to plummet. Smaller chips are available, enabling a microprocessor to be installed in the smallest of spaces.

In an automatic processor there are many tasks which should really be regularly monitored, for example:

- All solution levels
- All solution temperatures
- Dryer temperature
- *Area* of film entering the processor
- The transport speed, even the interrelationship between different speeds and replenishment.

A microprocessor is ideal for such mundane tasks. It can monitor all of the above with monotonous regularity and even has the ability to communicate the results in plain English to the operator on an LCD or LED display. In some automatic processors, the microprocessor even has the ability to communicate with an external service engineer's computer, and can run a programme to check the function of the electrical system of the automatic processor (Fig. 4.14B).

Perhaps the most important single development is the ability to monitor the *area* of the film entering the processor. Until recently, processors only measured the *length* of the film entering the processor, and replenishment was set as an average figure for the department throughput. With both length and width of the film being measured, a very high accuracy of replenishment can be achieved. The measurement is usually done by a series of switches, reed, microswitches or infrared light. The length of the film can easily be measured as in the normal processor; the special switches measure the width. It is then a simple calculation to determine the area.

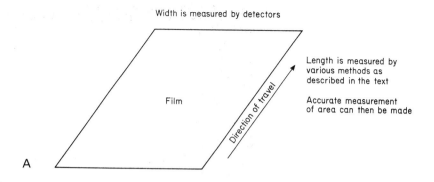

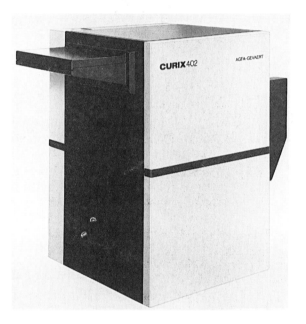

Fig. 4.14 (A) Determining area of film being processed. (B) Gevamatic 402 (photograph courtesy of D.I.S. Division, Agfa-Gevaert Ltd).

CINE PROCESSING

In cardiology suites there has been a demand for many years for a dedicated cine processor.

The cine processor has essentially exactly the same features as a conventional processor apart from its unique ability to transport small film in long lengths.

Cine processors are usually capable of handling:

16 mm film
35 mm film
70 mm film
75 mm film

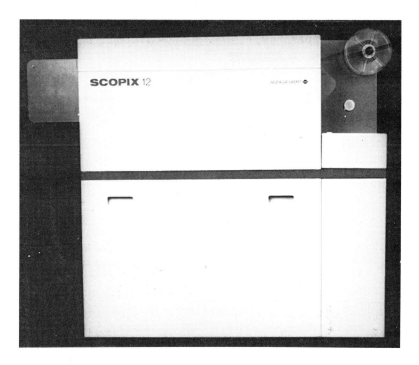

Fig. 4.15 Scopix 12 cine processor (photograph courtesy of D.I.S. Division Agfa-Gevaert Ltd).

100 mm film (roll and cut film)
105 mm film.

Figure 4.15 shows a cine processor which is totally microprocessor controlled, with a display communicating any faults occurring to the operator.

DAYLIGHT SYSTEMS

The term 'daylight system' was coined a few years ago and tends to be very misleading. Perhaps the name of these systems should be: 'A film handling system capable of loading and unloading cassettes in actinic light, without recourse to darkroom facilities'. All daylight systems on the market are capable of doing just this.

Different daylight systems have different design philosophies, but they all have one important factor in common. Without exception, they all use cassettes which are dedicated to that system. These cassettes are not interchangeable between different makes of daylight system.

Some makes are suitable for use easily as a manual cassette, but will transfer immediately for use in the daylight system. This gives the user the benefit of being able to purchase (and use) cassettes prior to the purchase of the actual daylight system.

Some makes have to use film which is in a dedicated package, to fit a particular daylight system. These packs can be loaded into the daylight system in actinic light. The films are notched to accommodate the mechanical requirements of the daylight system. Others use conventional NIF film, which must be loaded into a magazine in a darkroom prior to the magazine being inserted into the daylight system.

Daylight systems are split into two different types: dispersed systems and centralised systems.

Dispersed systems

The dispersed daylight system is in two parts. The first part is a series of loaders, of different sizes, which contain the film to be loaded into the cassettes. The second part is the unloader for the cassette, which is mounted on top of the processor (see Fig. 4.16).

The loaders can be distributed around the X-ray department, in varying areas, allowing easy access for the radiographers. The cassettes are then returned to a central processor (with unloader) for processing.

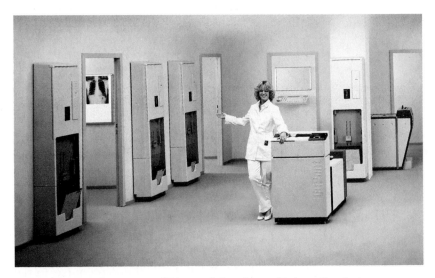

Fig. 4.16 Photograph courtesy of Diagnostic Imaging and Information Systems Division/Medical Products Dept, DUPONT (UK) Ltd.

Centralised systems

The centralised system contains the film magazines, the loading and the unloading mechanisms, all directly linked to the automatic processor.

In this case the radiographers return the cassette to the daylight

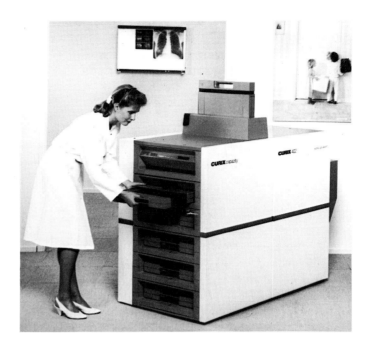

Fig. 4.17 Curix Capacity film handling system (photograph courtesy of D.I.S. Division, Agfa-Gevaert Ltd).

system, where the cassette is unloaded, the film fed into the processor and the cassette re-loaded.

In the more recent daylight systems, microprocessors have been totally incorporated. As well as looking after the routine day-to-day running of the automatic processor in the daylight system, they are also capable of keeping a record of all film used, all service interventions and of the electrical/electronic and mechanical state of the machine. In addition, they are also capable of communicating with external computers (notably the service engineer's) to produce a record and to run self test programmes.

Most of the recent daylight systems also communicate to the user by LED or LCD displays, giving details (for example) of faults occurring, size of cassette/film being used, etc. (see Fig. 4.17).

The mechanisms involved in each of the daylight systems are too complex and too varied to be included in a chapter such as this. It is sufficient to appreciate that the film is automatically unloaded from a cassette and transferred into the automatic processor. In a centralised system, the cassette is then reloaded with a correct-sized film. In the case of the decentralised system, the empty cassette is then taken to the correct-sized loader, where the film is automatically loaded into the cassette.

As in many areas of radiography, the choice of centralised or decentralised daylight systems is one of 'horses for courses'.

PROCESSING FAULTS

With the modern automatic processor, very few faults can be said to be typical, but most are connected with the transport system.

Longitudinal scratches

These are usually connected with the guide plates in the racks. The problem can sometimes be in determining which rack is responsible. The only solution is to remove the processor lid and override the cut-out switch, if one is fitted.

Film is then put through each area of the processor in turn.

Note: Care should be taken in this procedure, as the cut-out switch is there for protection.

It should be noted that *transverse* scratches, across the direction of travel, are almost impossible to cause in an automatic processor. They were almost certainly caused in the darkroom.

Pie lines

These are marks caused by chemicals partially drying out on rollers, or even by an eccentric roller in a chemical tank.

The term 'pie line' is applied because the marks repeat at intervals equal to the diameter of the roller causing them. This provides some clue as to how to trace the fault. There are sometimes different sizes of rollers within the processor; at least the diameter of the roller can be assessed and checks made.

White or black 'spots'

Usually caused by a breakdown on the surface of a 'hard' roller, sometimes due to excessive cleaning.

These types of marks can sometimes resemble calculi or phleboliths and can lead to misleading diagnoses.

To trace the fault can be a long and time-consuming job. Each roller must be checked for surface damage, unless the fault can be traced to a particular area as outlined above.

Drying marks

These can only be viewed by reflected light. They appear as dull longitudinal lines running down the film in the direction of travel.

These are caused by dirt or dust blocking part of the air knife.

Non-drying

Whilst not strictly a mark, non-drying can be the most troublesome fault in automatic processing.

It is almost never caused by a fault in the dryer; the fault tends to be in the fixer.

The first check to make should be a measurement of the pH and silver levels of the fixer. If these are high, then a check should be made of the replenisher pumps.

GENERAL FAULTS

Unfortunately, from time to time, faults occur on films which can eventually be traced to the way that the films have been handled or to the way in which they have been processed. Included below are some typical film faults and some ways in which it may be possible to decide how to cure them.

The list is equally applicable to manual and to automatic processing.

High density marks

Black 'splashes'

These generally have the appearance of a 'splash' on the film. They can have two separate causes:

1. The film has been splashed with developer *before* development. The area of the 'splash' now develops faster than the surrounding area and leaves an area of high density on the film.
2. The film has been splashed with water *before* development. The water softens the emulsion and allows developer to enter the area quickly, again leaving an area of high density on the film.

In both of the above cases, the marks can also be produced by liquid spills on the 'dry' bench.

Black marks

These can be of many and various shapes; because of this, only the major types have been listed.

Crescent shaped

Almost always caused by bad film handling techniques. They are usually caused by the darkroom technician gripping the film too tightly between the thumb and the forefinger. This presses the thumbnail into the film. This action sensitises the emulsion, as the silver halide crystal is sensitive to pressure. When the film is processed, the sensitised area will show up as a black, crescent shaped mark.

Note This mark can sometimes be *white*, if the film has been handled badly *before* exposure.

Black fingerprints

Usually caused by the darkroom technician having developer or water on his or her hands. This practice can lead to further problems if the intensifying screens are handled with wet hands, as the marks produced are not removable.

Static marks

These also can be of many and various shapes. However, if examined under a magnifying glass, the point of origin of the discharge can usually be clearly seen.

The worst example is 'tree static', where large discharges can cover large areas of the film. The discharge produces distinctive marks looking exactly like the branches of a tree.

Trying to cure static problems can be difficult and time-consuming. There are, however, some classic causes of static:

1. A combination of a 'formica'-type bench and vinyl floors can lead to static problems. The cure here is to cover the bench with an oil-based linoleum.

2. A very dry atmosphere in the darkroom can also produce static. The easiest way to prove that dryness is the cause is to boil a kettle in the darkroom.

3. A technician wearing a man-made fabric, particularly Nylon, can easily produce static.

4. The insertion and extraction of film into a cassette can produce quite high electrical charges. Screen cleaner, of the appropriate make, usually has anti-static properties. It is worth encouraging the regular use of screen cleaner.

Surface marks

These marks are usually single-sided and adhere to the surface of the film. They are obvious, but the causes are many; two examples are:

1. Algae in the wash tank. The wash tank is usually static overnight and is the perfect breeding ground for algae.

Some processors now incorporate an automatic drain for the wash tank if the processor is shut down to reduce this problem.

A simple way of retarding the growth of algae is to regularly rinse the wash tank out with a solution of Domestos (mixed half a litre of Domestos to three litres of water). Make sure to *thoroughly* rinse the tank out afterwards with clean water.

2. Bits of emulsion, etc., in the developer, fixer or wash tank.

If the surface marks persist, the only real cure is to check each tank in turn and clean it and also check the roller surfaces.

Pressure marks

As silver halide is sensitive to pressure, marks can be produced which are at first very difficult to trace. It should be noted that these can be *white* or *black*, depending on when the original mark was produced and how much pressure was exerted.

They have no special distinguishing marks and will appear randomly over the film. They can be caused by film being stored incorrectly (i.e. horizontally instead of vertically), or simply by poor film handling.

As a general guide, white marks are caused *before* exposure, black marks are caused *after* exposure.

The only procedure to follow is to check the handling and storage routine in the darkroom.

Radiation or light fogging

Again, these marks will appear at random over the film, but they will usually cover larger areas than marks resulting from other causes. Some identifiable causes are listed below.

1. If the film has been fogged through material, paper for example, a faint image of the material can usually be seen on the film.

2. If a similar mark occurs on a film of the same size, check to see if the marks can be superimposed. If they can, almost certainly the film has been fogged by X-radiation whilst in the box.

3. Black marks around the edge of the film point to light leakage in the cassette, or indicate that the film box has been opened in white light.

Overall high density

Possible causes are listed below.

1. Lead-based paint.
2. Some varnishes.
3. Formaldehyde.
4. Carbon monoxide.
5. Mercury. *Never* use a mercury thermometer in the darkroom.
6. Developer. Try to ensure wherever possible that films and photographic chemicals are not stored in the same room.
7. Heat. About 20°C is the maximum temperature acceptable for three months storage.
8. Time in storage. Films have a limited 'shelf life', and fog will increase with age.
9. Faulty or incorrect safelights can cause an overall fog. Check the wattage of the bulb (no greater than 25 W). Check the filter type to match the sensitivity of the film. Check for cracks, etc., in the filter.
10. Background radiation. There is a maximum level recommended of 7 μr/hr. This level can sometimes be exceeded in granite or breeze-block buildings. A simple check would be to leave an unexposed film, sealed in a light-tight envelope, in the suspect area for three weeks. If the film is fogged after processing, radiation should be suspected.

Low density marks

White 'splashes'

These can have two separate causes.

1. Fixer has been splashed onto the film before development. The area of the 'splash' is therefore cleared before the area can be developed.
2. There is grease or oil on the surface of the film. Although this may seem unlikely, if a darkroom technician eats a packet of crisps and then handles a film, oil is carried to the surface of the film. The oil acts as a barrier to the developer and a white mark is produced.

In both the above cases, the marks can be produced by liquid spills on the 'dry' bench.

White marks

These can be many and various in shape and cause; because of this, only the major types have been listed.

Crescent shaped

For details, see under High density marks, above.

White fingerprints

Usually caused by the darkroom technician having fixer or oil-based products on his/her hands. This practice can lead to further problems if the intensifying screens are handled with the fingers, as the marks produced are not removable.

Pressure marks

For details see under High density marks, above.

Sharply defined marks

These are usually associated with artefacts inside (or closely adhered to the surface of) the cassette. If any artefact is present on the screens, the light output from the screens is reduced or cut off completely. This, in turn, produces a white mark on the film. Screen marks always appear in the same position on the film, for obvious reasons, which means that the films can be superimposed with the marks in position.

It is worth stressing that developer, fixer and water can damage intensifying screens irrevocably, producing consistent, but ill defined marks on the films. Also physical damage (scratches, etc.) can produce marks on the films.

It may be necessary to view the screens under ultraviolet light to see the marks.

Other faults

There are various other faults which are not easy to categorise.

Dichroic fog

This appears as a pink stain if the film is viewed by transmitted light, and greenish blue when viewed by reflected light.

It is caused by development still continuing in the fixer. This will happen if the fixer pH is too high. This is usually caused by excess carry-over of developer into the fixer.

If using a manual system, check that intermediate rinsing is carried out between the developer and the fixer or, better still, that a stop bath is used in this position. Glacial acetic acid makes a very good stop bath. It stops development immediately and does away with intermediate rinsing.

Dichroic fog almost never occurs in an automatic processor.

Milky white stain

Due to the film being inadequately fixed, either because the film has not been in the fixer for long enough, or the fixer is grossly under-replenished.

Brown stain

The stain usually appears after a period of storage of the processed film. It is due to inadequate washing of the film. It can sometimes be cleared by refixing the film.

In both a manual and an automatic system it is always wise to do regular archival testing (see p. 216) to check washing efficiency.

The above list is by no means comprehensive, but it should help in identifying the more common faults which occur.

5

Intensifying screens

Introduction

Radiography as we know it today would not be a viable proposition without the use of intensifying screens; exposures would be too long, giving excessive kinetic unsharpness, and the amount of dose required to produce an acceptable image of most parts of the body would, to say the least, be too high.

It is interesting to note that Roentgen's discovery of X-rays on 8 November 1895 was due to him noticing, quite by accident, the fluorescence of a plate of barium platino cyanide whilst performing experiments with a Crookes tube. The first recorded instance of the use of a film and screen in combination to produce a radiograph was on 7 February 1896, only weeks after Roentgen first published a 'direct radiation film' of his wife's left hand; this was also of a hand and was taken by Professor Pupin of the Columbian University. Around June 1896 the now-famous inventor Thomas Alva Edison discovered the luminescent properties of calcium tungstate ($CaWO_4$) when exposed to X-rays, and along with other investigators concluded that this was the best phosphor for fluoroscopic and intensifying screens. Edison's factory commenced commercial production of these items soon after.

Many improvements have taken place since these early days but up until the early 1970s calcium tungstate intensifying screens were still the most widely used screens in radiography. This was because of the fact that although other phosphors had been used, calcium tungstate still remained the most suitable and its limitations prevented any major breakthrough in screen design.

In 1970 Wickersheim, Alves and Buchanan suggested the use of certain terbium-activated rare earth phosphors in intensifying screens and this proved to be the advance that screen technology had been waiting for, even though the early days were fraught with problems.

GENERAL CONSIDERATIONS

As both calcium tungstate and rare earth phosphors are now in common use, the remainder of this chapter is devoted almost entirely to their consideration. However, certain areas are common to both and these will be discussed before the specifics of each.

The need for screens

During exposure the X-ray beam is modified according to the structures through which it passes. The photons that have passed through the patient carry the information about that patient which then must be converted to a visual form.

Photographic emulsion exposed directly to these photons will record a suitable image. Unfortunately the sensitivity of film to direct X-ray exposure is very low and if used for all examinations would result in a prohibitively large X-ray dose and high kinetic unsharpness.

Intensifying screens convert the X-rays into visible light, which then exposes the film. This has the advantage of reducing the dose required for a particular examination, resulting in shorter exposure times and less kinetic unsharpness, but introduces other unsharpness problems due to screen structure (see screen speed, p. 185, and Chapter 7, Image quality). As a generalisation, a film that is exposed using screens has an image that is produced 95% by light and 5% by X-rays, although this obviously depends on the particular technique used.

Screens are commonly used as follows:

- Single screen technique, e.g. mammography; usually in special cassette (e.g. vacuum cassette)
- Double screen technique, e.g. conventional radiography with duplitised X-ray film (see Ch. 1) in a cassette
- Multiscreen techniques, e.g. tomographic multisection cassette.

What is a phosphor

This is probably the first question that needs to be answered. In the Dictionary of Science and Physics (Penguin 1979) it is defined as 'a substance that emits light at a temperature below the temperature at which it would exhibit incandescence'. This definition can be made more specific when considering phosphors for use in screens: a phosphor is usually a metallic crystalline solid, naturally occurring or artificially made, that exhibits the property of *flourescence* when exposed to X-radiation and can be manufactured in useful form to produce high image quality.

Fluorescence has two closely allied terms associated with it, both of which are very easy to confuse. These terms are *luminescene* and *phosphorescence*. In order to fully understand the differences it is necessary to have some knowledge of the basic physics involved in these processes (see Luminescence, fluorescence and phosphorescence, p. 175).

How does a screen work?

Screens work by a three-stage process:

- Absorption
- Conversion
- Emission or re-emission.

Absorption

A great deal is known about the absorption processes. Any good physics textbook will discuss in some detail the photoelectric effect, Compton effect and pair production. In screens, the incident X-ray photons are absorbed in the phosphor material by either the photoelectric or Compton effects. At energies used in diagnostic radiography the predominant effect is photoelectric. This occurs in the high atomic number elements of the phosphor and is further assisted by the fact that phosphors, being metallic crystalline solids, have a predominantly ionic structure which results in a low incidence of free electrons. In percentage terms the approximate number of photons absorbed by the photoelectric effect is 95%, to the Compton effect's 5%. In either case, secondary electrons are produced in relation to the exposure received (Fig. 5.1).

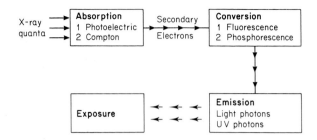

Fig. 5.1 Summary of screen function.

Conversion

In relation to the amount of knowledge about the absorption process, the conversion process is somewhat less clear. The energy available from the released electron is converted into light photons by either flourescence or phosphorescence (see p. 175), both of which involve the movement of electrons between 'electron traps' and 'holes' within the 'forbidden gap' and 'conduction band' areas of the crystal (see p. 173 and Fig. 5.1).

Emission

Very little is known of the mechanisms of re-emission; of the three processes this is the least understood. Photons released by absorption and conversion leave the phosphor material and expose the film, producing the latent image and, after processing, a density that is proportional to their intensity. The wavelength of the emissions is controlled in manufacture so as to match as closely as possible the peak sensitivity of the film it is exposing (see Fig. 5.1).

CRYSTAL PHYSICS

The solid state physics contained within the next section is without mathematical formulae and is simplified in order to facilitate an empirical understanding.

Crystalline solids comprise a regular three-dimensional array of atoms or molecules. Figure 5.2 is an example of pure silver bromide, which has a cubic arrangement. Many different shapes are possible depending on the nature of the substance. The predominant bonding type is ionic bonding: this involves the transfer of electrons between atoms, resulting in positive and negative ions which then combine in a regular pattern to give a relatively stable configuration.

Energy levels

Within the stable configuration there are only certain allowable

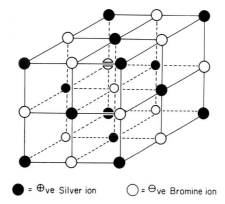

= ⊕ve Silver ion   ◯ = ⊖ve Bromine ion

Fig. 5.2 Cubic crystal lattice: silver bromide.

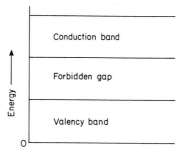

Fig. 5.3 Simplified energy level diagram.

energy levels, or bands. These are determined by quantum mechanics and in particular the Schrödinger equation. The three levels or allowed bands (Fig. 5.3) are:

- Valence band
- Forbidden band (or gap)
- Conduction band

Valence band

In this band the electrons are so loosely bound to their parent nucleus that they are free for sharing by adjacent atoms or molecules.

Forbidden band

Electrons within a system can only have a certain allowable range of energies (defined by the Schrödinger equation). The forbidden band is the range of energies outside this allowable range. Electrons may 'pass through' this gap if they are energetic enough, but cannot exist in any form within this area.

Conduction band

Any electrons within this band are free to move providing they maintain a certain minimum energy. If they fall below this minimum, they return to the valence band or other vacant electron site.

If a potential difference is applied to a substance with electrons in its conduction band, an electric current can be made to flow.

Crystal defects

No system is perfect and crystals are no exception to this rule. Indeed, it is this departure from the perfect that enables the fluorescent and phosphorescent effects to take place. Departures from the regularity of the ionic structure are called *defects* and are of two main types:

- Point defects
  — Frenkel defect (Fig. 5.4)
  — Schottky defect (Fig. 5.5)

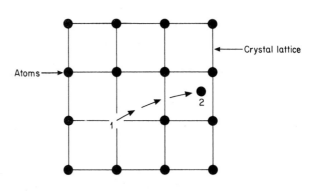

1. Vacant site
2. Interstitial ion/atom

Fig. 5.4 Frenkel defect.

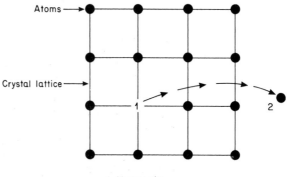

1. Vacant site
2. Atom out of position

Fig. 5.5 Schottky defect.

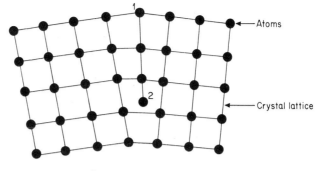

1. Extra plane of atoms
2. Dislocation extends into crystal

Fig. 5.6 Edge dislocation defect.

- Line defects
  — Edge dislocations (Fig. 5.6)
  — Screw dislocation.

These defects create areas of 'low energy' within the crystal, called 'electron traps' and 'holes'. Even supposedly perfect crystals contain some defects. The number of defects rises exponentially with temperature, typical values for point defects being 1 in 10^5 at 700°C for metals (i.e. 1 site in 1 000 000 is vacant). Defects can be produced by heating followed by rapid cooling, pressure and by ionising radiations.

Traps

These are areas of 'low energy' within the crystal that have the ability to catch and hold an electron for a period of time until it acquires the energy to escape.

The escape energy may be small (as in silver bromide) or very high (as in lithium fluoride). Traps are usually caused by two adjacent atoms attempting to share the charge of another atom, and are mainly the result of line-type defects.

Holes

A hole is the absence of an electron in the valence band; it is regarded as a mobile vacancy and has a positive electronic charge equal to that of a proton. Although it is a space left by an electron, it is regarded as a positive charge as the 'hole' has the ability to attract an electron.

Luminescence; fluorescence and phosphorescence

As previously indicated, these topics are central to the way a screen functions and are often confused due to their obvious similarity in pronunciation. It is as well to note that the actual mechanisms involved in the production of these three phenomena are still not clearly understood and therefore, any discussion is limited to theory only.

Luminescence

This can be radiographically defined as the ability of a substance to absorb short wavelength radiation and emit longer wavelength radiation, normally within the visible or near-visible spectrum. More generally it is the emission of electromagnetic radiation from a substance as the result of any non-thermal process.

Luminescence comprises two effects:

* Fluorescence
* Phosphorescence (or after-glow).

Fluorescence

A material is said to fluoresce when light emission starts when the exciting radiation starts and light emission stops when the exciting radiation stops. This, however, is somewhat simplified, as even in the quickest-responding phosphor there is some time lag before peak emission is reached and some light emission after the exposure has stopped. If this lag and continued emission is less than 10^{-8} seconds then the phosphor is said to fluoresce. The value of 10^{-8} seconds is

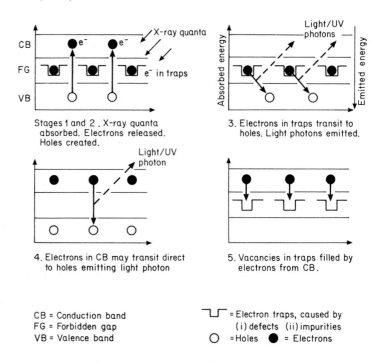

Fig. 5.7 Fluorescence: diagrammatic representation.

used as this approximately corresponds to the time taken for an electron transition between energy levels to produce a light photon (see Fig. 5.9).

The physical process of fluorescence can be described by considering Figure 5.7. Incoming X-ray energy is absorbed, producing secondary electrons. If these electrons have sufficient energy they transit the forbidden band and become free in the conduction band. This leaves 'holes' in the valence band. These 'holes' are immediately filled by electrons, either directly from the conduction band or from the electron traps within the forbidden band. The transition results in yet another energy change that produces a light photon. To complete the process, any vacant trap in the forbidden band is now able to capture free electrons from the conduction band.

This does not produce a light photon, as the energy change is too small.

Phosphorescence or after-glow

After-glow is the continuation of light emission even though the exciting radiation has stopped. Again, the threshold value is 10^{-8} seconds, and if a phosphor takes longer than this value to reach peak emission or if it continues to emit light after this period it is considered to phosphoresce (see Fig. 5.9).

The physical process can be described by considering Figure 5.8. As with fluorescence, the incoming X-ray is absorbed producing secondary electrons that, providing they possess sufficient energy, may become free in the conduction band. This creates 'holes' in the valence band. The free electrons then fall into traps where they are held for a period of time (determined by crystal type and inherent

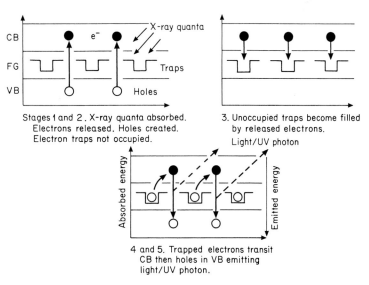

CB

FG

VB

e⁻   X-ray quanta   Traps   Holes

Stages 1 and 2. X-ray quanta absorbed.
Electrons released. Holes created.
Electron traps not occupied.

3. Unoccupied traps become filled
by released electrons.
Light/UV photon

Absorbed energy

Emitted energy

4 and 5. Trapped electrons transit
CB then holes in VB emitting
light/UV photon.

Fig. 5.8 Phosphorescence: diagrammatic representation.

impurities). If the trapped electron acquires enough energy it will escape from the trap and return to the holes in the valence band either directly or via the conduction band. In either case the energy change produces a light photon.

It is the holding of the electron in a trap for a 'period of time' that is the cause of the after-glow, as even when the exciting radiation stops there will still be some electrons waiting to transit between bands.

The length of delay in the emission is determined by the time taken for the electron to escape from its trap and return to a 'hole' in the valence band. It is logical therefore that this also determines how long light is emitted after excitation ceases.

Phosphorescence in screens is an undesirable effect, as it causes multi-imaging and occasionally film fogging. Unfortunately, it is not possible to differentiate completely between the two effects, and all screens have some after-glow (even though this may be so slight as to be insignificant from a practical point of view).

After-glow can sometimes be useful; for example, in an oscilloscope the path of a 'single dot' trace can still be seen even though the dot has moved on, it is the basis of so-called luminous dials on clocks and watches, and finally it is useful in dose meters where re-emission of the light photons does not occur until the material has been heated to a certain temperature (thermoluminescent dosimetry).

Some terminology

Figure 5.9 illustrates some of the common terminology associated with phosphor technology and also shows the fluorescent and phosphorescent processes in terms of a material that may be suitable for screen manufacture and one that it is not suitable. Both have a growth and decay period, and the duration of that period defines one criteria for a phosphor's suitability in screen manufacture.

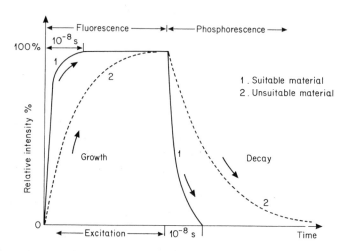

Fig. 5.9 Diagram illustrating suitable and unsuitable phosphor material.

Other factors would be spectral emission, resolution, speed, manufacturing suitability, etc.

Dopants

These are impurities that are introduced into the phosphor crystal structure in order to control its characteristics. Dopants are normally one of two kinds:

- Activators
- Killers.

Activators

Activators are impurities that stimulate the phosphor to emit light. Careful choice of the amount and type of activator enable the spectral emission of the phosphor to be controlled so it can be tailored to match the peak sensitivity of the film it is intended to expose. Only one phosphor in use in radiography does not require an activator; that is calcium tungstate, which is considered to be 'self-activating'. The rest all require the presence of a dopant in order to emit light; for example, lanthanum oxybromide (LaOBr) does not fluoresce unless it has a small percentage of activator present (usually terbium (Tb)). Conventionally the activator is written after the main phosphor formula and following a full stop, e.g. terbium-activated lanthanum oxybromide is written LaOBr.Tb.

Killers

This form of dopant is not used a great deal in screen technology. It is introduced to the phosphor structure to control the areas of the crystal responsible for phosphorescence and is therefore used to control after-glow.

Some phosphors may contain both activators and killers in order to produce a viable material.

SUMMARY: INTRODUCTION AND BASIC PHYSICS

1. Screens are used principally to reduce the amount of X-ray exposure the patient receives during his/her examination. Screens convert incoming X-ray photons into light. The image produced on the film is produced 95% by light and 5% by X-rays (approximately).

2. To be useful as a screen phosphor, a material must possess the property of fluorescence.

3. Screens function by a three-stage process; absorption, conversion and emission.

Absorption is mainly due to the photoelectric effect whilst conversion is either by fluorescence or phosphorescence. These involve the movement of electrons between traps and 'holes'.

Very little is known of the emission process except to say it is controlled so as to match the peak sensitivity of the film the screen is going to expose.

4. A simple discussion of crystal physics including energy levels, valence band, forbidden band, conduction band, crystal defects, traps, holes, etc., can be found in the text.

5. Luminescence is the ability of a substance to absorb short wavelength radiation and emit longer wavelength radiation in the visible or near-visible spectrum.

Luminescence comprises two effects, fluorescence and phosphorescence (after-glow). In fluorescence the light emission ceases when the exciting radiation ceases. In phosphorescence light continues to be emitted after the exciting radiation ceases. After-glow can cause unsharpness of the image.

6. Dopants can be divided into activators and killers. Activators are impurities that are added to a phosphor to stimulate it to emit light. Killers are added to try to control after-glow.

CONSTRUCTION OF SCREENS

An intensifying screen is constructed of various layers, as shown in Figure 5.10.

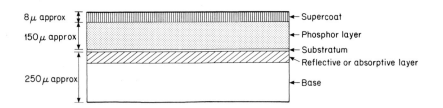

Fig. 5.10 Typical cross-sectional structure of a universal intensifying screen. All dimensions approximate.

Base

This acts as a support for all the other layers and is made of polyester. In many cases it is the same material as that used for film base but without the coloured tint. Base thickness varies but is approximately 250 microns (μ) for screens used in cassettes, and may be as thin as 175 μ for screens used in automatic film changers. Modern screen technology has led to the incorporation of the reflective or absorptive layer in the upper part of the base, although it is separated in Figure 5.10 due to its functional significance.

Most base materials are heavily protected by patents held by the various manufacturers, as they have been developed only by many years of expensive research.

Reflective or absorptive layer

This layer does exactly as its name suggests. As phosphor crystals emit light in all directions, a significant proportion of that light is going away from the film. The reflective layer redirects it towards the film, therefore ensuring that it contributes to exposure. This has the advantage of increasing the speed of the film/screen combination with a corresponding reduction in patient dose, but the disadvantage of increasing the amount of unsharpness produced (See Speed, p. 185, and Resolution, p. 195). In many screens the reflective layer is a thin coating (30μ) of titanium dioxide (TiO_2) or similar compound.

If the layer is absorptive, light travelling away from the film is absorbed by a dye and does not contribute to the formation of the image. Unfortunately this slows down the speed of the system, but has the advantage of improving the sharpness of the image. The dyes used in this layer are the subject of complicated patents, each manufacturer using its own particular development even though the chemical formulae may be very similar.

Substratum

This is effectively a layer of 'glue' that is used to attach the phosphor layer to the base. It is made as thin as coating technology will allow with regard to providing adequate adhesion between the two layers.

Phosphor layer

This is a suspension of the phosphor crystals within a suitable binder. It is approximately 150 μ thick in universal screens.

Binder technology is complex, and to be useful a binder must posses certain basic features. These are principally:

- Flexibility
- Inert to the phosphor crystals and the light they emit
- Provide even, known dispersion of the phosphor in the binder
- Phosphor plus binder must be able to be coated onto the base at the required thickness.

Most manufacturers use acetate acrylate as the binding agent, as this has all the necessary characteristics.

Even dispersion of the phosphor is vital, as areas of high concentration would lead to uneven light emission from the screen and consequent uneven exposure of the film. Each phosphor crystal is completely surrounded by the binder and the amount of phosphor per unit volume is known; this amount is called the coating weight, and is determined during manufacture.

The relevance of this is that a screen with a high coating weight (i.e. a high amount of phosphor per unit volume) can be made thinner, and therefore produce a sharper image, than a screen with a lower coating weight in the same speed class (see Speed, p. 185, and Resolution, p. 195).

Another factor to be considered is the specific gravity of the phosphor. In theory, the higher the specific gravity, the thinner the phosphor layer can be for any given speed class, but in practice the phosphor/binder relationship is found to be more significant in determining phosphor thickness. In universal screens, the ratio is approximately 9 parts phosphor to 1 part binder. Screen speed is also determined in the phosphor layer, the general rule being that, within limits, the thicker the phosphor the more light it will produce, and therefore the more exposure the film will receive for the same dose.

However, things are never quite that simple, and the addition of coloured dyes to the binder means speed and resolution can be controlled without altering the phosphor thickness (see Speed, p. 185, and Resolution, p. 195).

A final note is that at the time of writing (1985) the cost of phosphor is about equal to that of silver (approximately £6.50 per ounce). It will be interesting to see if this has remained the case when this material is published.

Supercoat

This is the top protective layer of the screen. It is usually a thin coating (about 8μ) of cellulose acetobiturate or other similar substance. Apart from the obvious function of protecting the phosphor layer from mechanical damage it provides a surface that is easy to clean and is a poor generator of static electricity. It has been estimated that a static charge of up to 4 kV can be generated by sliding a film quickly over the surface of a screen as it is removed from the cassette. The implications for static marks on the film are obvious.

The surface of the supercoat also has interesting features as it can be made with varying degrees of 'roughness'. For example, a smooth surface screen, i.e. one with a low friction co-efficient, would be of little use in an automatic film changer as the film would slide through the screens before they have a chance to close and 'trap' the film.

Also, a totally smooth surface tends to trap air between the film and screen in the cassette causing poor film/screen contact. Too rough a surface can seriously degrade image quality by increasing screen unsharpness factors. The degree of screen 'roughness' (or friction coefficient) is therefore carefully controlled to suit the situation the screen will be used in.

This is particularly important with the increased use of automated film handling systems such as 'film centres' and 'daylight systems'.

INTENSIFYING FACTOR (IF)

This is defined as the ratio of the exposure required to produce net density (ND) 1.0 without screens using a particular film, compared to the exposure required to produce net density 1.0 using screens with the same film, or more simply:

$$IF = \frac{\text{Exposure required to produce ND 1.0: No screens}}{\text{Exposure required to produce ND 1.0: Screens}}$$

Conventionally, net density 1.0 is used as this is a convenient point approximately halfway up the characteristic curve (see Sensitometry, p. 47); however, any density is a perfectly acceptable alternative providing that this is stated in the calculation, does not exceed the maximum useful density and is above the minimum useful density.

Effectively the IF of a screen tells you by how much you can reduce the exposure required to produce a particular film if you put that same film in screens. For example, assume a pair of screens has an IF of 5 and also that for some reason a radiograph has been taken using no-screen technique, and that the exposure required to produce an acceptable image was 50 kV, 25 mAs at 100 cm ffd.

If the film was now placed in a cassette with the screens the required exposure would be 50 kV, 5 mAs at 100 cm ffd, i.e. the mAs would be reduced to one-fifth of its original value. This technique also allows changes in exposure between two screens of known IF to be calculated, again providing the same film is used.

To be completely accurate IF should be quoted at a particular kV value or range of values. This is because the absorption of X-ray photons in the screen depends principally on the value, in photon energy, kiloelectron volts (keV), of the K absorption edge of the heavy element present in the phosphor. If the energy of the X-ray photon is at this value (or values for other significant absorption edges), then the degree of photoelectric absorption will be high and, in general, the amount of light emitted will also be increased compared to the amount released by photons with a marginally higher or lower energy (in most cases the higher the absorption, the higher the light output, the faster the screens and the higher the IF; see screen speed, p. 185).

This leads to the conclusion that all screens are kV dependent. As an example, Figure 5.11 shows the K absorption edge for calcium

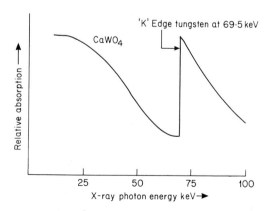

Fig. 5.11 Illustration of the photoelectric absorption properties of calcium tungstate and how it varies with X-ray photon energy.

tungstate. Between 15 and 69.5 keV there is a fall in the relative photoelectric absorption. At 69.5 keV there is a massive jump in absorption which again starts to tail off as the photon energy increases towards 100 keV.

In the practical situation the dependence of IF on kVp is well known to all radiographers. When using calcium tungstate screens in the 60–90 kVp range, an increase in exposure of 10 kVp allows an approximate reduction in mAs of one-half, and will still produce a film of similar density; i.e., 50 mAs, 70 kVp $\simeq$ 25 mAs 80 kVp in terms of film blackening.

In order to emphasise the importance of the intensification properties of screens, consider one X-ray photon falling on a direct exposure film. If this is absorbed by the film it will produce one development centre when the film is processed (see Chapter 3, Photochemistry). If the same photon is absorbed by a high speed $CaWO_4$ screen it will produce approximately 800 light photons; about half of these are absorbed in the screen before they reach the film, leaving 400 photons to expose the film.

If it takes, say, 10 light photons to produce one development centre then the number of development centres produced is approximately equal to 40. This does not mean exposure reductions of $\times$ 40 are required when going from no-screen to screen techniques, but illustrates that the amplifying power of screens is considerable. (See Screen efficiency, p. 185.)

SUMMARY: CONSTRUCTION AND INTENSIFICATION FACTOR

1. A cross-sectional diagram of the construction of a screen is shown in Figure 5.10. It consists of:

Base

Made from polyester, approximately 250 μ thick. Similar to film base.

Reflective absorptive layer

Either absorbs or reflects light emitted by the screen phosphor. This significantly affects screen speed and unsharpness. If reflective, it is a layer of titanium dioxide or similar compound.

Phosphor layer

This is a suspension of phosphor crystals in a suitable binder. Binder technology is extremely complex. Most manufacturers use acetate acrylate as the binding agent.

Supercoat

Top protective layer of the screen, it is a very thin coating of cellulose acetobiturate or similar material. The supercoat may be completely smooth or deliberately roughened, depending on the use to which the screen will be put.

2. Intensification factor is defined as the ratio of the exposure required to produce net density 1.0 without screens using a particular film, compared to the exposure required to produce the same density using screens with the same film: i.e. by how much you can reduce the exposure when moving from a non-screen to a screen technique.

SCREEN SPEED AND DETAIL

Screen speed and detail are inexorably linked. The general relationship is a reciprocal one; that is, as the speed of a film/screen combination increases, the amount of detail decreases (i.e. there is an increase in unsharpness: see Chapter 7, Image quality).

The main factors affecting speed are listed below; following this list, each is discussed in turn and its effect on detail is considered either within the section or (if more appropriate) at the end.

- Phosphor type — efficiency
- Thickness of phosphor layer/coating weight
- Presence of absorptive/reflective layer
- Presence of dye in phosphor binder or supercoat
- Exposure technique
- Phosphor grain size.

Phosphor type

It is common knowledge that different phosphors used in screens can affect their speed. For example, it is generally accepted that rare earth screens are 'faster' than $CaWO_4$ screens; however, this is an oversimplification. It is possible to make rare earth screens and calcium tungstate screens of the same speed class (see Speed Class, p. 191) but one will produce quite different results in terms of resolution compared to the other.

In order to be more precise it is necessary to consider a somewhat stylised situation; if the same amounts, in terms of volume, of calcium tungstate and a rare earth phosphor were subject to exactly the same X-ray exposure, and the light given off exposed a film that was of the correct spectral sensitivity to record the emission, it would be found, in general, that the film exposed to the rare earth phosphor would have a higher density than the film exposed to calcium tungstate.

The amount of light output from screens is normally examined by considering their efficiency. It has already been stated that screens work by the three stage process of absorption, conversion and emission. Total efficiency is the product of the efficiency of each of the processes, so that

$$N_t = N_a \times N_c \times N_e$$

where:
   N_t = Total efficiency
   N_a = Absorption efficiency
   N_c = Conversion efficiency
   N_e = Emission efficiency.

Absorption efficiency is also known as Quantum Detection Efficiency (QDE). Both terms are equally valid when considering the total efficiency of a screen system.

Occasionally the value of the emission efficiency is omitted, as this considerably simplifies quantitative evaluation due to the fact that this value is difficult to calculate.

Total efficiency can be increased by increasing any one of the three variables or any combination of them.

In general, the mother crystal determines the absorption whilst the dopant determines the conversion; therefore changing from a low absorption self-doped crystal (such as $CaWO_4$) to a high absorption deliberately doped crystal (such as LaOBr.Tb) results in increased efficiency, increased light output and apparently higher speed. Although still the subject for research it is probably worth saying that the type of re-emission from the crystal is determined by its shape — but precisely how, in most cases, is not clear.

The effect that changing the phosphor has on detail is best considered after discussion of the other factors.

Phosphor thickness

This is the factor that contributes most to screen unsharpness. The general rule is that, for the same phosphor type, the thicker the phosphor layer, the faster the screen but the greater the unsharpness it produces. Consider Figure 5.12

Suppose an incoming X-ray photon causes a phosphor crystal that is far away from the film to emit light. This light is given off in all directions but only some of it reaches the film. As can be seen from the figure, the area of film exposed is larger than the phosphor

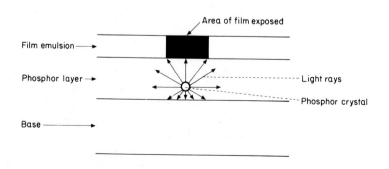

Fig. 5.12 Unsharpness due to screens: area of film exposed greater than that of the phosphor crystal.

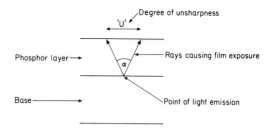

Fig. 5.13 Screen unsharpness: quantitative approach.

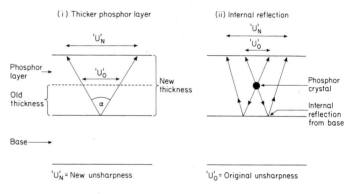

Fig. 5.14 Screen unsharpness (i) thicker phosphor layer; (ii) internal reflection.

crystal. This amount of spread of the light due to the distance it has travelled can be qualitatively expressed by the value 'u' in Figure 5.13. If the thickness of the phosphor is increased, the value of 'u' also increases (Fig. 5.14 (i)) and the unsharpness produced increases.

However, if the phosphor is thicker, more of the incoming X-ray photons will be absorbed, the total efficiency will increase and more light photons will be given off. Consequently, to produce a similar film density a reduction in exposure will be required, i.e. the screen has increased in speed. The converse is also true, in that for the same phosphor type, the thinner the layer the slower the screen but the less the unsharpness. It is not possible to go on increasing screen speed by this method indefinitely, as apart from the problems of unsharpness an optimum value of screen thickness to coating weight of crystal is reached which produces the highest light output. Exceeding this optimum eventually results in the screen absorbing its own light output with the effect that no increase in speed results from using a thicker phosphor layer.

Other relevant factors to be considered are the presence or absence of an absorptive dye in the phosphor binder or reflective layer. For example, if speed control is being exercised by dye tinting then two screens which have the same thickness may have different speed and unsharpness factors, due to the presence of the dye.

Coating weight

This is the amount of phosphor present per unit volume. The basic principle is quite simple, in that the more phosphor crystals there are in a given volume, the more light will be emitted due to the higher chance of X-ray absorption in that volume. Therefore, the higher the coating weight, the faster the screen. The amount of phosphor present depends on the specific gravity of the phosphor and the phosphor/binder ratio. In theory the higher the specific gravity, the higher the coating weight possible, but in practice the phosphor/binder ratio is more significant in determining speed and unsharpness.

Absorptive/reflective layer

As detailed earlier, these layers are coated on top of the base. If the layer is reflective any light going away from the film is redirected towards the film and contributes to its exposure. The effective speed of the screen is increased but so is unsharpness, due to the internal reflection increasing the 'u' value as shown in Figure 5.14 (ii).

The action of the absorptive layer is exactly the opposite of that of the reflective layer. It is normally a coloured dye that absorbs light going away from the film. This has the effect of reducing the speed of the screen (because of the reduction in light reaching the film) and also reducing the degree of unsharpness. The use of an absorption layer as described here is a relatively rare way of controlling screen speed.

It is quite possible for there to be neither of these layers present. When this is the case, some internal reflections still occur, due to the boundary between the base and the phosphor layer, and this still contributes to speed and unsharpness.

Dye tint in binder

This is probably the most common way to control screen speed and unsharpness. Its principle is based on the inclusion of a coloured dye within the binder of the phosphor layer and the effect that this has on the amount of light reaching the film. It is described quantitively by the Beer-Lambert Law which states that 'the proportion of light absorbed by a medium varies exponentially with the product of the path length of the light in the medium, the molar concentration and the molecular extinction co-efficient'. In simple terms, the greater the distance a ray of light travels in a coloured medium, the more it is absorbed (Fig. 5.15). The effect this has on screen speed and resolution is illustrated in Figure 5.16.

This shows a phosphor crystal producing a degree of unsharpness ('u') due to lateral diffusion of the light represented by angle α. The distance the light has travelled is represented by 'x'. If a coloured dye is added to the binder, the value of 'u' decreases because the amount of light absorbed by the dye in transiting the path length ('x') is such

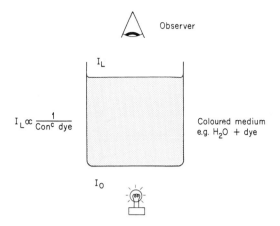

Fig. 5.15 Beer-Lambert Law: diagrammatic illustration.

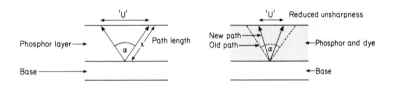

Fig. 5.16 Screen unsharpness: reduction due to dye tinting phosphor layer.

that only a very small fraction (or none at all) reaches and exposes the film. In order for sufficient light to reach the film to produce an appreciable image, the path length ('x') must decrease. This can only occur if angle α gets smaller and this in turn results in a reduction in the unsharpness ('u').

The result of this on speed is quite obvious; as the dye has a light-absorbing effect, it reduces the exposure reaching the film. This must be compensated for by an increase in exposure in order to obtain a similar film density, providing the same film is used.

A similar effect can be obtained by placing the dye in the super-coat; however, this is somewhat limited in terms of its effectiveness and is rarely used.

Exposure technique

It is relatively well known that the rare earth phosphors are 'kV dependent'. In practice this means that in order to make the best use of their total efficiency it is necessary to use them within a certain kV range.

Consider Figure 5.17. This shows how relative speed varies against kVp set for 5 different systems:

1. is a BaFCl.Eu system of speed class 350–400 (approx.)
2. is a Gd_2O_2 S.Tb system of speed class 150–400 (approx.)

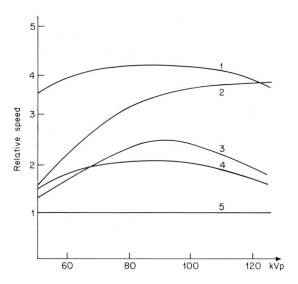

Fig. 5.17 System speed variation with kVp.

3. is a Gd_2O_2 S.Tb system of speed class 130–240 (approx.)
4. is a LaOBr.Tb system of speed class 150–200 (approx.)
5. is a $CaWO_4$ system (which is represented as a straight line for ease of comparison) of speed class 100.

As can be seen, system 3 has its maximum speed at approximately 90 kVp (speed class 240) with quite a marked fall off at kVs higher and lower than this. If this system was used in a situation requiring a set kV of, say, 70 kV, then its speed class will have fallen to 200.

System 4, however, has quite a flat top to its curve, illustrating that this system maintains its speed class of 200 quite well between 70 and 95 kV but either side of this limit it falls away until, for example, at 55 kV its speed is not much better than $CaWO_4$.

In practice it is important to know how the speed of a screen varies with the kV selected, as this could significantly influence the choice of what film/screen system should be used for a particular examination.

One final point to be considered is that Figure 5.17 implies that $CaWO_4$ screens are not kV dependent. This is not the case; but their dependency on variation in kV is not as marked as their competitors and is often represented as a straight line for comparative purposes.

Phosphor grain size

This factor is of *theoretical concern only*, the principle being that within certain limits the larger the phosphor grain the greater its absorption and therefore the more light it will emit. If a phosphor layer is made up of large grains it would be faster but produce more unsharpness than if the screen were made up of smaller grains, all other factors staying equal. In practice phosphor grains in screens have a range of sizes, which are usually between 4–8 μ in commercially available systems.

The fact that no matter what speed class a particular screen falls into it will have a phosphor grain size of 4–8 μ is quite reasonable, as the manufacture of even this range of accuracy of size is quite a complex process. Considering this with the previously listed factors affecting speed, it is easy to see that the use of phosphor grain size in speed control in practical systems is of little concern, providing they are small enough to provide adequate sharpness.

General interrelation of speed factors

The interrelationships of the factors affecting speed and detail are numerous, complex and the subject of much discussion. Complete consideration of them all is not within the scope of this chapter, but to illustrate the complexities involved consider the following question: two different film/screen combinations have the same speed class of 200. The first is a calcium tungstate system with conventional RP film, the second is a rare earth lanthanum oxybromide system with the same film. Which would you expect to produce the better image detail?

Both systems are the same speed class so they require the same exposure to produce similar image densities. The LaOBr.Tb has greater total efficiency than the $CaWO_4$ system, so in order to get the same amount of exposure to the film two options are open:

1. The phosphor layer can be made thinner or
2. The phosphor layer can remain the same thickness but have a dye introduced so as to reduce the speed to that of the $CaWO_4$ system.

In either case the amount of unsharpness produced by the rare earth system is less, so it appears to be the best choice. However, other questions also need to be asked such as, how thick is the supercoat? What about quantum mottle? What about the effect of other unsharpness factors such as focal spot size, ffd, etc.?

As can be seen, a relatively simple question such as which combination produces the best detail has a far from simple answer.

Speed classification

One of the major problems concerning film/screen combinations has been the difficulty in comparing different manufacturer's systems in terms of their speed. This has been accentuated with the introduction of so-called half speed film, orthochromatic and monochromatic rare earth systems and high speed barium fluorochloride phosphors.

The use of speed class considerably simplifies this problem and allows easy comparison of systems in terms of speed (but not necessarily detail rendition). It is based on an arbitrary scale with the value

Table 5.1 Speed classification: system basics

Speed class	50	100	200	400	800
Required mAs changes to produce similar densities (fixed kV + ffd*)	200 mAs	100 mAs	50 mAs	25 mAs	12.5 mAs
Exposure alteration compared to class 100	× 2	1	$\frac{1}{2}$	$\frac{1}{4}$	$\frac{1}{8}$

*All mAs valves are approximate.

of 100 being the bench mark to which all other systems are compared.

Table 5.1 illustrates the basis of the system. As can be seen, the speed classes range from 50 up to 800.

Values intermediate to those shown are often found, (e.g. speed class 350), as also are values higher and lower (e.g. 1200 and 25), but conventionally most systems fall into the range illustrated. The advantage of using speed class now comes into its own, as apart from showing relative system speed it also shows the variation in exposure required when changing from one system to another.

For example if you are at present using a speed class 100 system and the exposure required to produce a particular image is 70 kV 100 mAs 90 cm ffd, if you now wish to use a speed class 200 system then the exposure would be 70 kV 50 mAs 90 cm ffd; or if it were a 400 system the mAs would be 25 mAs, or if class 50, 200 mAs in order to produce a *similar* image. Therefore as the speed class goes up the amount of exposure required to produce an image goes down compared to lower speed class values.

A note of caution is perhaps required here. Firstly, as the relationships are only approximate it is not always possible to produce an exactly similar image in terms of the densities produced. This is mainly due to the kV dependency of the phosphors and other factors that are not relevant at this time. However, the approximations hold true for many practical purposes. Secondly, as previously stated, a lower speed class does not necessarily mean improved image quality, as phosphor type and screen structure are not considered. For example, a rare earth system speed class 200 may produce equal or better detail than a $CaWO_4$ speed class 100 due to factors previously discussed.

A *general* rule that seems to hold true is that rare earth systems, compared to other systems in the same speed class, produce better detail radiographs.

It is difficult to discuss speed class in abstract terms; Table 5.2 is included to show different manufacturers' film/screen combinations in terms of film type versus screen type and speed class produced. The bench-mark speed class 100 is taken as $CaWO_4$, universal-type intensifying screens and standard RP films such as Agfa-Gevaert Universal and Curix RP1. All results are in 'standard processing' which should be used throughout if consistent results are to be obtained.

A final note is that not all manufacturers use the designators 100, 200 etc.: some use 1, 2, 4, 8, etc., but the interrelationship is the same, i.e. 4–8 is halving the exposure.

SUMMARY: SCREEN SPEED AND DETAIL

1. In general as screen speed increases there is decrease in image detail, providing the same phosphor is being used. It must be remembered that this is not always the case.

2. The main factors affecting speed and detail are:

- Phosphor type
- Thickness of the phosphor layer and coating weight
- Presence of absorptive or reflective layer
- Dye tinting of the binder or supercoat
- Exposure technique.

3. *Phosphor type.* The higher the total efficiency of the phosphor the more light output the phosphor will produce, providing similar amounts of phosphor are being considered. The rare earth phosphors gain an increase in overall efficiency by having a high absorption efficiency compared to that of calcium tungstate (see Table 5.5). The more efficient the phosphor, the thinner it can be coated to produce the same speed class and as a result the higher the image sharpness it will give.

4. *Phosphor thickness.* In general the thicker the phosphor the faster the screen and the greater the unsharpness it will produce (see Figs 5.13, 5.14). However, dye tinting may alter this simple relationship.

Table 5.2 Examples of speed classifications

	Monochromatic systems ('Blue')						Orthochromatic systems ('Green')						
Speed class	Agfa-Gevaert Curix system		Kodak		Dupont		Kodak		3 M			Agfa-Gevaert Curix system	
Film	RP1	MR4	XRP	XG	CR4	CR7	OH	OG	XM	XD	XUD	ORTHO G	ORTHO L
50		UNIV									T2		
100	UNIV	SPEZ	MED SPEED	X-REG	PAR SPEED	HI PLUS		LAN FINE		T2	T4	ORTHO FINE	ORTHO FINE
200	SPEZ	MR400	X-REG		HI PLUS	QUAN II	LAN FINE	LAN MED	T2	T4	T8	ORTHO MED	ORTHO MED
400	MR400	MR800			QUAN II	QUAN III	LAN MED	LAN REG	T4	T8	T16	ORTHO REG	ORTHO REG
800	MR800				QUAN III		LAN REG		T8	T16			

SCREEN TYPES:	UNIV	= UNIVERSAL	T	= TRIMAX	REG	= REGULAR
	SPEC	= SPECIAL	MR	= MINIMUM RADIATION	MED	= MEDIUM
	QUAN	= QUANTA	LAN	= LANEX		

5. *Coating weight*. This is the amount of phosphor per unit volume. It depends on the phosphor's specific gravity and on the phosphor/binder ratio.

6. Reflective/absorptive layer. The reflective layer increases screen speed but also increases unsharpness, (due to internal reflection — see Fig. 5.14 (ii)). The absorptive layer decreases screen speed but also decreases unsharpness. These layers may or may not be present.

7. *Dye tinting*. This is the most common way to control screen speed and unsharpness. The addition of a coloured dye to the binder reduces screen speed and increases the sharpness by reducing the 'u' value as shown in Figure 5.16. It is based on the application of the Beer-Lambert Law. Occasionally the supercoat may be tinted to produce a similar effect, but this is done only rarely.

8. *Exposure technique*. This has no effect on screen unsharpness but can have effects on screen speed. Rare earth phosphors are 'kV dependant' and have their highest speed within a certain range of kilovoltages. Careful selection of exposure factors enables the highest speed to be obtained (see Fig. 5.17).

9. *Speed classification*. This is a method of comparing film/screen combinations in terms of their relative speed. It allows different manufacturers' systems to be classified in such a way as to make changing from one to another, in terms of what exposures to use, a simple process. Table 5.1 and 5.2 illustrate the basics of this system.

CROSSOVER EFFECT

This effect occurs due to the use of duplitised film emulsions and is a feature of single or multiscreen techniques. It produces a decrease in image quality caused by the light, which is not completely absorbed in the first emulsion layer, passing through the base and exposing the second emulsion layer (Fig. 5.18). This significantly contributes to unsharpness as can be seen qualitatively in the figure.

The widening light beam is the result of light diffusion within the

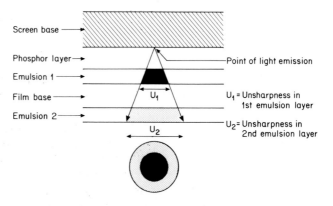

Fig. 5.18 Crossover effect: showing unsharpness reduced in two emulsion layers.

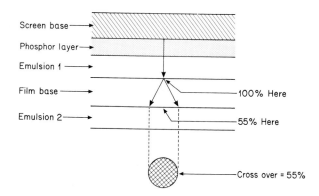

Fig. 5.19 Crossover effect: calculation of percentage crossover.

grains as it passes from one side to the other, causing a 'wider', less sharp image in the emulsion layer furthest away from the initial light emission.

The degree of crossover is usually expressed as a percentage, and varies from 15–25% in ultraviolet/blue systems to 60% in orthochromatic systems. More formally, crossover can be defined as 'the amount of light transmitted to the opposite side of the base expressed as a percentage' (Fig. 5.19).

Image degradation caused by 60% crossover is so great that it may necessitate the inclusion of an anti-halation layer or anti-halation 'in coating' as part of the film structure in order to reduce it to an acceptable level. In turn, this may mean that there is a requirement to use only a particular film with a particular screen in order to obtain the best results. This makes the film screen combination a so-called 'closed system'.

RESOLUTION

This is an often-quoted value and is frequently used, quite erroneously, to support claims of how much detail a particular film screen combination will provide. It is measured in *line pairs per millimetre* ($lp\ mm^{-1}$) but is quite often seen as line pairs per centimetre or even line pairs per inch.

A line pair is a line of a particular width followed by a space of the same width; so, for example, if the quoted resolution for a particular system is $4\ lp\ mm^{-1}$, this means that there are 4 lines and spaces contained within 1 mm, therefore each line is 1/8 mm wide and each space is 1/8 mm wide.

In simple terms, resolution indicates the size of the smallest object that the system will record and, therefore, the smallest distance that must exist between two objects before they are seen as two separate objects. Typical values for resolution are shown in Table 5.3. Unfortunately, resolution gives no indication of a system's performance in recording the detail of objects larger than the limiting resolution, nor

Table 5.3 Resolution values

System	Speed class*	Resolution (lp mm^{-1}
Curix Universal** + Curix RP1 film	100	6–8 approx.
Curix Special** + Curix RP1 film	200	4–6 approx.
Curix MR 400** + Curix RP1 film	400	4–6 approx.
Human eye	N/A	At 4 ft, in average illumination conditions, 2–4 appox.

* Speed class included for information only. Increasing speed class does not necessarily mean decreasing resolution. Generalisations are only useful when considering the same phosphor type. Values vary depending on many factors, e.g. processing conditions and exposure conditions, to name but two.
** Products of Agfa-Gevaert Ltd.

how it copes with high or low contrast details. Additionally it is often difficult to discover whether published information is for system resolution (i.e. the X-ray equipment + film/screen combination + processing, etc.) or whether it is a theoretically calculated value. Finally, it is important to distinguish between resolution (which is objective) and definition (which is subjective). For more detail see Chapter 7, Image quality.

MOTTLE

This is the apparent 'granular' appearance in areas of apparently even density in the radiographic image. Contributers to this can be conveniently divided into three sections:

- Film grain
- Quantum mottle
- Structure mottle.

Film grain

This is due to the coarse structure of the silver crystals forming the overall density in the emulsion. Even though the silver halide crystals are small (10^{-6}m), development tends to make them aggregate together (clumping) and form a small but visible unevenness in density. Many factors can affect this, ranging from film speed to processing conditions. True film grain in modern emulsions is so small as to be almost imperceptible, but it can be seen on magnification.

A fuller description of grain is to be found in Chapter 7, Image quality.

Quantum mottle

Sometimes called 'noise', this is due to the random distribution of image-forming X-ray quanta producing non-uniform light emission from the screens. This light subsequently exposes the film, producing a developable silver halide grain or grains. In general the faster the film/screen combination is, the higher the quantum mottle will be, because the lower the dose required to produce a given density, the fewer X-ray quanta there will be and the higher the chance that these will be recorded on the film as a separate 'density spot'.

However, this does not take into account the fact that one film may have high quantum mottle compared to another film but it may be less well 'imaged', i.e. unsharp, and consequently less visible.

True quantum mottle is a significant degree coarser than true film grain.

A fuller description of quantum mottle is to be found in the Chapter 7, Image quality.

Structure mottle

This is a feature of the screen manufacturing process and is caused by the fact that it is not possible to evenly disperse the phosphor crystals throughout the binder medium.

No matter how efficient the mixing and coating process, areas of high phosphor crystal density occur. When exposed these areas produce a higher light output than the surrounding areas and consequently a higher film density. This contributes to the overall mottled appearance.

In practice, however, coating technology is so far advanced that structure mottle in modern screens is negligible. Occasionally it is possible to have two screens with similar mottle characteristics. When this occurs there is a tendency for one to reinforce the other; in this case the mottle may become obtrusive.

RECIPROCITY AND RECIPROCITY FAILURE

The reciprocity law was first proposed by Bunson and Roscoe in 1862. In simple terms, it states that the amount of density produced on a film is dependent only on the total amount of light energy employed. This means that if the exposure (E) remains constant then the amount of density produced will also remain constant (all other factors being equal). Exposure is the product of Intensity (I) and Time (t):

$$E = It$$

If the reciprocity law holds true then, providing E is constant, any combination of I and t may be used to produce the same density. For example, say 100 'units' of E are required to produce a density of 1 then

$$E = It$$
$$100 = 10 \times 10$$
$$= 100 \times 1$$
$$= 1 \times 100$$
$$= 2 \times 50$$

All produce D = 1.0

and so on.

However, this simple relationship does not hold true, as was proved by a researcher called Abney. He discovered that at very long or very short exposure times, the resulting density value was somewhat less than was expected. This is reciprocity law failure.

In practice this means that the use of very high mA and short exposure times, or very low mA and long exposure times, will not produce the same result in terms of density as a set of exposure factors between the two extremes. In practice, reciprocity failure seems at a minimum for times of 0.1 s and is so small as to be insignificant for exposure times between about 0.002 s and 3 s.

There are a number of ways of illustrating reciprocity failure; one of the most common is to plot speed variation against exposure time, (Fig. 5.20). As may be seen in the figure, a decrease in speed indicates reciprocity failure, as decreasing speed would give lower densities for a given amount of exposure.

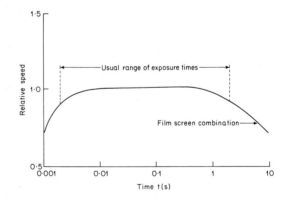

Fig. 5.20 Reciprocity failure: diagrammatic representation only.

Different films have differing reciprocity characteristics. Figure 5.21 illustrates the two extremes encountered in radiographic departments. Film directly exposed to X- or gamma radiation shows little or no variation in speed, whilst the monitor photography film shows no speed loss at short exposure times but some loss at longer exposure times. From this it can be deduced that to a large extent, reciprocity characteristics can be controlled in emulsion manufacture.

Finally, it is interesting to note that it is possible, with the aid of an engineer, to calibrate the mA settings of the X-ray set to hide the effects of selecting high or low mA values, providing that the timer is known to be accurate. This would apparently make the reciprocity law hold true.

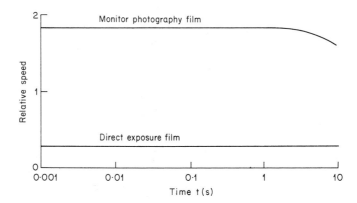

Fig. 5.21 Examples of reciprocity characteristics: diagrammatic only (actual data available from manufacturers).

SCREEN ASYMMETRY

This is a feature of some manufacturers' screens: it involves the provision of pairs of screens, i.e. front and back screens, which must be attached to the front and back of the cassette.

If the two screens in a cassette are identical then the screen closest to the X-ray tube absorbs a proportion of the arriving X-ray beam and produces a certain amount of light. The back screen does not receive as many X-ray quanta, due to the fact some have already been absorbed, and therefore the amount of light output will be less. The front screen therefore produces a higher density on the film than the back screen. In order to counter this asymmetric production of density; the back screen is made slightly faster, so that even though it receives fewer X-ray quanta its light output is the same as the front screen, thus producing the same density on both sides of the emulsion. This is normally achieved by the back screen having a slightly thicker coating of phosphor.

In calcium tungstate systems this asymmetry was of little practical significance. However, with the highly X-ray absorbent rare earth systems this has taken on some degree of importance. Failure to mount the screens in the cassette in the correct order can lead to significant speed reduction compared to that expected. However, it should be noted that not all screens are supplied in this front, back combination.

SPECTRAL EMISSION

Matching spectral output

The following subsections deal with the wavelengths of light (i.e. the colours) that are emitted by the various commonly-used screen phosphors. Accurate knowledge of this is essential, as it is vitally important to match the spectral output of the screen to the spectral sensitivity of the film. In general, failure to do this will result in a loss of system speed and a loss of information transfer from the emergent beam from the patient to the film. However, occasionally a deliberate mismatch of screen and film sensitivity is used in order to reduce system speed and improve image quality. This is a particular feature of the rare earth film/screen systems and is more fully discussed below.

Calcium tungstate (CaWO₄)

This has been the commonly used phosphor for intensifying screens up until recent history. Calcium tungstate requires no activator and produces a continuous spectrum principally in the blue part of the visible spectrum, with a peak output at approximately 425 nm. Figure 5.22 illustrates the spectral output of the phosphor; superimposed on the same figure is the sensitivity of conventional monochromatic ('blue') film. As can be seen the film is sensitive to the majority of the screen output and therefore records all but a small proportion of the available information.

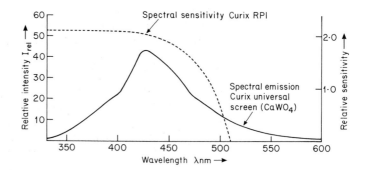

Fig. 5.22 Spectral sensitivity: Agfa-Gevaert Curix RPI film. Spectral emission: Agfa-Gevaert Curix Universal (CaWO₄) screen.

Rare earths

A good deal of misinformation has been circulated about the rare earth phosphors. The following few paragraphs are included to give the reader some background into this most recent addition to screen phosphor technology.

The elements known as rare earths are neither rare nor earths. They are soft, malleable metals and not at all in short supply. Cerium, the most abundant, is more plentiful than tin or lead. Thulium, the scarcest, is only slightly rarer than iodine. The misnomer arose because their oxides were at first taken for the elements themselves.

At an atomic level all the fifteen rare earths have two outer electrons, and in the penultimate shell they have eight or nine electrons. Their greatest difference is in the N shell. In atoms, this difference is very minute and so we find that the rare earths form a very close family. A mineral containing one of them contains all the others.

The rare earths are so nearly identical that separating them can involve thousands of steps. Because of this the individual elements did not become available until the late 1950s. However, the family has been used industrially since the early 1900s in the form of naturally-occurring mixtures.

Perhaps one of the most common uses of these mixtures is an alloy called misch metal, i.e. mixed metal. Combined with iron, misch metal produces cigarette lighter flints. Its main role is in iron and steel-making, where it absorbs impurities and improves texture and workability. A mixture of rare earths combined with carbon produces the intense carbon arc lights. Numerous rare earth compounds go into high quality glass, making it completely colourless or adding a deep colour depending on the combination used. Additionally they are used in the phosphors of television cameras and in advanced technology lasers.

The following rare earths are those most commonly found in phosphors used in radiology.

Lanthanum (La)

Atomic No. 57   Atomic weight 138.91
Electron configuration 2, 8, 18, 18, 9, 2

Comes from Greek *lanthanein*, to lie hidden. Discovered in 1839, it is highly reactive. Because it gives glass special light-bending properties, lanthanum is used in expensive camera lenses.

Lanthanum is involved in many rare earth screen phosphor patents. An original report by Buchanan, Finkelstein and Wickersheim in 1972 and released by AEC/NASA in the same year concerned terbium-activated gadolinium and lanthanum oxysulphides.

Europium (Eu)

Atomic No. 63   Atomic weight 151.96
Electron configuration 2, 8, 18, 25, 8, 2

The name is derived from *Europe*. Discovered in 1896, it is the most reactive rare earth. Atom for atom, europium can absorb more neutrons than any other element. This factor makes it very valuable for nuclear reactor control rods. In intensifying screens it is one of the principal activators.

Gadolinium (Gd)

Atomic No. 64   Atomic weight 157.25
Electron configuration 2, 8, 18, 25, 9, 2

From the mineral gadolinite. Discovered in 1880, it comes in the middle of the rare earth series and divides the lighter metals, which impart pliancy to alloys, from the heavier strengthening metals. It is the principal element in many orthochromatic ('green') screen systems.

Terbium (Tb)

Atomic No. 65   Atomic weight 158.92
Electron configuration 2, 8, 18, 26, 9, 2

Named after Ytterby, in Sweden where it was discovered in 1843. Its principal use in screens is as an activator.

Yttrium (Y)

Atomic No. 39   Atomic weight 88.905
Electron configuration 2, 8, 18, 9, 2

Again, the name comes from the Swedish town of Ytterby. Discovered in 1794, it is *not* a rare earth but is a first transition metal. It is included because it has been used as an activator in some rare earth phosphor combinations.

Rare earth spectral emission

All the rare earth phosphors used in intensifying screens produce a line spectrum, the position and intensity of each line being dependent on the type and amount of dopant (i.e. activator) that has been added to the mother crystal. Somewhat conveniently, they can be divided into those that are suitable for use with orthochromatic ('green') sensitive film and those that are used with monochromatic ('blue') sensitive film. Table 5.4 illustrates three of the main phosphors. It should be noted that whilst not strictly a rare earth, barium fluorochloride has a rare earth activator.

Table 5.4 Rare earth screens: principal phosphors; symbols; emissions

Phosphor name	Chemical symbol	Principal emission
Lanthanum oxybromide	LaOBr.Tb	Blue
Gadolinium oxysulphide	$Gd_2O_2S.Tb$	Green
Barium Fluorochloride	BaFCl.Eu	Ultraviolet

As with calcium tungstate, it is vital to match the peak spectral lines with peak spectral sensitivity of the film to ensure maximum speed and information transfer. Figures 5.23, 5.24 and 5.25 show the spectral emission of lanthanum oxybromide (LaOBr.Tb), gadolinium oxysulphide ($Gd_2O_2S.Tb$) and barium fluorochloride (BaFCl.Eu) along with a film of suitable sensitivity superimposed on the same diagram.

A point to notice is that the line emissions of the true rare earth phosphors extend throughout the whole of the visible spectrum (i.e. LaOBr.Tb emits both green and red light), but only the most intense (i.e. the blue) lines are recorded by the film.

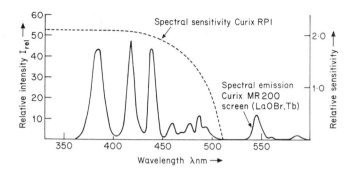

Fig. 5.23 Spectral sensitivity: Agfa-Gevaert Curix RPI film. Spectral emission: Agfa-Gevaert Curix MR200 (LaOBr.Tb) screen.

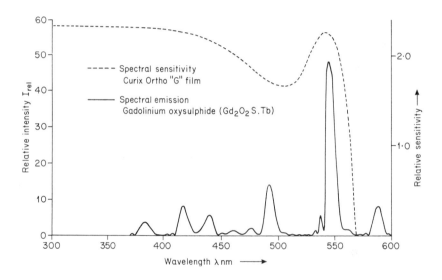

Fig. 5.24 Spectral sensitivity: Agfa-Gevaert Curix Ortho G film. Spectral emission: gadolinium oxysulphide.

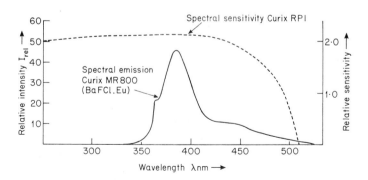

Fig. 5.25 Spectral sensitivity: Agfa-Gevaert Curix RPI film. Spectral emission: Agfa-Gevaert Curix MR800 (BaFCl.Eu) screen.

A similar situation exists for Gd_2O_2S.Tb which has its highest light output in the green part of the spectrum with only a small light output in the blue. It is this factor that allows a mismatch of film and screens to produce an image even though the system will have low speed due to the relatively low intensity of the non-predominant spectral lines.

Also, it will be seen that the BaFCl.Eu phosphor produces essentially a continuous spectrum, with its peak in the ultraviolet at about 385 nm.

A final close examination of the lanthanum and gadolinium spectra will reveal that the spectral lines of each are roughly at the same wavelengths, the variation being in the relative intensity of each spectral line. The intensity of each line is controlled by the amount and type of dopant. In general, increasing the concentration of dopant alters the peak emission towards the red end of the spectrum. Consequently there is no reason why LaOBr.Tb cannot be used to produce green-emitting screens providing the amount of terbium dopant present is high enough. In practice, this is not done as this has a detrimental effect on overall efficiency. The same is also true of the gadolinium phosphors.

KILOVOLTAGE RESPONSE

The speed of all screens is to some extent kV dependent. Even the speed of calcium tungstate screens alters with changing kV; however, in this case, the change in speed is so small as to be negligible for all practical purposes.

Unfortunately, this does not apply to the rare earth screens. Figure 5.26 is a plot of relative speed versus kVp for four different speed classes, ranging from a calcium tungstate class 100 to a barium fluorochloride class 800 system. This shows peak speed for the rare earth systems at 80–85 kVp, with a fall in speed down to 60–65 kVp and a sharp decline at kVp lower than 60.

Between 80 kVp and 105 kVp (approx.) speed is more or less constant, this being followed by a decline after about 105 kVp. Therefore, in order to obtain the best use of the speed offered by rare earth screens, careful selection of the appropriate kV factors is necessary.

OTHER INFORMATION

Frequent mention has been made of various factors throughout this chapter with no reference to actual values, e.g. absorption values, etc. This was done to try and keep non-essential numeric information out of the main text. However, for those interested Table 5.5 may prove to be useful.

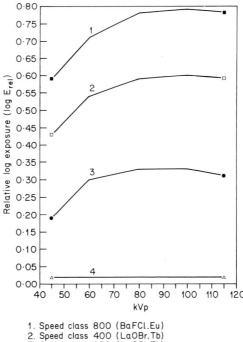

Fig. 5.26 kV response rare earth screens.

1. Speed class 800 (BaFCl.Eu)
2. Speed class 400 (LaOBr.Tb)
3. Speed class 200 (LaOBr.Tb)
4. Speed class 100 (CaWO₄)

Table 5.5 Phosphor data

	Ortho Gd₂O₂S.Tb	Blue LaOBr. Tb	UV BaFCl.Eu	Blue CaWO₄
% Absorption 80 kV	40.5	43.5	39.0	26.7
% Conversion	18.0	17.0	16.0	5
Specific weight	7.4	6.2	4.6	6.8
Phosphor thickness (μ)	207	228	347	250
Efficiency	7.3	7.4	6.2	1.7

Advances in technology

Screen technology is advancing all the time and this inevitably means that a book such as this will not contain the very latest information. However, the following advances, although not at present in commercial production, seem certain to take place.

At present in many 800 class systems, the phosphor of choice is barium flurochloride, europium-activated. As previously stated this is often erroneously referred to as a rare earth phosphor. At least one manufacturer intends to change this to a true rare earth phosphor by using lanthanum oxybromide, thulium-activated (LaOBr.Tm). Thulium has the advantage that it is more stable than terbium and induces a

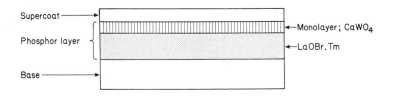

Fig. 5.27 Cross-section of screen using rare earth and calcium tungstate phosphor.

higher production of ultraviolet light, which leads to a reduction in crossover unsharpness.

One of the most interesting developments that will occur is the use of calcium tungstate and rare earth phosphors in combination. A patent for such a screen has been registered by Agfa-Gevaert NV (Antwerp) since 1976 and is illustrated in Figure 5.27. It is for lanthanum oxybromide, thulium-activated, with a monolayer of calcium tungstate coated on top of the rare earth layer. The thulium activator has the advantages previously stated whilst the single layer of calcium tungstate crystals does not fluoresce but acts as a filter, allowing normal light rays to pass through yet absorbing or reflecting angular rays (Fig. 5.28). The calcium tungstate does not fluoresce, as the single layer of crystals has practically no absorption or conversion properties. This method of controlling light scatter produces a significant gain in sharpness and is a unique concept.

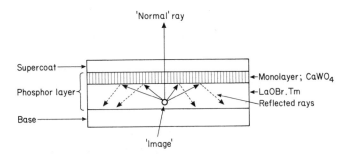

Fig. 5.28 Effect of $CaWO_4$ monolayer increasing sharpness.

Care, cleaning and testing

These items are fully covered in Chapter 6, Quality assurance, so no further mention will be made here except to say that screens must always be cleaned using the manufacturer's recommended cleaning agents. Never use soap and water.

SUMMARY: CROSSOVER TO CLEANING AND TESTING

1. Crossover causes a reduction in image quality and is caused by light which is not absorbed in the first emulsion layer passing through

the base and exposing the second emulsion layer. It varies from 15–60%, depending on the systems in use (see Fig. 5.18).

2. Resolution is a definite quantitative value and is measured in line pairs per millimeter ($lp\ mm^{-1}$). It defines the smallest object, or distance between two objects, that must exist if they are to be recorded as separate entities. Film/screen combinations have resolution ranges from 2 $lp\ mm^{-1}$ to 15 $lp\ mm^{-1}$ (approx.) (see Table 5.3).

3. Mottle is the apparent granular appearance in areas of 'even' density on the film. It comprises three contributing factors: film grain, quantum mottle, and structure mottle. Quantum mottle is the largest influence on this granular appearance.

4. The reciprocity law says that the amount of density produced will be constant providing the exposure reaching the film is constant. The law fails, however, for very long or very short exposure times. Reciprocity law failure means that the density produced is less than expected.

5. Screen asymmetry occurs when both screens in a cassette are identical. The back screen receives slightly less exposure than the front screen and therefore has a lower light output and contributes less to film exposure. In fast rare earth systems this can be a significant problem, therefore manufacturers sometimes provide screens in matched pairs, one marked front and the other back. The back screen is slightly faster to balance the fact that it receives less exposure.

6. The colour of the light output from screens must be matched to the peak spectral sensitivity of the film. This ensures maximum system speed and maximum information transfer. Occasionally a deliberate mismatch of screen output and film sensitivity is used in special cases.

7. Calcium tungstate produces a continuous spectra with a peak light output at about 425 nm (blue) and is used with monochromatic film (see Fig. 5.22).

8. The rare earth phosphors produce a line-type spectrum with the major peaks in either the green or blue parts of the visible spectrum. The position of these peaks depends on the phosphor and dopant being used. Three of the most common phosphors are lanthanum oxybromide, gadolinium oxysulphide (both terbium-activated) and barium fluorochloride, europium-activated.

Green-emitting phosphors are usually used with orthochromatic films (Figs 5.23, 5.24, 5.25). Advanced technology phosphors may include lanthanum oxybromide, thulium-activated, and the use of a monolayer of calcium tungstate with rare earth phosphors to improve screen sharpness (Figs 5.27, 5.28).

9. The speed of all phosphors is to some extent dependent on the kV used during the exposure. Rare earth phosphors are particularly kV-dependent in terms of their speed (Fig. 5.26).

10. Screens should only be cleaned using the manufacturer's recommended materials and techniques.

BIBLIOGRAPY

Jacobson R E, Ray S F, Atteridge G G, Axford N R 1978 The manual of photography, 7th edn. Focal Press, London
James T H 1979 The theory of the photographic process, 4th edn. Collier Macmillan, London

6

Quality assurance

Introduction

The term 'quality control' was borrowed from industry a few years ago. In industry, quality control simply means sampling random parts (for example) and subjecting them to tests to check that they have reached a required standard.

In radiography the term has been widened to imply a routine which provides a means of producing high quality radiographs on a day-to-day basis. This of course means that a variety of control procedures must be undertaken. Perhaps in radiography, the term 'quality assurance' would be more accurate.

The World Health Organization has defined quality assurance in X-ray medical diagnosis as:

An organised effort by the staff operating a facility to ensure that the diagnostic images produced by the facility are of sufficiently high quality so that they consistently provide adequate diagnostic information at the lowest possible cost and with the least exposure of the patient to radiation.

The objective of a quality assurance programme in an X-ray department is to monitor the performance of all the factors which could influence the quality of the image and to try to reduce any film wastage within that department.

In a variety of studies that have been prepared on film wastage, it is often suggested that in some departments wastage can be as high as 20%. In any department, this represents a significant sum of money. Allowances must be made for teaching departments where, of necessity, there must be a higher rejection rate of films. However, an average wastage figure would be of the order of 12%, in a department with no form of quality assurance.

If a quality assurance programme is designed for an X-ray department it should ideally fulfil four main criteria:

1. It should be simple. The programme should not require sophisticated equipment or advanced scientific techniques.
2. It should be inexpensive, for obvious reasons. No programme should cost more to run than the saving in film costs!
3. It should be quick. All the basic checks should be done in a matter of minutes rather than hours.
4. Perhaps most important of all it should be semi-quantitative, so that repeatability of results is assured. In a quality assurance programme it is important that the results achieved in January can be reproduced the following November.

REJECT ANALYSIS

Preparatory to starting quality assurance in a department it is wise to do a pilot study, or reject (or repeat) analysis of film wastage (i.e. why were films repeated?) to try to establish the 'norm' for the department. Obviously the longer the period for these analyses, the better the statistical values obtained.

Stage one

The initial preparation for reject analysis must be to inform *all* the staff that the survey is starting. It is vitally important that all the staff appreciate that co-operation from everyone is essential, otherwise reject analysis will become meaningless.

The aims of the project should be stressed:

1. To try to identify where, and why, the wastage is occurring.
2. To try to reduce the overall costs within the imaging department.

It is also very important for the staff to appreciate that the analysis is not a 'witch hunt', to identify poor radiographers, but is merely an assessment of the current conditions.

Stage two

A period of 8–10 weeks is set aside to conduct the survey, ideally starting on a Monday morning and finishing on a Friday night.

Prior to the Monday morning start, *all* film in the department must be identified, counted and the *details recorded.*

The easiest way of achieving this is to empty all cassettes, the film hopper and any partially empty boxes. This film is then set aside until the end of the survey, when it can be used again.

To ensure accuracy of the records, a check must then be kept, on a daily basis, of all films removed from the film stores.

Stage three

It is advised that all film analysis should be conducted on a daily basis. The volume of films which may be rejected, and then have to be sorted, should deter anyone from attempting to do a weekly check.

The rejected films should then be sorted out into categories. Some suggested categories are:

1. Positioning
2. Movement
3. Too light
4. Too dark (unknown whether films are over- or under-exposed: may be machine/processor/screen problem)
5. Processing (marks, scratches, etc.)
6. Others (i.e. screen artefacts, LBDs, etc.)
7. Rejects by room.

These are not the only categories that can be used. These are merely suggestions; the user may wish extra categories inserted. It may be wished, for example, to identify the cassettes used for the rejected films. There is a lot of information to be gained from a survey such as this. The statistical evidence produced can be interpreted and used in many ways. Of course, it also means that the statistics have to be gathered correctly and interpreted wisely.

Information can be gained about rooms which may be consistently faulty. Cassettes and screens may be identified which are outside speed tolerances. Persistent faults in a room may point to a mis-understanding of the equipment, perhaps even to more 'in-house training', for example. The survey may not just prove how costly the department is to run. It can also be used to justify extra staff, for example, if records can prove this need.

Analysis

At the end of the period, all films remaining in the department must be counted. The films used will be known, because of the record of movement of film from the film store. The total number of films used can now be obtained.

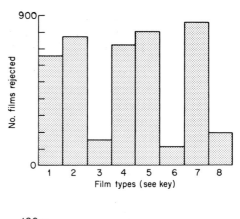

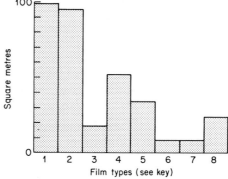

Figs 6.1 and 6.2 Key to the histograms.

Size	Number of films	Square metres
1. 35 × 43	660	99.33
2. 35 × 35	777	95.18
3. 30 × 40	153	18.36
4. 24 × 30	727	52.34
5. 18 × 24	807	34.86
6. 18 × 43	113	8.75
7. 100 mm	863	8.63
8. Other*	200	24.06
Total	4300	341.51

* CT, duplicating film, copy films, occlusals, etc.

If possible, weekly analyses should be obtained of film usage. This will give an even better statistical evaluation.

Figures 6.1 and 6.2 indicate just one way in which the statistics obtained from a reject analysis survey may be presented. The figures obtained are from an actual survey conducted in a large imaging department.

Many books advise the analysis is produced by taking the percentage of *films* rejected. Whilst this is adequate, there is a major flaw in this argument (which is illustrated in the Figures). If the aim is to assess the wastage of film, the best guide is to find the total *square meterage* rejected. This final figure will give a very good guide to the actual cost: 20 18×24s do not represent the same cost as 20, 35×43s!

Table 6.1 shows the square meterage of film in boxes of 100 films.

Table 6.1 Square meterage per box of 100 films

Film size × 100	Square metres
13 × 18 cm	= 2.34
15 × 40 cm	= 6.00
18 × 24 cm	= 4.32
20 × 40 cm	= 8.00
24 × 30 cm	= 7.20
30 × 40 cm	= 12.00
35 × 35 cm	= 12.25
35 × 43 cm	= 15.05
$6\frac{1}{2}$ × $8\frac{1}{2}$ in	= 3.56
8 × 10 in	= 5.16
10 × 12 in	= 7.75
12 × 15 in	= 11.62
7 × 17 in	= 7.74
15 × 6 in	= 5.79

It is only reasonable to point out that the percentage figures arrived at do not always tell the whole story. Dr. J. Gore of Hammersmith Hospital suggested that reject analysis did not take into account two important factors.

1. Diagnostic criteria

In this case the radiologist accepts a film for diagnosis, even though it would normally be unacceptable, because it would be very difficult or impossible to repeat it.

2. Compensation

In this case the radiographer makes allowances for a room which is known to take 'the extra five kV', or a faulty cassette which needs a 'little bit more'. In other words the radiographer compensates for an already known fault.

The problem outlined in 'diagnostic criteria' is a root problem unique to medical radiography. It effectively means that there is no 'standard' radiograph for each examination. To compare medical radiography with industrial radiography illustrates this point completely. In industrial radiography full specifications are given about densities to be achieved on the film and on the area to be examined. If these are not reached, the film will be automatically rejected. Of course, criteria like these cannot be applied in medical radiography, but this demonstrates a major problem in reject analysis.

Having established the percentage rejection/square meterage rate, other factors in the department must be investigated. This will then lead to a complete quality assurance programme.

AREAS TO MONITOR

There are four main areas which need to be monitored closely if quality assurance is to be undertaken. They are as follows.

Image producers

The image producers are obviously the X-ray set and the associated chain of equipment. It might, of course, mean a ciné radiography unit, in which case tests must be done on the image intensifier, etc.

Tests on X-ray equipment are many and varied and can be open to a number of interpretations. The scope of these tests is well outside a book such as this. Most equipment manufacturers are only too willing to help and advise with testing, and approaches should be made to them.

Image receptors

These could be a monitor television, for example. However, the image receptors which we are concerned with are the X-ray intensifying screens and film.

Image processors

Could be magnetic tape, for example. Our concern is with the conventional processing machine found in the X-ray department.

Viewing system

This could be a screen or a cine viewer. Our concern is with conventional viewing boxes.

APPARATUS REQUIRED

There is a minimum requirement for apparatus if a quality assurance programme is to be undertaken in the department:

1. A densitometer
2. A contact test grid, made to BS 4304/1968 specifications
3. An ultraviolet light, the output to be 250 nm or below
4. A calibrated step wedge, *or* a sensitometer, *or* manufacturer's pre-exposed step wedge film.
5. Alcohol thermometer, plus a maximum–minimum thermometer
6. Hydrometer
7. There are other minor items required, such as pH papers or a pH meter, relative humidity strips or meter, and silver estimating papers. A light meter would also be an ideal accessory. These can usually be begged, or borrowed, from other sources in the hospital.

Whilst every hospital may not have all the above items, they may be found in another hospital within the group.

To give some idea of the preparations involved in the setting up of a quality assurance programme, the document issued by Agfa-Gevaert preparatory to starting the programme is included. Each section of the programme is dealt with in much greater detail later in the chapter.

SETTING UP A QUALITY ASSURANCE PROGRAMME
(Extracted from the Agfa-Gevaert Diagnostic Imaging Systems Division document.)

On the first day, the major processor in the department will be needed to find the optimum temperature for this processor. This is a time-consuming exercise and the processor will most probably be required for the whole day. *It should not be switched on for this morning.*

Following this evaluation, an X-ray room will be required to complete the cassette/screen evaluation. This room *must* produce consistent reproducible exposures, otherwise the tests will be invalid. This can only be assessed by testing. The length of time taken for the cassette/screen survey is dependent on the number of cassettes to be surveyed. As a guide, a full survey of 150 cassettes will require about 4 working days.

The rest of the survey will be conducted around the work of the department.

A full report will be produced at the end of the quality assurance evaluation.

Note It is not considered that X-ray machine evaluation is part of the responsibility of a film manufacturer. However, if faults are suspected, this information will be communicated to the department head for further action.

PROCESSOR EVALUATION

The objective of these tests is:

1. To ensure that the processor is operating at peak performance and optimum temperature.

2. To identify any possible problems, so that any corrective action may be taken to ensure that the processor remains at peak performance.

Test equipment

Electric pH meter

This meter is calibrated on site to standard solutions. Its primary use is to establish accurate pH readings and thereby to ensure correct replenishment rates.

Silver estimating papers

When these papers are immersed in fixer they change colour. This colour change is matched against a colour chart. This match gives an indication of the quantity of silver in the fixer in grammes per litre (g/l). Too high a silver level can be caused by under-replenishment or blockage and will certainly result in incomplete fixing of the film.

Residual thiosulphate test solution

When a drop of this solution is placed on each side of the film, a stain appears. The shade of this stain is matched to a colour chart to indicate whether all the residual chemicals have been washed from the emulsion. This gives an indication of the archival life of the film, which certainly should be in excess of ten years.

Alcohol thermometer

Used for direct measurements of solution temperatures. A mercury thermometer is *not* recommended in a photographic area as accidental breakages can cause numerous photographic faults.

Sensitometer

The sensitometer used is calibrated to a standard wedge. The unit is capable of producing a green light emission, suitable for orthochromatic films, as well as a blue light source.

The sensitometric strip produced is a 21 step wedge, also known as a 'root 2' wedge. This image is particularly suitable for quality assurance, as it offers a detailed 21 step wedge for accuracy, but for regular use it can be used for a three step system.

SCREEN/CASSETTE EVALUATION

The objectives of the tests are:

1. To determine any loss of film/screen contact.
2. To determine the presence of any scratches or abrasion damage to the screen.
3. To determine any speed variations due to the age and condition of the screen.

Test equipment

Screen contact tester

This is a perforated zinc grid enclosed between two pieces of perspex. The grid is laid flat on the face of the cassette and an exposure is made at approximately 55 kV at 6 feet ffd, the processed film being viewed at 12 feet. If contact is uniform, the film in turn will show overall uniform density. Areas of high density will indicate a loss of screen contact in the area of the dark patches.

Ultraviolet (UV) light

This UV light emits light at a wavelength of 250 nm. This particular wavelength is extremely suitable for activating the screen phosphors. When the screen is scanned with the UV light, the surface phosphors are excited and artefacts and abrasions are readily discerned.

Densitometer

The densitometer used is calibrated on site to a standard step wedge.

VIEWING BOX EVALUATION

The objectives of this test are:

1. To achieve correct and constant light output throughout the department.
2. To achieve the correct balance between viewer light output and ambient light in the viewing room.

Test Equipment

Light meter

The light meter is a calibrated Weston Master 4.

Specification

The light output from each viewing box is measured according to the ANSI specification for viewing conditions.
  These state that a light meter set at 100 ISO (21 DIN.) held one foot away and facing the viewing box should record a minimum value of 13 EV. When the meter is now reversed to face the room light there should be a maximum value of 8 EV.

DARKROOM SAFELIGHTS

Optimally, a darkroom should be bright enough to handle films in safelight for about 45 seconds.
  The darkrooms will be tested using a standard safelight test.
The above extract is reproduced courtesy of the DIS division, Agfa-Gevaert Ltd.

  As can be seen, the setting up of a quality assurance programme involves considerable effort. It should be remembered that quality assurance is an ongoing programme. The biggest problem encountered is that the results produced are 'negative', i.e. nothing untoward happens. This is the result wanted. Unfortunately, this can sometimes lead to the conclusion that quality assurance is a waste of time and the tests become less and less frequent. This is the time to take care!

The preceding pages offer a brief summary of quality assurance, which may prove useful to the student. The full details now follow.

It is not the aim of this book to advise on tests which are to be run on the X-ray apparatus itself. This requires specialised knowledge and equipment, and the student is advised to consult other publications which deal with these tests.

Safelights

Before commencing the tests, it would be wise to perform a check of the safelights in the darkroom. See Chapter 2, Sensitometry, for details of how to conduct the test.

IMAGE PROCESSORS

It is perhaps wisest to consider first the apparatus which processes the image, the automatic processor.

The automatic processor is an essential piece of apparatus in virtually every X-ray department, and almost every film produced passes through it.

In the days of totally manual processing, there was a great deal of flexibility in the procedure, and temperature or time could be adjusted to accommodate variations in processing solutions. Not so with an automatic processor. Time, temperature and replenishment are closely controlled and certainly will not cope with a grossly overexposed film which 'only needs 2 minutes'.

Moreover, even very large X-ray departments may have only two processors, so any faults which develop can affect a large number of films over a fairly short time.

So much of quality assurance is the practical application of the knowledge of photochemistry and sensitometry in addition to the basic understanding of screens and phosphors. It is recommended that the relevant chapters (Chs 2,3 and 5) should be read before continuing this chapter.

Processor checks

As well as checking the purely mechanical side of the operation of the processor, there are other chemical checks which must be done to ensure the smooth running of the unit.

After considering what are basically mechanical checks on agitation, temperature, speed and replenishment, other checks must be done on the chemical and sensitometric performance of the processor. In this case the following must be monitored:

1. Developer, in terms of pH variations and sensitometric performance. Specific gravity measurements should also be considered.
2. Fixer, in terms of pH variations and silver levels within the fixer. Specific gravity measurements should also be considered.

Mechanical checks

The suppliers of the automatic processor will have available literature which will advise on how to carry out routine mechanical inspections. It is of course very important to note replenishment rates and, even more importantly, know how to correct them! Whilst no piece of mechanical apparatus can be considered to be perfect, the modern automatic processor is basically a very reliable unit.

One point should be mentioned here. With the advent of area scanning of film, replenishment rates have become very accurate as now the *area* of the film is measured, rather than only the *length*.

Chemical checks

pH

Each chemical manufacturer supplies details of the pH operating levels of the developer and fixer.

Two sets of pH papers will be required, to cover the ranges for developer and for fixer. Automatic processing developers, with few exceptions, range between 9.0–10.6, whilst automatic fixers range between 4.0–5.0.

Ideally pH should be measured daily, although many departments settle on weekly measurements, measuring replenishment rates at the same time.

A note of realism could be added here. In large processing laboratories, where amateur colour film is processed, it would not be unusual to see routine sensitometry and chemical measurements being done every *hour*. These laboratories simply cannot afford to release poor quality films as customers would complain in profusion.

No matter how often measurements are made, it is most important to record the measurements in a log book. Many people consider that as the measurements are always the same, it seems unnecessary to do them and even more unnecessary to record them.

The routine measurement of pH is not a very time-consuming task, but if it is logged regularly it can provide some very important information. Whilst pH papers are adequate for most measurements they do require an accurate estimate of colour change to be made by the user, ideally in daylight. An electric pH meter is the most suitable way of obtaining accurate pH measurements. In the graphs of pH the following parameters apply.

1. The developer pH is assumed to be a norm of 10.00 in the machine tank and the replenisher pH is 10.3.

2. The fixer pH is assumed to be 4.4 in the machine and replenisher tanks.

3. It is assumed that daily measurements are made.

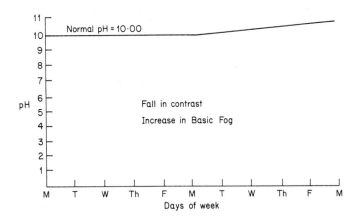

Fig. 6.3 Developer grossly over-replenished.

Figure 6.3 illustrates what would happen when there is gross over-replenishment of developer over a period of days. There is a gradual increase of pH, due to the fact that the replenisher has a higher pH than the machine tank developer. Gradually, the basic fog will begin to rise, as the machine tank developer is now becoming unselective due to its increased activity. The rise in basic fog will cause a fall in average gradient as the slope of the curve will be altered.

Gross under-replenishment causes the pH to drop (Fig. 6.4). This produces a fall in average gradient, now due to the fact that the developer is not as active (low pH), so maximum densities are not reached on the film. The change in the slope of the curve also gives an apparent decrease in the film's speed.

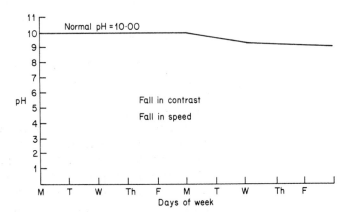

Fig. 6.4 Developer grossly under-replenished.

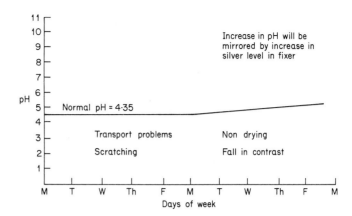

Fig. 6.5 Fixer grossly under-replenished.

When fixer pH is measured with gross over-replenishment, there is no discernible effect. However, with gross under-replenishment (Fig. 6.5), many problems can be caused. The pH now increases, due to carryover of the developer which cannot be buffered by an under-replenished fixer. The higher the pH, the worse the problems become, but they are typically:

1. Transport problems due to the film swelling excessively in the wash water because of inadequate hardening.
2. Scratches due to a very soft non-hardened emulsion.
3. Non-drying because of excess water in the emulsion.
4. At the very worst, a fall in average gradient due to a milky white overall fog shown on the film due to non-fixation.

The following has been mentioned before, but no apologies are included for mentioning it again. Many people assume that, because results do not vary, the quality assurance system is not working. The whole point of quality assurance is that the measurements *should* always be the same. The results *should* always be negative. The aim of these measurements is to spot a trend, and if the trend occurs, to stop it.

Specific gravity

The measurement of specific gravity can be very useful if there are any doubts about too much, or too little, water being added to a mix. Again, manufacturers will supply details of the specific gravity of their chemicals.

If the measured specific gravity is too low, then the solutions are too dilute, i.e. somehow too much water has been added. If the specific gravity is too high, not enough water has been added.

Be aware of one major trap if specific gravity has to be measured. All hydrometers are calibrated according to temperature. If the hydrometer is calibrated at 20°C then the liquid must be brought to that temperature before making the measurement.

More information on the behaviour of developer and fixer is contained in Chapter 3, Photochemistry.

Fixer silver level

The most accurate way of checking that the fixer is being replenished correctly is to measure the silver content of the fixer. This can be done very quickly and easily using silver estimating papers.

These are dipped into the fixer tank, and the colour change is compared to a colour chart supplied with the papers. For a 90 s processor the level should be about 6–7 g of silver per litre of fixer. Some simple sums will indicate that a typical processor will contain about 120–140 g of silver, which is all recoverable. The user should be aware that these papers are called silver *estimating* papers and only provide a guide to the silver content. The papers should be renewed regularly; about once a year is sufficient.

Sensitometric checks

The automatic processor should process a film correctly. This seems a trite statement, but the only way to find whether this is happening is to do some form of sensitometric check and compare the results with the manufacturer's published figures.

The performance of the film in the automatic processor should be maximised. This can be done fairly simply, although the tests themselves are very time-consuming.

Fog, speed, average gradient

The automatic processor should be started from cold and then a series of measurements are made at 1°C intervals. The range of temperature measurements will depend on the type of chemistry in use, i.e. whether it is 'cold' or 'hot' developer.

Sensitometric strips are then fed through the machine at the 1° intervals. Plots are then made of:

1. Basic fog versus temperature.
2. Speed versus temperature.
3. Average gradient versus temperature.

It can be considered that the chemistry and processor performance will be maximised when the fog is at an acceptable level, i.e. below D0.22, and the speed is as high as possible when compared to the average gradient. It should be noted that the average gradient will climb gradually and then begin to fall as the basic fog increases. The optimum temperature will be about 1 °C below the maximum average gradient achieved, with acceptable fog level (Fig. 6.6)

In Chapter 2, Sensitometry, the advantages and disadvantages of different methods of producing a characteristic curve are considered.

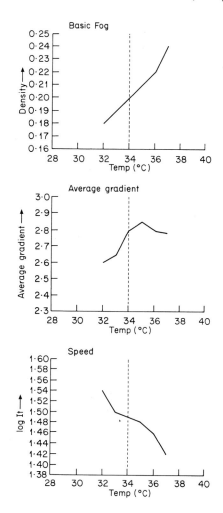

Fig. 6.6 Plots of basic fog, average gradient and speed against temperature.

One of these methods should be chosen to produce sensitometric strips for testing.

Once the optimum settings are obtained, the ongoing tests can be done very simply. It is not necessary to do complete 21 step curves; a three patch system can be adopted for routine tests.

Perhaps the most useful tool now required is a densitometer, although some qualitative estimates can be made.

For the simplest method of sensitometry which is still accurate, three areas are required for measurement. These are detailed in Figure 6.7.

These three areas can be considered as the following:

1. *Basic fog.* As measured at patch A.
2. *Speed index.* Value of density at patch B.
3. *Contrast index.* Value of density at patch C.

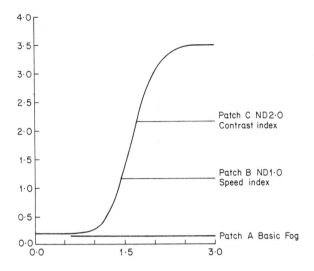

Fig. 6.7 Three patch system: basic fog, speed index and contrast index.

Note that points 2 and 3 are *indices* and only represent a point on the curve and not an absolute value for speed and contrast.

Once the curve is produced on a day-to-day basis, these same three values are always measured and recorded. It is now that trends may be observed (Fig. 6.8).

If the speed index goes up or down, it means that the apparent

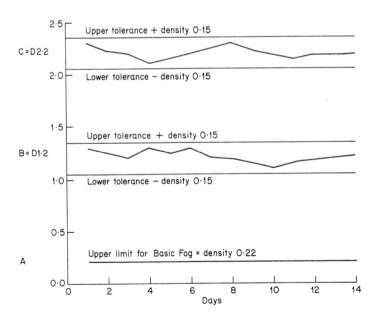

Fig. 6.8 The start at C is the measured density of patch C; the start at B is the measured density at patch B; the value of A is the measured value of basic fog. The maximum and minimum values around these values are shown. The starting density values of all three patches will vary, according to types and batches of films used.

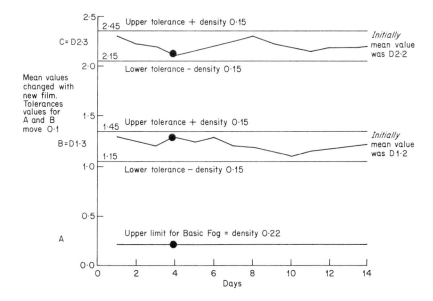

Fig. 6.9 ● represents the change at day 4 to a new batch of film. The old values at A, B, and C are changed to the new values on the new film. The only proviso is that an old and new film should be processed together (see text).

speed of the film has done the same. If the contrast index goes up or down, so has the average gradient on the film.

Ideally, if the curves are being produced on film from the department, a specific box should be designated for such tests. When the changeover to a new box of film occurs, a film from the old box and the new box should be exposed together. This precaution is necessary, as there might be a difference in sensitivity between different emulsions. Any difference in densities should be noted and the resultant differences recorded. This slight change is important to note. If, for example, the starting density at B was D1.2, as in the graph, and at changeover the value was D1.3, then this is the *new starting point* for B (see Fig. 6.9). Exactly the same rules would apply to Patches C and A.

Agfa-Gevaert Ltd make a pre-exposed sensitometric film for just such a purpose. The film incorporates a 21 step (root 2) step wedge and a three patch system. If using a film such as this, exactly the same precautions apply. If a different box of film is used then the results have to be amended.

Figure 6.10 shows the changes that can occur using this method. It is important to realise that it is a trend that is being looked for, not a massive sensational swing.

Using a densitometer, the results can easily be achieved and certain defined limits can be made for allowable swings. Variations of D0.15, either up or down, will mean a move which is out of tolerance. Most radiographers find a basic fog much greater than 0.22 unacceptable. The variations allowable for both speed and contrast indices above and below the starting value are D0.15 (Fig. 6.10).

Trends exhibited		Possible causes of trends
/	Basic Fog	Excess developer in fixer
/	Speed index	Faulty developer preparation
\	Contrast index	Insufficient mixing
/	Basic Fog	Insufficient starter added to developer
\	Speed index	Over-replenishment of developer
\	Contrast index	Completely oxidised developer
—	Basic Fog	Developer over-diluted
\	Speed index	Under-replenishment of developer
\	Contrast index	
/	Basic Fog	Developer temperature too high
/	Speed index	Faulty preparation of developer
/	Contrast index	Insufficient mixing
\	Basic Fog	Developer temperature too low
\	Speed index	Exhausted or under-replenished developer
\	Contrast index	Faulty developer preparation
/	Basic Fog	Fixer in developer
—	Speed index	Under-replenished fixer
\	Contrast index	

Fig. 6.10 Trends of basic fog, speed index and contrast index, and some possible causes of those trends.

Without a densitometer, some guesswork has to be done, but fairly accurate results can still be obtained. An increase or decrease in basic fog can be estimated, as can the speed index. Unfortunately, because the contrast index is above density 2, it is impossible to make a reliable estimate of increase or decrease in density. Even so, 70% of potential problems can be spotted using purely visual qualitative estimates.

IMAGE RECEPTORS

This is perhaps the most important area of quality assurance. It covers three main topics; film, intensifying screens and the cassette.

X-ray film

Although the performance of the film can be monitored by the consumer, there is very little that can be done about the quality of the film. All film manufacturers have stringent quality assurance procedures which involve detailed batch sampling and close monitoring of production and packing, etc. It would be incorrect to say that film faults are not produced in the manufacturing process, but they are few and far between.

There are, however, two areas where the consumer can take care of the quality of the film *after* it has reached the X-ray department.

Stock control

A great deal has been written about stock control of film. There are some simple, basic rules to follow.

All film has a 'shelf life'. This simply means that the film has a useful life during which it can be expected that it will maintain its manufactured quality. After this period, usually indicated by an expiry date on the box, the quality of the film begins to deteriorate and the overall basic fog will begin to increase. It is therefore essential to make absolutely sure that X-ray film is used in strict rotation.

This can be done very simply:

1. When films are received into the department they should be date stamped, or identified in some way so that the date of entry into the department is known.

2. They should then be used in strict rotation, i.e. First In are First Out, or Last In Last Out. Two useful mnemonics are FIFO and LILO. If this practice is followed, there should be no possibility of finding three-year-old boxes of film on the shelf.

Storage conditions

There are a number of points which are worth remembering when storing film. Further details are available under 'basic fog' in Chapter 2, Sensitometry.

1. Always store film vertically, not horizontally. If they are stored horizontally, it is almost certain that pressure marks will be produced on the films at the bottom of the pile.

2. Try to maintain an even temperature in the storage area. An ideal way to check the temperature swings is to use a maximum–minimum thermometer. The swing should be relatively low, perhaps of the order of 1–2°C. The ideal temperature would be 10°C if the films are to be stored for a period greater than three months. Of course film can be stored in temperatures much lower than this with no detrimental effect. Significantly higher temperatures will only hasten the aging process.

3. Make sure that the storage area is not damp. For example, hot water pipes passing through a storage room can cause condensation. A value of about 50% relative humidity should be aimed for.

4. Avoid storing photographic chemicals in the same area as the film. Spillage of the chemicals can obviously cause problems. There

is an additional hazard as well: a number of developers contain minute quantities of a radioactive isotope of potassium. If films have to be in the same storage area as chemicals, keep the film at least 2 m away from the developer.

5. Certain fumes are known to fog films, carbon monoxide (car exhausts), formalin and formaldehyde (typical laboratory chemicals) and certain types of paint, to name but a few.

6. Mercury vapour will also fog film. *Never* use a mercury thermometer in a photographic darkroom. If a mercury thermometer is broken inside an automatic processor, the problems are enormous. Mercury 'kills' developer and also forms an amalgam with stainless steel. The processor will require a great deal of cleaning, possibly even a replacement tank.

7. Finally, consider carefully the building materials used in the construction of a film storage area. Avoid materials like breeze block if possible, as some constituents may well be minutely radioactive from relics of the old H-bomb tests in the atmosphere. As a point of interest, it would be unwise to consider building with Aberdonian granite. Aberdeen has the dubious honour of having the highest background radiation in the United Kingdom! The maximum recommended background radiation level is 7 $\mu r/h$, for a prolonged storage period.

After having checked stock rotation and storage, it is time to move on to the next major area for investigation.

INTENSIFYING SCREENS AND CASSETTES

Screens and cassettes are interlinked in such a way that it is foolhardy to divide the testing procedures for each of them. The quality assurance procedures for both are therefore described together. Many radiographers find it strange, when repeating a 'thin' film, that after giving a reasonable increase in exposure, the new film is grossly overexposed. The X-ray set is blamed, then the processor, even the film itself, but very rarely is the intensifying screen suspected. It is quite possible that the repeat film was done on a different cassette, with screens theoretically the same but in fact with a different age. It is in cases like this that quality assurance comes into its own.

Numbering

It is very important to number cassettes, both inside and out. This makes identification of a faulty screen, for example, very easy. Various types of numbers exist commercially to do just this job.

Routine cleaning

In any photographic procedure cleanliness really is next to godliness, and cleaning of screens is no exception. However, in a case as simple as this, mistakes can still occur. It is worthwhile looking at some 'do's' and 'don'ts' of screen cleaning.

1. *Always* clean screens with the cleaning solution recommended by the manufacturer of the screens. Some screen cleaning solutions from manufacturer A will damage screens made by manufacturer B.

2. *Never* use soap and water. Even after apparently thorough washing some soap can be left on the supercoat. Eventually this can discolour, and will then act as a filter for the light emitted by the screen. In addition, accumulated layers of the soap can become radio-absorptive. These two factors, emission down and X-ray reduction, can produce a much slower screen system. Cleaning with water may lead to other problems when dealing with rare earth screens (see p. 200). *All* rare earths are hygroscopic. If the screen supercoat is damaged, water may be absorbed by the phosphor, causing discolouration of the supercoat and therefore a reduction of the light emission and subsequent loss of speed.

3. Normal everyday dust and dirt should be removed with a soft brush, such as a camera lens cleaning brush. For more ingrained dirt, use a lint-free cloth and screen cleaner, rubbing in a circular motion without undue pressure. If a great deal of effort is required to remove the dirt from the screens, it is almost certain that the dirt is already too far embedded into the supercoat of the screen.

4. Once the screens have been cleaned, leave the cassettes partially open so the screens can dry naturally.

The act of using a screen cleaner has two specific benefits. The cleaner obviously cleans the screens, but most screen cleaners contain an anti-static element. A considerable amount of static can be generated simply by the act of inserting and extracting the film from the cassette. Static in turn will attract dirt and dust.

Drying the screens is essential, as some components of screen cleaners, when in contact with film, can fog the emulsion if the screen is still wet.

Inspection

Stage one

After the screens have been cleaned thoroughly, they have to be inspected in white light. If the screens are examined by reflected light, any bad surface marks and scratches will usually show up quite readily. Any screens with marks in the central area should be put to one side for further tests.

Stage two

There is another visual inspection that can be carried out on all cassettes. All X-ray screen phosphors operate by converting short wave energy into long wave, usually visible, energy. If a short wave source can be found that will excite the phosphors, they will fluoresce. An X-ray tube performs this service admirably, but is extremely impractical for prolonged testing. Fortunately, ultraviolet light, with a wavelength of about 250 nm, will also excite X-ray phosphors. The test procedure is as follows.

The cassettes are laid out flat on a darkroom bench and then all the lights in the darkroom are switched off. The intensifying screens are then scanned, using the ultraviolet light source. As the UV light actually makes the phosphor fluoresce, any defect, such as fingermarks or areas of diminished light output, will be clearly seen.

Warning Prolonged exposure to ultraviolet light can cause conjunctivitis. UV light of 250 nm is readily absorbed by the glass in a pair of spectacles and should be safe for most users, but care must be taken.

If any faults are demonstrated on this test, particularly if they lie in the central area of the screens, the screens are moved on to the next test procedure.

Stage three

It is possible that screens were rejected in the first stage; these are collected with the rejected cassettes from the second stage and are now examined using X-radiation. This part of the test increases quite dramatically the cost of a quality assurance programme. It should only be used as a 'last resort' to confirm that the marks demonstrated visually are confirmed by X-radiation. It is possible that the cassettes could be passed on to the screen contact test, but sometimes small artefacts are not visible on a screen contact test. Essentially this test should be used with considered judgement.

These cassettes are loaded with film and placed under the X-ray tube. In this instance, distance is not so critical and the tube can be raised to the limits of its vertical travel to provide the largest area coverage possible. A 'flash exposure' is then given, about 10 mAs and 55 kV for 'universal'-type screens and the films are then processed.

When the films are viewed after processing, any artefacts will be clearly seen as the films will have a density of somewhere around 1.0. It is then that the difficult decision about which cassettes to reject must be made. Obviously any artefact which resembles phleboliths or calculi must be immediately suspected and rejected. The rest of the marks remain with the conscience of the user.

Screen contact

In the inspection stage, it is quite possible that a number of cassettes have been rejected on the basis of unacceptable marks on the screens. The remaining cassettes must now be tested for screen contact. Fortunately, the screen contact test also has an inbuilt test for the speed of the screens.

Reproducibility

Before commencing the test there is one precaution which must be observed. As the screen contact test can also be used as a speed test it is imperative that the X-ray set used for the tests is working correctly. This can be checked by making a number of exposures on one cassette, carefully masking the film for each exposure. When measured with a densitometer each exposure should have produced the same density. A deviation in density of about 5% is acceptable. If the deviations are greater than this, the set is not giving reproducible exposures and another set must be found and the tests done again.

To confirm reproducibility during the tests, one cassette, ideally of a small format, should be chosen as a control cassette. This cassette, loaded with film, should be placed in the centre of every group of cassettes which is exposed during the tests. The same density should be recorded on this control cassette after every exposure.

Problems also occur with the anode heel effect. As a precaution, a record should be kept of the position of every cassette during the tests. If density variations are found from 'north' to 'south', but are similar in all test exposures, the variations can be assumed to be caused by a similar effect.

METHOD OF TEST FOR CONTACT BETWEEN THE X-RAY FILM AND THE INTENSIFYING SCREENS

B1. Test object
The test object shall be a sheet of zinc, 0.036 in (20 SWG; 0.91 mm) thick, continuously perforated with $\frac{3}{32}$ in (2.4 mm) diameter holes at a pitch of 7 per inch. To facilitate the measurement of the density of the film exposed during the test, the test object shall have a clear area, not less than $\frac{1}{2}$ in (13 mm) diameter, near to its centre. The test object shall be of such a size as entirely to cover the effective area of the cassette.

B2. Method of test
The cassette shall contain two salt intensifying screens and be loaded with screen-type X-ray film.

The test object shall be laid flat and in contact with the top of the cassette, which shall then be exposed at a focus-film distance of 1.5 m (59 in) using an X-ray tube with a focal spot between 1.0 and 1.5 mm, the tube focus being centred over the cassette. The operating voltage shall be 50 kV, the total filtration shall not be more than 2 mm A1 equivalent, and the exposure time shall be such as to produce a maximum diffuse transmission density of from 2.0 to 3.0 on full standard development.

B3. Criteria of contact
The developed film shall be viewed against a film illuminator of the fluorescent tube type from a distance of not less than 12 ft, or through a reducing lens which gives an image equivalent to that of a film viewed at a distance of 12 ft.

If the contact is uniform the appearance of the film when viewed under these conditions will be that of having an overall uniform density. Areas which appear dark will indicate the areas where there has been lack of contact in the cassette between the film and the intensifying screen.

Fig. 6.11 British Standard (BS 4304:1968, part B) Test for screen contact. **NB** BS 4304 1968 has since been withdrawn and no alternative has replaced it.

British standard

The test for screen contact is part of a British Standard, BS 4304/1968, Appendix parts A and B. Part B covers screen contact; part A, light leakage. The British Standard is outlined in Figure 6.11.

When conducting the test it is wise to expose a number of cassettes at the same time, but they must always be of the same speed class. Increasing the numbers saves time and also reduces any chance of errors due to variations in output of the X-ray set. The control cassette will act as confirmation of reproducibility.

The important points to note in this test are:

1. The construction of the perforated metal (Fig. 6.11).
2. The kV used. Greater than 55 kV will cause significant over-penetration of the zinc.
3. The density which must be achieved. This is used for the speed measurements as well.
4. The viewing distance. It is impossible to see the defects at close range.
5. Make sure that screens *of the same speed class* are exposed together, along with the control cassette.

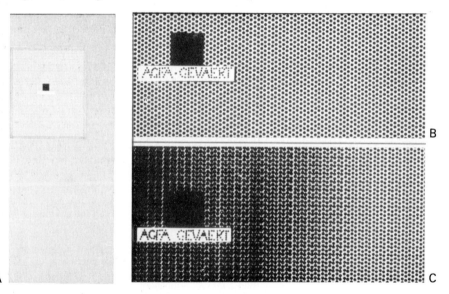

Fig. 6.12 Results from a radiographic test grid (A) 17″ × 14″ test grid (B) radiograph produced in a cassette with good screen contact (C) radiograph produced by a cassette with poor screen contact.

When the films are viewed it will be readily apparent which cassettes have a loss of screen contact. A cassette with good screen contact produces films with an overall even density. Poor contact shows up as patches of high density areas (Fig. 6.12).

Obviously cassettes that show poor screen contact in the central area should be rejected. Loss of contact in other areas should be evaluated by the individuals concerned.

Speed tests

The British Standard asks for a density of greater than 2.0 to be produced in the central area of the grid. This density measurement also permits a measurement of the relative speed of the screens.

After the films of the contact test have been reviewed, the density of the central cut out is measured and all the values recorded. The average is then taken of the highest density values recorded within every speed class. Cassettes which have recorded significantly less than this average density should be rejected on grounds of unacceptable speed loss.

There are two main objections to this test which are worth noting.

1. Exposing at different positions in the X-ray beam can cause variations in exposure.

The only way to overcome this would be to expose a single cassette at a time, on a rotating turntable, so that the cassette was exposed north, south, east and west to the X-ray beam.

This is, to say the least, very time-consuming, costly and tedious, but it does represent the most accurate way of testing.

One way to reduce this work would be to take the precaution outlined earlier, whereby a note is kept of the position of every cassette in the X-ray beam. Noticeable errors, e.g. anode heel effect, will show up as consistent errors by virtue of position.

2. The 'decision point' for rejection on grounds of speed.

Perhaps the safest decision to be made is to take an average of two speed classes, e.g class 100 (universal) and class 200 (special). If the densities recorded on any class 200 approach class 100 densities, then the cassette can safely be rejected in terms of speed achievement and re-allocated to another room.

Light leakage

The description of this test in the British Standard is clear. The chances of light leakage occurring in modern cassettes is very slim. Light leakage will be well demonstrated without recourse to this test. The necessity of being cost-effective precludes the use of this test as a routine.

It can now be assumed that all the cassettes have been tested and those which do not conform have been rejected.

Cost-effectiveness

It was asserted at the beginning of the chapter that quality assurance should not cost more to perform than it saves. The above series of tests are, to say the least, expensive, as full size film is used for every test. Quality assurance must be cost-effective. This can be achieved in a number of ways.

For example, contact testing should only be undertaken if loss of screen contact is suspected. For routine speed checks, a small size film could be used in the centre of the cassette. This can provide a very accurate method of checking speed, but obviously will not give any guidance in detecting artefacts, etc. However, the UV light will help with this.

When it comes to outright rejection of cassettes it might be worth considering putting all cassettes of the same *measured* speed in the same X-ray room. Many screens can reduce in speed considerably over a period of time. There is no objection at all to matching measured speeds of cassettes together in the same room, as long as the cassettes and screens have passed all other tests. For example, some class 200 screens may actually achieve only class 100 speeds. These, if all other tests are passed, are now used in the room with other *actual* class 100 screens.

The cost of staff to run the quality assurance programme is more difficult to quantify. It is safe to say that a programme will require minutes per day of staff time, rather than hours. Nonetheless, even these figures will add up to a noticeable time in a year. The benefits of such a programme must be weighed carefully.

The decision of which cassettes to reject is always a problem, due to the cost of any replacement. Low speed screens can be used in the way outlined above; artefacts and contact are much more of a problem. It should of course be noted that rejections due to artefacts and screen contact are the personal decision of the department head.

THE VIEWING SYSTEM

The remaining part of the chain to check is the viewing boxes themselves. These are still perhaps the most ignored piece of equipment in the department, and yet one of the most important.

Cleaning

First and foremost the viewing boxes must be clean. This, of course, means both outside and inside the box. An amazing amount of dirt can gather in the inside of a viewing box, which in turn can reduce the light output. There are many varieties of anti-static polish available for cleaning viewing box screens.

Colour temperature

Most X-ray films used in the department have a blue base. This base, amongst other things, produces a much more aesthetically pleasing film. However, a blue base, combined with a yellowish viewing box light, can produce a film which looks very unpleasant and dirty.

It is most important, therefore, to use fluorescent tubes with a wavelength of about 6500 K. This colour temperature is found in tubes with brand names such as 'Northern Light' or 'Tropical Daylight', both of which produce bright, 'blue/white' light. Colour temperature meters are available, but at a significant cost. The eye, however, can be used as an extremely good judge of the colour temperatures required.

If at any time tubes have to be changed due to discolouration or failure, it is best to change all the tubes in that particular viewing box. In addition, the ideal would be to have all the fluorescent tubes throughout the department exactly the same.

Balance of light

The final (and very useful) test, which can improve viewing conditions considerably, is to balance the ratio of room light to viewing box light.

An ANSI specification makes the following recommendations:

A standard photographic light meter, without a diffuser attached, is set at 100 ISO (21 DIN). The meter is then held one foot away from the viewing box, with the photo cell pointing towards the viewing box.

A *minimum* value of 13 EV should be recorded on the meter. This corresponds to about 5500 lux.

The meter is then reversed, with the photo cell pointing away from the viewing box and towards the normal room lighting used for viewing.

In this position the light meter should record a *maximum* of 8 EV. This figure corresponds to 86 lux.

It should be stressed that these are not extremely stringent criteria. If these can be improved upon, a significant gain will be made in the quality of viewing. Additionally, films can be read much more easily (see Ch. 7, Image quality).

Interestingly the output of the viewing box can be measured in foot candles using the same meter. In this case the meter should be set at 64 ISO; the shutter speed is then read for an aperture of f 8.

If, for example, the shutter speed is 1/500 of a second, then the output of the viewing box is 500 foot candles; 1/400 th, 400 foot candles; 1/300 th, 300 foot candles, etc.

An average viewing box should produce readings similar to the specifications quoted. An output 15–20% lower than this is insufficient. It is also important to note that this output should be recorded fairly evenly over the surface of the viewing area.

CONCLUSIONS

It is realised that the ideal and the practical can differ considerably, particularly when the expense of such an exercise is considered.

Nevertheless, quality assurance is becoming a very important factor in the modern X-ray department.

With the advent of legal Ionising Regulations (1985) as opposed to a voluntary code of practice, coupled with the current EEC directive, the onus is more and more on department heads to prove that equipment is working optimally and correctly.

Quality assurance can be looked upon as another tool in the armoury of an X-ray department. It is a means of assuring all interested parties that the equipment within the department is working at optimum efficiency. If records are kept correctly, they will demonstrate the performance of all the equipment used in the department. This certainly enables fault finding to be conducted much more quickly. If a manufacturer has to be contacted because of a fault, a detailed report can be given of the behaviour of the equipment prior to the breakdown. The statistics derived from any analysis within the department can be utilised in many ways, the scope being solely determined by the imagination of the user.

Last but not least, quality assurance enables a department to produce high quality radiographs at the minimum dose to the patient and radiographer, at a minimum cost to the department.

REFERENCES

Hospital Physicists Association 1977 Quality assurance measurements in diagnostic radiology. Conference Report Series 29.
Harris D St Hellier Hospital, Carshalton, Surrey. Personal communication.

7

Image quality

Introduction

At the end of the day, the patient is the reason for the technology of imaging. The radiologist or clinician requires the highest quality images available to enable the most accurate diagnosis and treatment. It is the radiographer's job to produce that image.

To identify a high quality image is not easy. In the following pages an attempt has been made to lead the reader through the complex subject of assessing image quality. Frequent reference will be made to other topics more fully covered by other chapters. Hopefully this, plus some new information, will help 'tie the loose ends together'.

SIGNAL TO NOISE RATIO

Image quality may be defined as the signal to noise ratio:

$$\text{Image quality} = \frac{\text{signal}}{\text{noise}}$$

The signal is the information required from the imaging system, e.g. the radiograph, whilst the noise is anything that may detract from that signal.

The signal can be defined as the minimum size of object that must be visible, whilst the noise, in the conventional film/screen system, could be defined as the graininess of the image. The formula may be used to assess image quality in any system, providing the signal and noise can be measured. This is possible with very sophisticated equipment.

To put this formula in simple terms, it means that if the signal level is very high the object will be clearly seen, but if the signal level is similar to the noise level, the object will be very difficult to see, as it will be partially obliterated by the noise. A simple analogy is the television system. With the old 405 line transmitters, scattered over quite wide distances, there was very often 'snow' visible on the TV picture, i.e. a low signal:noise ratio. With the improved 625 line transmitters, usually covering a small area, the picture is considerably improved. In other words, the signal:noise ratio has been increased. The remainder of this chapter is concerned with assessing the photographic quality of a conventional film/screen image.

However, there is a problem which raises its head in radiographic imaging. It would be very tempting to call it the 'eternal compromise'.

Looking at Figure 7.1, the compromise becomes very clear. If the sharpness of the system is increased the visually disturbing noise will also increase, as now the system is resolving the noise better as well as giving a sharper signal. If the contrast is increased the signal will appear to be clearer, but so will the noise. To try to compensate for all the factors is impossible. It has to be a compromise.

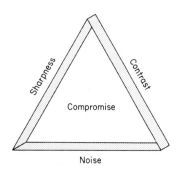

Fig. 7.1 Image quality is a compromise between sharpness, contrast and noise.

RESOLUTION AND MTF

There is one basic question that can be asked: *'How sharp does a radiograph have to be?'* The question can be supplemented by: *'How is sharpness measured?'*

Normally sharpness, usually referred to as resolution, is measured using a line pair (lp) phantom. The line pair phantom is made up of strips of lead separated by an air gap equal to the width of the preceding lead strip. Starting at low frequencies (perhaps 1 line pair per millimetre, or lp mm^{-1}), the phantom then progressively decreases the width of the lead strip and the following air gap until high frequencies, perhaps as high as 10 or 14 lp mm^{-1}, are reached (Fig. 7.2).

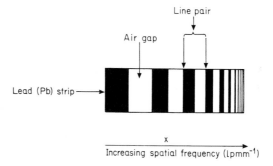

Fig. 7.2 Example of one type of line pair phantom.

Resolution

Resolution can be defined as the size of the smallest object or distance between two objects that must exist before the imaging system will record that object or objects as separate entities. It gives no indication of how the system will record objects of larger dimensions or whether they will be visible to an observer. Usually measured in line pairs per millimetre (lp mm^{-1}), resolution has a limited value in assessing system performance. Ensure that no confusion exists between the words 'resolution' and 'definition'. Definition is a subjective impression of the details that can be seen in the radiograph and is difficult to quantify.

Modulation Transfer Function (MTF)

This allows assessment of system performance at different spatial frequencies (i.e 'object sizes'). In a perfect world it would be expected that the differences in density of the line pair phantom would be recorded in exactly the same way as the original phantom, with the sharp edges clearly delineated, as illustrated in Figure 7.3.

Because of transition density within the film, distinct transition

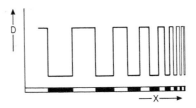

Fig. 7.3 Reading from an image of a perfectly transferred line pair phantom (100% transfer at all frequencies).

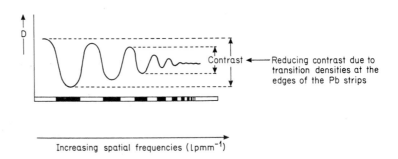

Fig. 7.4 Example of an actual density profile obtained from a line pair phantom showing decreasing information transfer at higher lp mm^{-1}, due to transition densities.

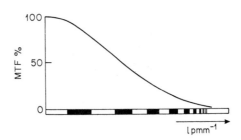

Fig. 7.5 Example of MTF curve, showing loss of information transfer at high spatial frequencies, e.g. at high 1p mm^{-1}.

edges are formed which produce a density reading similar to the one in Figure 7.4 when scanned with a microdensitometer.

It can be seen that at low frequencies the transfer of the signal through the system is quite good. As the frequencies get higher the contrast begins to drop rapidly and the pairs of lines become impossible to see.

If a number of calculations are done, figures can be obtained for the percentage of accuracy of the transfer of the signal through the system. In this way the modulation, or altering, of the signal through the system has been measured. In other words, the Modulation Transfer Function (MTF) for the system has been obtained (Fig. 7.5).

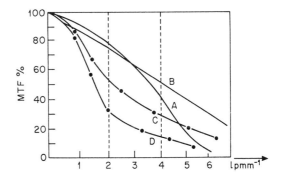

Fig. 7.6 Example of four different MTFs.

That answers the question of how sharpness is measured. It is only fair to mention that many authorities do not consider this to be a perfect way, but it suffices for many circumstances.

The *degree* of sharpness required, however, raises many questions.

Illustrated in Figure 7.6 are four different films, each with markedly different MTF characteristics. It would appear at first glance that film A is the one that should be chosen for work in a general radiographic department, as this transfers most information at low and high frequencies.

EFFECT OF SCREENS

Now is the time to draw on more imaging technology. Consider Figure 7.7.

It is generally accepted that in a *general* radiograpic department, the maximum resolution required is about 2 lp mm^{-1}. For *mammography*, for example, the demands are greater, and perhaps 4 lp mm^{-1} are required. The minimum size of object it is required to see has

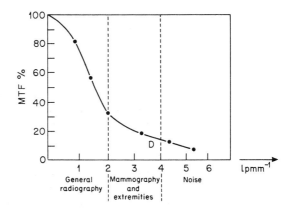

Fig. 7.7 Suggested limiting resolutions shown on an MTF curve (curve D from Fig. 7.6).

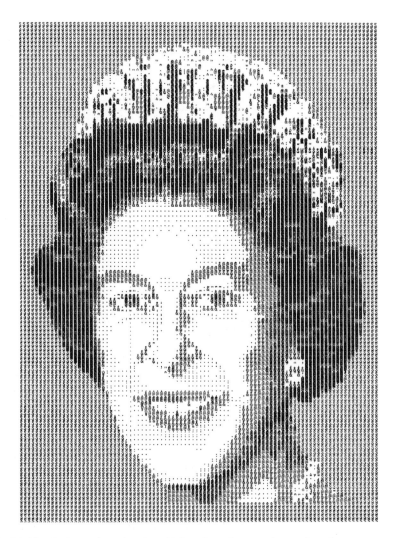

Fig. 7.8 The Queen's face showing 'high noise'. See text for explanation.

now been defined (i.e. the signal). Therefore, everything smaller than this size is information that is not required and is considered noise (Fig. 7.7).

Many years ago it was suggested that if a sheet of acetate was inserted between the film and screen, it would be enough to 'defocus' the system and perhaps reduce the noise in the image.

An idea of this effect can be obtained using Figure 7.8. In the illustration of the Queen, which is made up of letters and symbols, there is a large amount of noise. If the figure is covered with tracing paper the image, although 'defocussed', takes on the appearance of a continuous tone print. In other words, the noise on the signal has been reduced.

Of course, it would be correct to question deliberate unsharpness created in this way, and this poses a somewhat controversial question

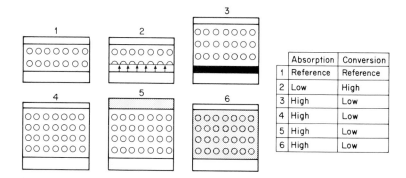

	Absorption	Conversion
1	Reference	Reference
2	Low	High
3	High	Low
4	High	Low
5	High	Low
6	High	Low

Fig. 7.9 Six different screen constructions, all with the same speed class. Which produces the best image quality?

worthy of some consideration. But first, consider how an intensifying screen achieves its efficiency.

Total % efficiency = absorption % × conversion %

In every case it is better to go for a high absorption of the *image forming quanta* than to rely on conversion to gain speed, as this reduces the noise. Consider Figure 7.9.

All of the screens in Figure 7.9 are class 200 and yet they achieve their total efficiency in many different ways. The best choice for image quality would be screen 6. This would be the sharpest, as it has the lowest quantum mottle (because of its high absorption) and the lowest lateral light scatter, because of the dye tint. Having now established the construction of the screen and its ultimate sharpness, more questions can be raised.

- Should the phosphors be conventional calcium tungstate?
- Should the phosphors be rare earth?
- Should the phosphors emit green, blue or UV light?

The question of which phosphors to use is complex and requires a fairly detailed explanation.

Calcium tungstate is an established phosphor and with modern coating techniques can be a very useful phosphor in a range of intensifying screens.

When rare earth phosphors are considered, a number of points are worth raising.

If the man in the street is asked what benefits have accrued from the NASA space programme his usual answer is 'non-stick saucepans', i.e. Teflon. However, few people realise that rare earth phosphors originated as a direct by-product of the NASA programme.

Buchanan et al, from the Palo Alto Research Laboratories, published a paper in 1972 that pointed out that to improve the performance of the (then) current intensifying screens, a review of conversion and absorption efficiency must be undertaken.

The suggestion of the group was that elements from the lanthanide series could be used in place of calcium tungstate.

The absorption efficiency of the rare earth phosphors is at least 50% better than calcium tungstate. Conversion efficiency is at least 4 times better than calcium tungstate. Thus, the total efficiency of a rare earth system is many times better than calcium tungstate. The advantages of rare earth phosphors have been listed many times, but it does no harm to do so again.

1. They offer decreased radiation exposure to both staff and patients.
2. There is reduced kinetic unsharpness, as shorter exposure times are usually available.
3. There can be reduced geometric unsharpness as longer ffds can be used without an increase in exposure.
4. There will be lower tube loadings.
5. There is the availability to use fine focus more often, again decreasing geometric unsharpness.
6. There is the ability to use grids with a higher grid ratio, thereby producing better quality images.
7. It is possible to produce increased contrast, by reducing the kV instead of the mAs.

Interestingly, in 1977 Taylor, of the National Radiological Protection Board, made a cost/benefit analysis of rare earth screens. On the basis that the use of these screens would reduce the overall exposure by a factor of 2, she suggested that the cost of reducing public exposure by a generally-applied rare earth programme would be £1 per man rad. She went on to say that the current (1977) costs to prevent radioactive detriment in the nuclear industry were approximately £420 per man rad. It would seem that a rare earth screen programme is the most cost effective way for protection against hazardous radiation exposure.

When film/screen combinations are first designed there are a number of image quality parameters to take into account. They are, of course, *contrast, sharpness* and *noise*: the compromise needed between them was mentioned at the beginning of this chapter.

Statements are made about the benefits or otherwise of green or blue/UV-emitting systems, many without scientific foundation. It might be worth taking an unbiased look at the three systems (Table 7.1).

Table 7.1 Factors to be considered when comparing differing screens

	UV/Blue	Ortho	
1. Contrast	?	?	— Film
2. Sharpness	?	?	— Crossover
	?	?	— Phosphor
3. Noise	?	?	— Absorption

1. It is obvious that films can be made to virtually any reasonable sensitometric profile: therefore, in terms of contrast, orthochromatic and monochromatic films can be identical.

2. When sharpness is considered, two factors come into play, crossover and phosphor.

Crossover

Film acts as a natural absorber for UV and blue light. Therefore, crossover in both of these systems is low, for blue less than 50%. In the UV systems it can be as low as 20%, which is negligible.

In orthochromatic systems, crossover is much higher unless the film is specially treated. Crossover can be measured as high as 70%, which leads to a less sharp image.

It can be said that, in terms of sharpness caused by crossover, the UV/blue-emitting systems are better.

Phosphor

Table 7.2 lists the varying characteristics of three rare earth screen systems. The UV-emitting barium fluorochloride screen reaches its efficiency by having absorption and conversion in the correct ratios. Because of the very low crossover associated with UV, this screen is eminently suitable for very fast systems.

Table 7.2 Characteristics of different phosphors

Characteristics	Ortho (Gd_2O_2S)	Blue (LaOBr)	UV (BaFCl)
% Absorption 80 kV	40.5	43.5	39.0
% Conversion	18.0	17.0	16.0
Specific weight	7.4	6.2	4.6
Phosphor thickness (μ)	207	228	347
Efficiency	7.3	7.4	6.2

It can be seen from Table 7.2 that gadolinium oxysulphide gains its efficiency by its higher conversion, relative to lanthanum oxybromide. This would lead to greater unsharpness, as it is higher absorption that always leads to better sharpness and image quality. However, as the specific weight of gadolinium is greater than lanthanum, the coating weight can be less. The gadolinium screen can be made thinner, thus leading to better sharpness. If Table 7.1 is redrawn as Table 7.3, it can be seen that the net result indicates that overall the systems are virtually equal in performance.

There might be a preference for the monochromatic system, as silver halide is naturally sensitive to UV and blue light and therefore does not have to be sensitised. Also, no special darkroom lighting is required.

Table 7.3 Comparison of UV/blue systems with orthochromatic systems

	UV/Blue	Ortho	
1. Contrast	=	=	— Film
2. Sharpness	+	−	— Crossover
	−	+	— Phosphor
3. Noise	+	−	— Absorption
Net result	(+) =	=	

EFFECT OF FILM

Most manufacturers produce both full and half speed film. It is sometimes not clear as to why half speed film is required in a film assortment.

Half speed film really came into being with the emergence of rare earth phosphors. The film was necessary, particularly with the very fast systems, as it markedly reduced quantum mottle. There was also another reason: the image quality improved when this film was used. Takano, Sonada, Sakamoto and Simiya produced a paper which showed that the dominant factor affecting the granularity of a film system is quantum mottle, contributing from 65–80% of the total noise. They also say that the use of a more sensitive screen gives less graininess than using a highly sensitive film, because the lower MTF of the screen cancels out the quantum mottle.

The following examples, although simplistic, may help the reader to understand why the combination of a slow film and a fast screen helps to produce high quality images (see Table 7.4).

In the Agfa-Gevaert range of monochromatic film and blue-emitting screens, Curix RP1 and universal screens are a class 100 system. Let us now assume that 100 X-ray quanta are required to produce a density of 1 on the film (it should be noted that the numbers used in Table 7.4 are examples only, and realistically they should be raised by many powers). In this case (Table 7.4, column one), 20 original information-carrying X-ray quanta have been absorbed, producing 1000 light photons and raising Curix RP1 film to density 1.0.

The next case (Table 7.4, column two) would be a class 200 system,

Table 7.4 Comparison of three film/screen systems

	Class 100	Class 200	Class 100
Number of X-ray quanta	100	50	100
Type of screen	Universal	Special	Special
Percentage absorption	20%	40%	40%
Photons emitted	1000	1000	2000
Film type	Curix RP1	Curix RP1	Curix MR4
Net density	1.0	1.0	1.0

i.e. Agfa-Gevaert special screens plus Curix RP1. This system will require exactly half the exposure of a class 100 system.

Special screens are class 200 and therefore require only half the exposure of the universal screens, hence only 50 X-ray quanta are needed. However, because special screens have an absorption of 40%, 20 quanta are absorbed, exactly the same number as universal screens.

The final example (Table 7.4, column three) reverts to a class 100 system, using special screens and a half speed film, Agfa-Gevaert Curix MR4.

Using Curix MR4 the system becomes half speed, i.e. it returns to a class 100 system and requires 100 X-ray quanta again. Because a special screen is used, 40 information-carrying quanta are absorbed. These absorbed quanta produce 2000 light photons and, because MR4 is a half speed film, raise it to Density 1.

It can be seen that starting with a Class 100 system, only 20 of the information-carrying quanta are absorbed (in other words, over 80 of these quanta are not used).

The easiest way to increase the absorption of the screens would be to substitute a faster screen, which must be able to absorb more quanta, as the usual way to increase screen speed is to increase the coating thickness of the phosphor.

In the class 200 system exactly the same number of quanta are absorbed because, although the number of X-ray quanta is halved, the absorption is doubled.

When a class 100 system is realised using Curix MR4 film and a special screen, 40 of the information-carrying quanta are absorbed, only 60 are lost. This simple fact explains why such high quality/low noise images can be produced using half speed film.

Naturally, the above arguments would hold true for orthochromatic systems as well.

CONTRAST

A radiograph is the product of a transfer of information. During this transfer it is exposed to a number of different influences. Contrast goes a long way to determining the quality of the radiograph. There are four principal 'types' of contrast:

- Subject contrast
- Film contrast
- Radiographic contrast
- Subjective contrast.

Subject contrast

This is caused by differential attenuation and absorption of the X-ray beam as it passes through the patient (i.e. the subject). It is responsible for the differing intensities of the emergent X-ray beam, and

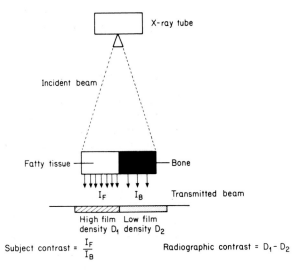

Fig. 7.10 Diagrammatic illustration of subject contrast.

therefore the exposures that eventually reach the film. Consider Figure 7.10. This represents the same thickness of bone and fatty tissue. The bone attenuates more of the beam than the fatty tissue and therefore the emergent intensity in the area below the bone is less than the surrounding fatty tissue. The film receives less exposure and produces a lower photographic density when compared to the fatty tissue areas. In this case the subject contrast can be defined as the ratio of the emergent intensities, i.e.:

$$\text{Subject contrast} = \frac{I_F}{I_B}$$

The factors affecting subject contrast are:

1. Different thicknesses of the same tissue
2. Different densities of the same tissue
3. Different atomic numbers of the tissues
4. Radiation quality (kVp, anode material, etc.)
5. Use of contrast agents.

Different thicknesses

Consider two different thicknesses of the same tissue type. The thicker of the two will attenuate more of the beam and allow less exposure to reach the film. Subject contrast is the ratio of the intensity that has passed through the thin part, compared to the thicker part.

Different densities

Consider the same tissue with the same volume but at a higher density (i.e. higher mass per unit volume). The higher density will attenuate more of the beam. This will reduce the intensity of the emergent beam and thus affect the subject contrast.

Different atomic numbers

The higher the atomic number of a substance, the higher the attenuation of the incident X-ray beam. At the energies used in diagnostic radiography, photoelectric absorption predominates and is the largest contributing factor to subject contrast.

Radiation quality

In this case, radiation quality means the kilovoltage (kV) set for the exposure. For the same subject, increasing the kV decreases the difference in intensities of the emergent beam and therefore decreases the subject contrast. Low kV will produce high subject contrast, but the kV must be high enough to adequately penetrate the area being examined.

Further examining the influence of kV we find that:

1. Changing kV gives a high contrast variation in bone work.
2. The influence of kV is smaller on soft tissue rendition.
3. In the low kV range, 10 kV has more effect on contrast than in the higher kV range.
4. In the middle kV range, 20 kV is needed to give an appreciable change in contrast.

Other factors also determine the radiation quality and therefore the final subject contrast:

- The anode material, e.g. mammography
- Varying voltage ripple components
- Tube filters and supplementary filters
- Scattered radiation.

The anode material, voltage components and tube filtration are determined by the X-ray equipment in use and are beyond the control of the radiographer in a normal situation.

Scattered radiation, however, can be controlled to a certain extent, and deserves a brief mention in its own right. The influence of scatter is mainly felt in two ways:

- Radiation fog, which increases the overall photographic density of the film
- Reduction in the image latitude.

Limiting these effects is of prime importance, if high quality images are to be obtained. In general, the higher the selected kV, the higher the amount of scatter and the higher the radiation fog and reduction in image latitude. However, as previously stated, the kV must be high enough to penetrate the area being examined. Therefore the use of grids, collimators, compression bands, and other methods of reducing the production of scatter, is of singular importance.

Use of contrast agents

These may be positive agents, such as an iodine compound or barium, or negative agents such as carbon dioxide or air. In either case, they are normally used to fill a cavity or space in the body that usually has a low subject contrast when compared to surrounding structures. The agent alters the subject contrast by either increasing the X-ray absorption properties of the structure concerned (e.g. IVP), or decreasing the absorption properties, with the obvious effect on the intensity of the emergent beam. They can also be used in combination, for example double contrast barium meals and enemas.

Film and radiographic contrast

Film contrast

This is defined by the average gradient of the film (see Ch. 2, Sensitometry). It is a measure of the film's ability to amplify the subject contrast (see Fig. 7.11).

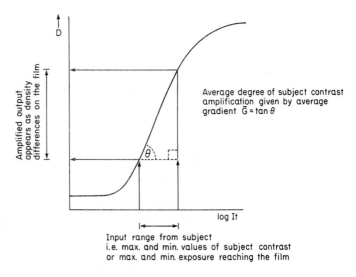

Fig. 7.11 Effect of film contrast on subject contrast.

Radiographic contrast

This is simply the Photographic density difference between two adjacent areas on the film. These differences in density may or may not be observable to the naked eye.

Subjective contrast

This is the last link in the chain of contrast factors; it is the observer's opinion of the contrast that he or she sees on the film. It is a combination of all the other factors listed, plus viewing conditions, the performance of the eye, the observers ability and perhaps their personal opinion. (see Perceptibility, p. 262 and ROC, p. 264).

The eye analyses the structures in the radiograph and will select details. The success rate depends on the different degrees of brightness. This ratio of difference is expressed as:

D detail minus D surroundings

This variable indicates the difference in logarithmic form which suits the physiology of the eye.This measurement is also the measurement of subjective contrast, i.e..

Contrast = D detail − D surroundings

There are other influences on contrast which must be considered:

1. Processing conditions
2. Darkroom lighting
3. Viewing box and viewing conditions.

Finally, the importance of masking the film should not be understressed. Masking improves the range in the higher densities, whilst reflected light and glare can seriously decrease contrast and thereby decrease the speed of perception (further details in Perceptibility, p. 262).

Summary

All the contrast factors exhibited on a radiograph can dictate two important variables:

- Perceptibility
- Speed of perception.

In addition, subject contrast is initially determined by:

- kV selected
- Voltage ripple components
- Anode material
- Filtration
- Scatter
- Contrast agents.

Scatter will be reduced and contrast will be increased by:
- Collimation
- Compression
- Use of grids
- Air gap technique.

Film contrast is influenced externally by:

- Processing conditions
- Darkroom lighting
- Viewing box and viewing conditions.

Finally, subjective contrast can be influenced by the viewing conditions themselves (see Ambient light, p. 260).

GRAININESS

Graininess is the perception of the apparent granular structure of the image (see Ch, 5, Intensifying screens). Three factors could be responsible for the apparent mottled appearance on a radiograph. These are:

1. The relatively coarse structure of the silver halide grains
2. Structure mottle
3. Quantum mottle.

Film grain

It must be remembered that the silver halide grains in the emulsion are of microscopic size. Typically a silver bromide crystal will be of the order of microns in size.

When the latent image is formed, the alteration to the crystal is not visible, even under an electron microscope. It is only developer that can amplify this effect.

Developer + silver bromide = an amplification factor of 10^9

After development, the exposed silver bromide crystal splits and threads of metallic silver merge with the threads of neighbouring crystals, in turn causing visible graininess. The graininess is increased due to the superimposition of the two emulsions. It can also be exacerbated by short development times, requiring high temperatures. In general it can be said that:

The higher the speed of the film, the greater the inherent film grain.

Consider Figure 7.12. Here an arrowhead is illustrated as the object, and represents a macroscopic view of density 1.0. A slow film (a) achieves this density by using 20 image-forming quanta and interacts with the silver halide to produce two developable grains per collision.

Using a film which is twice as fast (b), it must necessarily use only half the number of quanta, by definition (i.e. 10 quanta). The only way that density 1.0 can be reached is by doubling the number of developable grains. Now there are four per quanta collision. Comparing the two arrowheads it is clear that (a) shows the object clearly, whereas in (b) the object is not outlined as well.

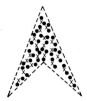

The perfect system images the 'arrowhead' perfectly with no grain. D = 1·0

(a) A 'slow' system absorbs 20 quanta → 40 developed grains → D = 1·0
Note: Some definition of arrowhead is lost

(b) A fast system. Film is now 2x the speed ∴ only 10 quanta must produce 4 developed grains per collision to reach D = 1·0. Even more definition is lost. The image is 'grainy'

x = Quanta collision
• = Developed grain

Fig. 7.12 Diagrammatic illustration of film grain in relation to film speed.

This diagram shows, in simple terms, the effect of film grain. It should be appreciated that this effect would only be visible with significant magnification.

However, if a high speed radiographic film is exposed to *light*, grain is barely visible. It can therefore be assumed that the *largest significant factor* in the production of graininess is quantum Mottle or screen mottle.

Structure mottle

This subject is fully discussed in Chapter 5, Intensifying screens. It is sufficient to state here that structure mottle, particularly with modern screens, is insignificant.

Quantum mottle

It is worth looking at what happens when the film is exposed to two different sources of energy, light only and X-radiation.

Light

The energy of light is relatively low, therefore several light photons are needed to render silver bromide developable. The grain size of the film in this case is the cause of the graininess of the image.

X-radiation

The high energy of X-ray photons enables them to render a complete silver bromide crystal developable. This may require only one collision. Additionally, the production of secondary electrons by the photoelectric effect may expose neighbouring crystals, in turn rendering them developable.

The higher the energy of the radiation, the fewer photons are needed to produce a given density. Decreasing the number of quanta gives a more irregular statistical variation of the location of the quanta. This random distribution of the X-ray flux density gives the image a granular appearance which is known as quantum mottle.

Of course sensitivity also plays a part. A low speed film/screen system needs a higher dose, i.e. the statistical distribution of the X-ray quanta is more even.

A simplified formula to express this can be given as:

Quantum mottle = 1 / square root of exposure

In other words, if the exposure is quadrupled the quantum mottle will be reduced by one half.

Measurement of graininess

Graininess can be measured as density fluctuations in an area that should appear homogeneous. The measurement is made using a scanning microdensitometer (Fig. 7.13)

Figure 7.13 shows the variations in readings which can be obtained with a small or large aperture. There seems to be no standard for the dimensions of the reading aperture, therefore only comparative values are possible. For those interested in formulae:

Graininess = $\theta \times \sqrt{F}$
where θ = variable field compensation actor. F = field size.

Obviously, graininess represents the variable noise in the system and thus is a factor affecting signal to noise ratio.

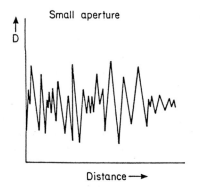
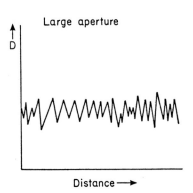

The larger aperture evens out the density variations giving an apparently lower 'graininess'

Fig. 7.13 Density profile for the same area on a film but using a different size aperture in the microdensitometer.

Summary

1. Graininess in a radiograph is chiefly a product of exposure.
2. Graininess impairs perception of small details far more than large details.
3. The contrast of details must be higher on the film if significant graininess is present.
4. The largest constituent of graininess on screen film is quantum mottle.
5. Graininess reduces image quality and perceptibility.

UNSHARPNESS

The causes of unsharpness are sometimes difficult to assess. The purpose of this section is to try to put some values in place of abstract concepts.

Unsharpness on a radiograph is caused by the following four factors:

1. Photographic unsharpness (Up)
2. Movement of the object (Uk)
3. The intensifying screens (Us)
4. The radiation geometry (Ug).

This is traditionally summarised in the following formula:

$$Ut = \sqrt{Uk^2 + Us^2 + Ug^2}$$

although some sources suggest the cube root of the sum of the cube of each factor should be used.

It is best if, when examining a radiograph, the major cause or causes of unsharpness are identified and reduced if possible.

Photographic unsharpness (Up)

In theory, it is quite possible to predict the expected unsharpness. However, several values must be known. For example, with a very small focal spot, large ffd, no screens, an immobile object and non-screen film the predicted result would be a sharp image. But, due to electrons released in the film, and the effects of processing, there will be a transition density at any edge: in other words, unsharpness. Knowing that photographic emulsions are capable of resolving up to 5000 lp mm^{-1}, this effect can be considered to be negligible.

Movement of the object (Uk)

Kinetic unsharpness (Uk) is the result of the object speed (v) in any direction other than perpendicular to the film plane, in mms, multiplied by the exposure time (t) in seconds.

$$Uk = v \times t$$

Strictly speaking, this value should be multiplied by the enlargement ratio, i.e. the *focus film distance* (ffd) divided by the *focus object distance* (fod). The geometric factor involved, e.e. ffd/fod, can be assumed to be about 10%–20%, providing macro techniques are not used.

$$Uk = v \times t \times ffd / fod$$

To take a particular example: with organ movement of about 5 mm and an exposure time of 0.2 s, the predicted unsharpness will be 1 mm. This could only be improved significantly by reducing the exposure time to 0.02 s.

It is likely that if a decision was made actually to reduce the exposure, a faster screen would be chosen. The question is, 'is it worth it?'

Screen unsharpness (Us)

Quoting absolute values for screen unsharpness is difficult, because so many factors are involved. It is well appreciated that screens must reduce the sharpness of the image by the mere fact that light is scattered throughout the phosphor coating.

If we use a fast film/screen system to try and reduce kinetic unsharpness (Uk), then the risk is that the inherent screen unsharpness may be greater than the reduction in Uk and thus no advantage is gained. In addition, if we used high definition screens we might be forced to use longer exposure times, because of the use of lower speed screens. This, in turn, could cause an increase in kinetic unsharpness. In other words, a truly vicious circle!

Geometric unsharpnes (Ug)

This is caused by the fact that the focal spot in the tube is not a point source. Figure 7.14 shows that for a point source, the edges of an object will be recorded as sharp edges on the film. However, for an extended source, each edge of the object receives a ray as if it were two separate points, causing the penumbra effect shown, which produces unsharpness. Likewise, if the fod is reduced, then the unsharpness is increased. To counter this the fod needs to be increased, to reduce Ug, but this will mean increasing the mAs and perhaps the exposure time. This in turn increases Uk. If the *object film disstance* (ofd) is increased Ug is increased, and an increase in exposure will be required which may increase Uk. Alternatively a faster screen may be used, thus increasing Us. The vicious circle has returned!

It is worth considering a practical example of the geometric unsharpness caused by the size of the focal spot and the ffd. To calculate Ug in this instance, we require the ratio of the object film distance to the distance between the focal spot and the object.

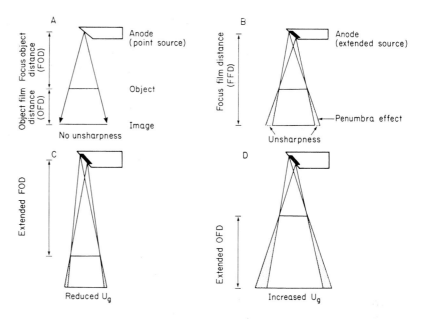

Fig. 7.14 Effect of (A) point source, (B) extended source, (C) focus object distance, and (D) object film distance on geometric unsharpness (Ug).

This means that, the larger the focal spot, the greater the distance between the object and the film, and the closer the focal spot is to the object, the more Ug will increase. If a simple example is taken where:

ffd = 100 cm and fod = 80 cm ∴ ofd = 20 cm

then

Ug : focal spot size = 20 : 80

therefore

Ug = 1 / 4 of the focal spot size.

If we take a typical focal spot size of 1.2 mm, then

Ug = 0.3 mm.

Finally, it is worth remembering that:

To achieve as low a value for unsharpness as possible, a number of compromises must be made.

VIEWING THE IMAGE

Much has been said about quantitative evaluation of the performance of the imaging system, but little has been said about the performance of the observer who uses the image to perform diagnosis.

Performance of the eye

A complete discussion of the physiology of the eye's performance is best found in a suitable textbook, and is not necessary to understand the factors that affect the eye's ability to perceive. The main factors affecting the performance of the eye are:

- Spectral sensitivity
- Visual acuity
- Recognition acuity
- Detection acuity.

Spectral sensitivity

The spectral sensitivity of the human eye is shown in Figure 7.15. However, this sensitivity depends on whether rod or cone vision is predominant and therefore also depends on the degree of illumination. With cone vision in low levels of illumination (e.g. twilight), the peak sensitivity is shifted towards the blue part of the spectrum at 500–560 nm, whereas at high illumination levels (e.g. a sunny day) it is shifted towards the yellow part of the spectrum. Rod vision comes into its own only at very low levels of light intensity, e.g. starlit night. Taken together, this gives the eye a dynamic range in terms of illuminance of about 10 to the power 11.

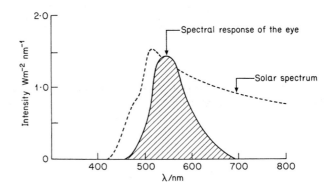

Fig. 7.15 Spectral sensitivity of the human eye.

Visual acuity

Visual acuity can be defined as our ability to perceive spatial detail. It depends on visual angle, luminance and contrast. Figure 7.16 illustrates visual angle (α). In simple terms, it is not the distance of an object that governs whether it will be seen, but the angle that the object subtends to the eye that is important. If the angle exceeds some critical value, the object will be seen. Luminance and contrast are also important factors. If you tried to see the object in Figure 7.16

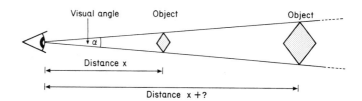

Fig. 7.16 The principle of visual angle. Providing the object at the greater distance subtends the same angle (α) and α is greater than α_{min} then the object will be visualised. It is independent of distance.

at twilight, it would be considerably more difficult to see than in bright sunlight. Likewise if the object were a snowball in a snowfield it would be impossible to see due to the lack of contrast. The equation of visual angle, luminance and contrast poses an almost infinite number of variables that prove impossible to simulate in experiments.

Sources suggest that with a 4 mm diameter pupil and a light source of 560 nm, the eye's resolution at 600 mm distance would be approximately 3 lp mm^{-1}. Obviously this resolution would alter with distance, and with the use of a magnifying glass. To take a 'reductio ad absurdam' situation, if all the cones and rods were evenly distributed across the retina, the eye would have a resolution of 10,000 × 10,000 pixels. Compare this theoretical resolution with a 'high' resolution monitor! It has been suggested that the eye can resolve significantly better than the 3 lp mm^{-1}. Further information, if required, should be sought from specialist publications.

Recognition acuity

This is the ability to recognise a series of standard characters such as letters or specific shapes. Previous experience of the observer can play a significant part in recognition acuity, as practice reduces the time required to 'spot' a particular shape.

Detection acuity

Detection acuity is the ability to detect the presence of an object. Experiments in this area are restricted to detecting simple objects of easily specified structure, as real situations are too complex to model (see Receiver operating characteristics, p. 264). Detection acuity depends on visual angle, contrast and luminance. For example, large objects with low contrast can be seen easily in high levels of illumination. As the object gets smaller and the luminance decreases, the contrast must increase if the object is to remain visible. This leads to the conclusion that in order for an object to be perceived it must exceed some 'perception threshold' that depends on visual angle, contrast and luminance. This threshold must vary from individual to individual, as it depends on the observer's own physiology.

Viewing box

The viewing box must provide an even illumination of the correct colour temperature so that the film being viewed is provided with the best conditions to ensure the highest perceptibility. The light source should be of the Northern or Tropical daylight type, with a colour temperature of 6500 K. This provides an intense blue/white light which is particularly suitable for use with blue base films. Balance of the intensity of the viewing box light to the ambient room light can significantly improve image quality, and the reader is referred to Chapter 6, Quality Assurance for exact values in this area, and to the next section, Ambient light, for problems that may arise.

Ambient light

Over recent years, arguments have been presented saying that viewing conditions can have an adverse effect on diagnosis.

In 1981, Dr Bollen, from the Agfa-Gevaert Research Department, presented a paper in San Francisco on this very problem. The paper offers mathematical and visual proof that there is indeed a very serious effect caused by high ambient light: the following explanation is offered as a simplified version of a complex topic.

Behind the patient, the emergent beam will vary between very high and very low levels of intensity. The logarithmic value of these differences can be called the Total Radiation Intensity Range (TRIR).

The aim of the recording system is to convert the TRIR into a range of densities. The exposure levels are a product of intensity and time.

Dr Bollen suggested that three 'phenomena' can be recognised as interfering with perception:

1. The noise of the human visual system, due to the limited number of light photons in the visual detection system at low light levels.
2. Dazzling of the observer by extraneous light.
3. Visual sensitometric properties caused by reflection on the film surface.

When using a conventional densitometer the light falls specularly on the film.

The 'proper' density is arrived at by measuring the transmitted light (It) and comparing it with the incident light (Io). From this we derive:

'Proper' density = $\log Io / It$

If an observer views a radiograph, the densities recorded by the eye are correct only if:

1. The spectral sensitivity of the human eye is equal to that of the densitometer.
2. The spectral emissions of both light sources are equal.
3. There is *no* ambient light.
4. Only that particular area is visible to the observer.

If, however, ambient light of intensity Ia falls on the radiograph, part of the light will be reflected back into the observer's eye. This is denoted as Ir.

The 'visual density' will be less than the 'proper density' due to reflection of the ambient light at the film's surface. If ambient light levels are zero, Ir is equal to 0 and there is obviously no lowering of visual density. However, the following list of figures will give some guide as to the drop which can occur.

Ir/It = 0.5, density drop = 0.2
Ir/It = 1.0, density drop = 0.3
Ir/It = 5.0, density drop = 0.6
Ir/It = 10.0, density drop = 1.1

In order to test this theoretical approach, Dr Bollen carried out the following experiment. The apparatus used was a Gamma Scientific Spotmeter, which is a telescopic photometer. This was used to measure the visual densities. A Macbeth densitometer was used to measure the proper densities. Both instruments were equipped with an optical filter to match the spectral sensitivity of the eye.

A masked density step wedge was mounted on a viewing box. Using the photometer, light coming from an area of 3 mm^2 was measured at a distance of 1 m. The intensity of the viewing box (Io) was kept at 1700 lux. The ambient light level (Ia) was varied by a dimmer attached to the room lights. Io and Ia were measured by a conventional light photometer.

A number of film types were tested, ranging from grey-dyed gelatine film through conventional black and white films to Medichrome.

It is interesting to note that the black and white films of different types and containing different sizes of silver particles behaved identically. The grey-dyed gelatine film followed the same law as silver bromide films. Some anomalies were found with Medichrome which were mainly due to the differences in colour temperature of the viewing box and the Macbeth light source.

The predicted results, calculated theoretically, coincided almost exactly with the results achieved experimentally. It was discovered that all the films seemed to have a total reflectance of the order of 5% to 7%. In fact, it meant that 'proper' densities could be converted to 'visual' densities without any need for the telescopic apparatus.

Taking Agfa-Gevaert Curix MR4 as the film, the following changes in average gradient were noted.

0.0 lux, Average gradient = 3.12
50.0 lux, Average gradient = 3.06
100.0 lux, Average gradient = 2.94
200.0 lux, Average gradient = 2.78
500.0 lux, Average gradient = 2.59

It should be stressed that these figures were obtained using net density (ND) 0.25 and ND 1.5, as ND 2.0 was barely achieved at the higher ambient light levels.

In addition to these drops in 'visual' contrast, dramatic losses were noted in the perceptible radiation intensity levels, i.e. perceptibility was drastically reduced.

Dr Bollen made some recommendations which, whilst obvious, point out the poor way in which films are viewed.

For example, many radiologists gather round a viewing box in white coats to view an 'interesting case'. This effect is then exacerbated by pointing, with a finger, at the radiograph.

Perceptibility

It is appreciated that there are essentially three major influences on image quality. They are:

- Contrast
- Unsharpness
- Graininess (noise).

Each of these factors has been explained independently, but it is now time to add all of the information together to produce a common denominator. This is possible because we can reduce the influence of graininess and unsharpness to compensate for changes in contrast. The human eye is capable of perceiving low contrast, but if contrast falls below a certain value the image structure is totally invisible. This value is called the 'contrast threshold' or sometimes the 'minimum contrast'.

A number of other factors also play a part:

- Luminance of the image detail
- Accomodation of the eye
- Glare from the side
- Reflected glare.

As soon as the contrast of the image reaches, or passes, contrast threshold, then in theory the image is clearly seen. This is perceptibility. A knowledge of various contrast thresholds has a deal of relevance, as perceptibility can be derived for all parts of the radiographic image.

We can say simply that an image structure can be perceived when:

Contrast is equal to, or greater than, the contrast threshold.

If the value of contrast is significantly greater than contrast threshold, then the image structure is easily seen. This is perception. Perception in this context can be defined as:

The act of discerning the details on the radiograph.

The more the contrast of the image structures exceeds contrast threshold, the higher is the speed of perception.

If the topic of subject contrast is referred to in Chapter 2 (Sensitometry), it should be clear that the *subject contrast* must remain within the *film latitude* to give the best potential for the contrast threshold to be exceeded. If it is not within this range, i.e. in the toe or the shoulder of the curve, the potential for reaching contrast threshold is never realised, simply because there is no amplification of subject contrast by the film.

A perceptibility curve

A perceptibility curve provides quantitative data about real system performance by using a suitably designed phantom. From the phantom a number of observers can determine the minimum perceptible radiation contrast at a number of different exposure levels. Average values of all observers are calculated and a graph is plotted using minimum perceptible radiation contrast, (Δ log E)$_{min}$ against log E. Figure 7.17 is an example of such a graph.

Mathematically, it is the distribution function of the number of just perceptible steps. The area under the curve is a measure of the perceptibility. Other graphic measures have also been suggested, such as a plot of minimum perceptible density difference (Δ D$_{min}$), versus density (Kanomori, 1966).

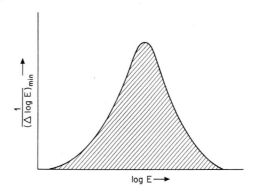

Fig. 7.17 Perceptibility curve.

Summary

The perceptibility curve derived for a film will depend upon a number of factors, some of which are listed below.

1. The characteristics of the observer.
2. The luminance of the viewing box.
3. The reflected light and glare conditions.
4. Graininess can affect the level of the contrast thresholds.
5. The effects of graininess in general radiography are slight.
6. Unsharpness can be interpreted, with the help of an MTF curve, as a change in detail contrast.
8. It is possible, in certain cases, to manipulate the contrast threshold by altering the contrast factor of the film, or by dropping the kV. This is only possible if the drop in contrast is *not* due to unsharpness.

A perceptibility curve can completely define image quality, as it takes into account all the parameters which influence diagnosis.

RECEIVER OPERATING CHARACTERISTICS (ROC)

One method of assesing total image quality has been discussed in considering perceptibility, above. Other methods are available but many, whilst giving values for system or part system performance, ignore the final link in the chain of 'image production', that of the observer who views the radiograph and makes the final diagnosis. It is essential therefore that some system is developed to evaluate the performance of both the system and the observer, to enable a more rational decision to be made on what system suits which observer, and if any particular system consistently gives better results no matter who observes it. Receiver operating characteristics may be of some assistance in this area.

Principles or ROC

ROC is based on signal detection theory. Simply, it is a method of quantifying the ability of an observer to make a diagnosis based on the detection and recognition or failure to detect and recognise some feature in the radiographic image. In the language of *signal detection theory* (SDT), the observer makes a decision as to the existance of a signal in the presence of noise. The decision the observer makes falls into one of four categories:

1. *False positive* (FP) 'The signal is there' when it is not really there, i.e. observer 'thinks' he/she can see something.
2. *True positive* (TP) 'The signal is there' and it really is there.
3. *True negative* (TN) 'The signal is not there' and it is really not there.
4. *False negative* (FN) 'The signal is not there' when it really is.

These four categories are summaries of how the brain's decision mechanism works; the brain, when confronted with a stimulus that it knows may be noise only or signal + noise, has to decide whether the stimulus contains the real signal. When the difference between the signal and noise is large the brain makes few mistakes. However, when it is small and at the threshold of perception, many mistakes may occur. Obviously the second case is the most important (e.g. in the early stages of calcification in, say, the breast) and to this end it is in this area, i.e. at the threshold of perception, that SDT experiments are carried out.

Problems in SDT

There are many problems in setting up SDT experiments, a few of which are outlined below.

1. Difficulty in simulating the real situation.

2. It is not possible to use real radiographs as they are too complex an item regarding signal and noise (thousands of signal to noise ratios exist on the radiograph). In addition it must be known which radiographs contains noise only or signal + noise.

3. The observer's previous experience of recognition and classification of the object used (i.e. the signal) significantly improves the results obtained. Not surprisingly, more practise = better results.

4. Time to view each radiograph. If given sufficient time, there is little difficulty in detecting the signal. To elliminate this a limited viewing time is set.

As can be seen, this list could be significantly extended, and is included only to give the reader a 'feel' of the problems.

In order to overcome some of the difficulties, a simplified situation must be created that can be controlled, measured and any conclusions transferred to the real situation.

The simplified situation

In SDT experiments associated with ROC and radiography a situation is created where noise (quantum mottle) varies randomly whilst the signal (the image of a plastic bead) does not change. The observer being tested is given a number of radiographs, 50% containing noise only, 50% containing the signal + the noise. The signal to noise ratio varies from film to film, so that in some cases the object is easily seen whilst in others it is at the perception threshold (i.e. the object can look like noise and the noise can look like the object).

The brain now has to make a decision, 'is there an image there or not?', for each film. Whenever the signal strength reaching the brain exceeds some critical value (Cv), the brain decides there is an object present. When below Cv the brain responds 'object (signal) not present'. This critical value varies from observer to observer and determines how many mistakes the observer makes.

The decisions the brain can make have been discussed earlier, and are summarised in Figure 7.18.

Stimulus ⟶

	Noise only	Signal and noise
Positive	FP	TP
Negative	TN	FN

(Response)

Fig. 7.18 Summary of ROC possible decisions.

It is important to note that a large Cv, i.e. strict criterion level as in a careful observer, reduces the number of FP responses but also reduces the TP responses. A low Cv, i.e. a lax observer, will correctly pick out nearly all the TP reponses but will also make large numbers of FP responses. It has been shown that a person's Cv level varies throughout the day, according to work load, viewing conditions, etc.

The number of responses in each class is recorded and calculated to give:

1. P(S/s) = Probability that a positive response is obtained when there is a signal.
Therefore: P(S/s) = TP/TP+FN
2. P(S/n) = Probability that a positive response is obtained when there is only noise.
Therefore: P(S/n) = FP/FP+TN

A graph is now plotted of P(S/s) vs P(S/n): this represents the ROC curve as Cv varies. One observer with a fixed Cv gives one value of P(S/s) and P(S/n), and one point on the graph. Several observers, or criterion levels of Cv, are needed to produce a curve. An example of a curve is shown in Figure 7.19.

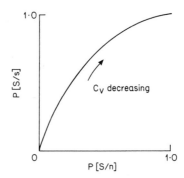

Fig. 7.19 Typical ROC curve.

Practical procedures of ROC analysis

Procedure 1

The test procedure is the same as in 'The simplified situation' (described above), using 200 radiographs, with 50% noise only and 50% signal plus noise. Only a single observer views each film in normal viewing conditions. The results are recorded on a separate card for each radiograph, which is numbered to correspond to the number on the film. Observers record on the card where they think they see the object on the radiograph by means of a cross or circle. Several observers perform the test and a curve is drawn as previously described. It is important for each observer to keep his/her criterion level (i.e. Cv) the same throughout the experiment.

Procedure 2

This is probably the best method as it allows a curve to be drawn for a single person or group of people.

The test is carried out as before except that the observer required to make a decision as to the degree of confidence he/she has about his/her response according to the following list:

5 = completely confident object present
4 = probably present
3 = don't know
2 = probably not present
1 = definitely not present.

This provides each observer with five different criteria levels, enabling a personalised ROC to be drawn.

Table 7.5 and 7.6 are examples of how the rating procedure is carried out. This in turn can produce a table of values for $P(S/s) + P(S/n)$ (Table 7.7). The ROC curve is now constructed plotting $P(S/s)$ vs $P(S/n)$; this is shown diagramatically in Figure 7.20.

Table 7.5 ROC results

| | Category | | | | |
	1	2	3	4	5
Number of signal films in category	3	12	35	35	15
Number of noise only films in category	15	35	35	12	3

Table 7.6 ROC results

	Categories 1+2+3 +4+5	2+3 +4+5	3+4+5	4+5	5
Number of signal films in category	100	97	85	50	
Number of noise only films in category	100	85	50	15	3

Table 7.7 ROC results

| | Category | | | | |
	1	2	3	4	5
P (S/s)	1	0.97	0.85	0.50	0.15
P (S/n)	1	0.85	0.50	0.15	0.03

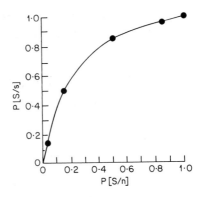

Fig. 7.20 An actual ROC curve (data from Tables 7.5, 7.6 and 7.7).

Interpretation of results

The closer the curve approximates to a right angle, the better the system. This is easily seen by studying Figure 7.21.

As the graph moves from right to left and upwards, the chance of making a positive response when there is a signal is increasing, and the chance of making a positive response when there is only noise, is decreasing; therefore, as previously stated, the closer to a right angle the graph is, the better.

Various ways of quantifying this 'right-angledness' have been proposed, with no firm conclusions to date.

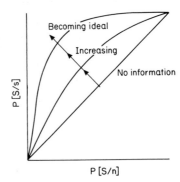

Fig. 7.21 ROC curve — interpretation of results.

General comment

The preparation of radiographs for this procedure is not a complex process.

Finally, it is important to note that the ROC curves are not confined to one particular situation of, say, low contrast sharp bordered particles but can be drawn for numerous other situations, such as high contrast 'fuzzy'-edged strand objects. ROC curves are very versatile and can assess a system and an observer in almost any situation.

An experiment in ROC analysis

Normal ROC experiments involve the use of one set of radiographs being seen by one observer. It is obvious that this is a time-consuming and labourious process. However, a technique for demonstrating the principles and problems of setting up and taking part in such an experiment has been developed by Dr J. Gore, formerly of the Medical Physics Department of the Hammersmith Hospital. Dr Gore's technique enables quite a large audience to participate in a useful experiment.

The experiment produces a large number of decision matrices at one time, but it is not strictly valid for a number of reasons.

A large number of specimen radiographs with noise and signal + noise are made, and then either mounted directly onto a large format slide carrier or (more practically) copied onto standard 35 mm film.

The resulting slide is projected onto a white screen from several feet (to suit the projection conditions) and viewed by the audience in as dark a condition as is practical. Each participant in the test is asked to decide if the slide being viewed is noise only or signal plus noise, to record this, and to indicate where he/she thinks the signal is (if any) on a card with the slide number.

The observer is told that the signal is a round object and that there may be up to 3 signals in any one film. The time allowed to view each slide is kept constant at approximately 8–10 seconds.

In order that each participant may produce his/her own personalised ROC and to give the experiment a greater range of results, the observer, as well as indicating the position of the signal, can be asked to show how confident he/she is that the signal is or is not there, using the 1–5 scale outlined in procedure two.

A few of the problems of this experiment are listed below:

1. When using the 35 mm format, the ROC is a function not only of the radiographic system but also of the projector system used.
2. The nature of the viewing screen material; 'daylight' screens tend to increase the noise level.
3. The angle of view of the observer.
4. Distance the observer is from the screen.
5. Degree of background lighting.
6. Production of results for a group of people.
7. The fact that the observers know that there are no more than 3 signals on any one film.

Some advantages of the technique are:

1. Allows a large number of participants.
2. Demonstrates how fatiguing the experiments are to take part in.

3. Easy to demonstrate the effect of adding or taking away noise or signal by use of a second projector.

4. Easy to demonstrate effect of change in contrast.

5. Easy to demonstrate effect of change in object size.

These are just a few of the advantages and disadvantages of ROC analysis on a large scale.

The method used for recording the observers' responses to the test depends on which test is being performed, and can range from a simple 'signal present or not present delete one not appropriate' to the more popular 'position and certainty' sheet.

REFERENCES

Bollen R 1981 The influence of ambient light. The Proceedings of the S.P.I.E. Conference (Medicine), San Francisco 3: 22–24

Buchanan R A, Finkelstein S I, Wickersheim K A 1972 X-ray exposure reduction using rare-earth oxysulphide intensifying screens. Radiology 105: 185–190

Buchanan R A 1971 Lockheed develops method to reduce X-ray exposure. Nuclear Science Symposium of the Institute of Electrical and Electronic Engineers, San Francisco, 3–4 November

Christensen E, Curry T, Dowdey J 1978 An introduction to the physics of diagnostic radiology, 2nd edn. Lea & Febiger, Philadelphia

De Belder M, Bollen R, Duville R 1971 A new approach to the evaluation of radiographic systems. (Presented at New Trends in Radiography: a conference of the Royal Photographic Society.) Journal of Photographic Science 19

Gore J 1978 Personal communication (ROC analysis)

Kanomori H 1966 Determination of optimum film density range for roentgenograms from visual effects. Acta Radiologica 4: 463

Open University 1978 Images and information (ST. 291). Open University Press, Milton Keynes.

Taylor F E 1977 Cost and benefits of rare earth screens. Letter to the editor. British Journal of Radiology 50: 294

8

Monitor photography

Introduction

Monitor photography may be defined as the filming of images from a cathode ray tube (CRT). Although in its infancy in the early 1970s, it has now become a major part of diagnostic imaging departments throughout the world. In fact, monitor photography has expanded at a rate which was totally unexpected by many people.

Initially, monitor photography was associated with the early CAT scanners where a simple camera was simply bolted on to the diagnostic monitor, and films were then made of the images on the diagnostic monitor. These cameras merely took one exposure at a time, usually on 5 × 4 inch film.

There are now much more sophisticated video imagers available which contain their own monitor and camera and are totally dedicated to monitor photography. These imagers come in a variety of guises and can make as many as twenty five exposures on one film. These imagers are known as multiformat cameras.

With the advent of ultrasound, computed tomography, digital radiography, MRI, and other technologies, where the only image available is displayed on a monitor, a dedicated video imager is now a necessity, as the images themselves are becoming more and more sophisticated. Very high resolution is being demanded by the latest generations of scanners, resolution unheard of in the early days of scanning.

All of the newer technologies demand a 'hard copy' to be produced, either on paper or on film. Usually the patient's notes carry a paper copy of the image and the original film is used either as a 'master' in the filing system, or for higher quality imaging. This statement is not meant to denigrate images on paper, it is merely a photographic fact of life that film *must* produce a better quality image than paper.

All of these new technologies have created demands for film (and paper) capable of recording these high quality images, and which responds to the phosphors used in the imagers. The purpose of this chapter is to discuss briefly the way the image is produced on the monitor itself and to consider the way the film is designed to cope with the stringent demands placed upon it.

THE CHARACTERISTICS OF THE VIDEO IMAGE

The detailed technology of the production of the video image is well outside the scope of this book: indeed, many books are available which are dedicated solely to examining the subject in detail. However, the basic principles can be covered fairly simply.

The following descriptions relate to the imaging process from the television camera to the monitor. The principles obviously apply equally to the image production on the imaging camera monitor.

Persistence of vision

The moving video image relies on the principle of persistence of vision, the same principle used in cinema photography. To produce a flicker-free, moving image, 25 frames a second are required.

Interlacing

Consider first of all one still picture of one frame. This frame is made up of two fields which consist, in a 625 line system, of 312 lines each. The two fields when combined add up to the one complete frame of 625 lines.

It will be noted that if the picture is observed very closely, it is made up of minute dots along the horizontal scanning lines. These dots are the resolutions of individual pixels along the line. If the pixel is considered as having depth, it is referred to as a voxel.

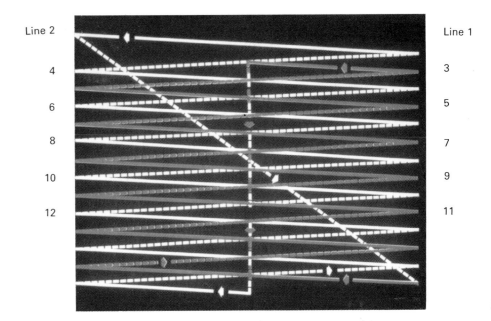

Line 2

Line 1

4   3

6   5

8   7

10   9

12   11

Fig. 8.1 Odd, then even lines are scanned.

The field is constructed by an electron beam scanning the tube phosphor from top left to bottom right in a series of horizontal lines, as illustrated in Figure 8.1. First the odd lines are scanned, then the even lines. In this way the composite (the frame) is completed.

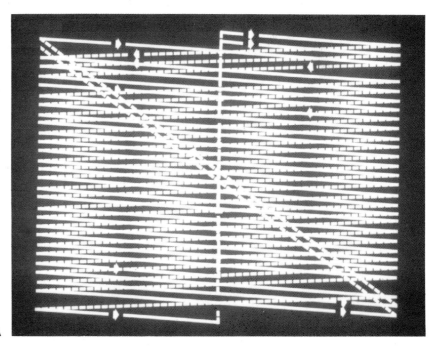

A

Fig. 8.2 Multiple interlacing: (A) × 2 interlacing; (B) raster lines almost disappear.

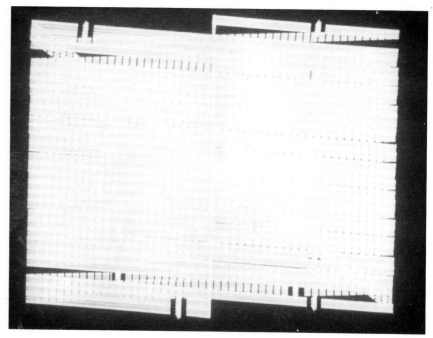

Fig. 8.2B

This system of constructing the frame is called 'double interlacing', and requires sophisticated electronic circuitry to achieve the accurate spacing of the lines which is imperative for high quality images.

This interlacing can be carried still further. For example, × 4 and × 8 interlacing are not uncommon and will produce images which, to all intents and purposes, are line free (Fig. 8.2).

Image display

The display system used in most imaging departments is usually referred to as a monitor, which bears a strong family resemblance to a television set. There is a main intrinsic difference between the two, apart from the obvious fact that a diagnostic system is usually a closed system (i.e. the images arrive by wire, rather than by an aerial). In a television set, the video signal arrives at the tube through various electronics and RF circuitry. In a monitor, the video signal is fed directly to the processing circuitry uninterfered with. On some colour monitors an RGB input is often available (this input accepts directly the *Red*, *Green* and *Blue* signals offered by the colour video signal).

THE TELEVISION CAMERA

Two of the most popular cameras are the Videcon and Plumbicon cameras. Again, these cameras are very complex electronically. In basic terms the image is formed in a similar way to the monitor image. In this case, the electrons generated have to scan the signal plate of the tube and gain information about the amount of light and dark areas formed on the signal plate. The plate is scanned in a similar way to the monitor, in regular horizontal lines. The video signal is generated in pulses which correspond to the image formed on the signal plate. This signal is formed in a complex way by (in the Videcon) tiny globules embedded in the signal plate, discharging like condensers. This description is again simplistic, but information on this technology is readily available.

BANDWIDTH AND RESOLUTION

The bandwidth of a system is defined as the difference between the maximum and minimum frequency that the system has to cope with. In a 625 line system, a *horizontal* resolution of 300 lines, which approaches equal horizontal and vertical resolution, is a fairly good system (Fig. 8.3).

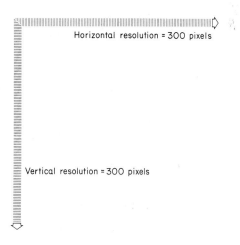

Horizontal resolution = 300 pixels

Vertical resolution = 300 pixels

Fig. 8.3 A monitor which could offer equal horizontal and vertical resolution would produce reasonable resolution.

The maximum frequency can then be calculated by multiplying the maximum number of cycles (300) by the number of scan lines per frame and the number of frames per second, i.e.

$$\frac{300}{\text{cycles}} \times \frac{625}{\text{lines}} \times \frac{50}{\text{frames}} = 4\ 687\ 500$$

The resultant figure is quite remarkable, a *maximum* frequency of almost 5 million hertz is required i.e. 5 MHz!

The minimum frequency required will be when only one cycle is to resolved, i.e. when the screen is half black, half white — a highly unlikely occurrence but a good theoretical concept (Fig. 8.4). In this case the calculation is:

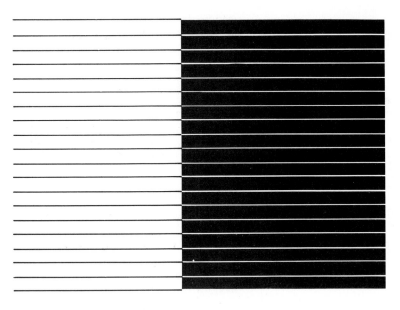

Fig. 8.4 The simplest possible signal would be half the screen white and half black, i.e. 1 hertz.

$$1 \times 625 \times 50 = 15\ 625$$

This figure represents the *minimum* frequency to be dealt with.

Therefore, the bandwidth required to cope with the maximum and minimum frequencies is:

$$4\ 687\ 500 - 15\ 625 = 4\ 671\ 875$$

or 4.67 MHz.

It is important to realise that this figure is for an uncomplicated black and white image. If the image were coloured, for example, then the figure for bandwidth would be much greater. Brightness and colour levels would also have to be taken into account, which increase the demands for bandwidth.

PHOSPHORS

There are a number of phosphors commonly in use as the coating for the monitor tube. They each have a characteristic light emission, when stimulated by the electron beam. The most common are listed below.

P45	'White' (a mixture of blue and green)
P11	Blue
P31	Both green-emitting phosphors
P24	

P4
P40
} Both 'white' phosphors, i.e. blue and green.

THE IMAGING FILM

The film used for monitor photography has some features which are unique. It is well worth while looking at the individual features which make up this film. The obvious place to start is the base.

Base

The base material is generally polyester, with all the attendant advantages of this material. The base can either be coloured or clear. It should be appreciated that the choice of colour for the base material is not arbitrary, but has a sound scientific basis.

Blue base

If a blue-based film is chosen it can give some distinct benefits.

1. In general, a blue base gives a more aesthetically pleasing image. Although this is obviously subjective, large numbers of people choose a blue-based material in preference to clear base.
2. In continuous viewing, blue-based material is much more restful on the viewer's eyes.
3. Blue-based material also produces a slightly higher visual contrast than clear base.

One disadvantage of blue base is that if it is viewed on a poor quality, yellow-light emitting viewing box, the film will have an apparent high base fog.

Clear base

1. Clear base has a very low base fog when compared to a blue-based film. This is due to the fact that density is contributed by the base *only* and it is usually extremely low.
2. The basic fog of clear-based film remains low even when viewed on poor viewing equipment. There is also a slight increase in perceptibility in the toe of the curve due to the lower base fog, which makes this type of base particularly suitable for ultrasound work.
3. Clear base does, however, produce slightly lower visual contrast.
4. Continued viewing of a clear-based film may be more tiresome for some viewers.

The emulsion

The characteristics of the emulsion are determined by the phosphors used in coating the monitor. As can be seen from the earlier listing,

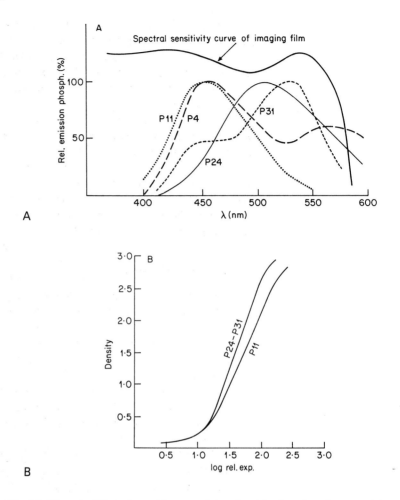

Fig. 8.5 Characteristics of emulsion are determined by the phosphors used in coating the monitor: (A) Spectral sensitivity curve of a typical imaging film superimposed onto the emissions of P4, P24, P31 and P11 phosphors; (B) contrast changes significantly depending on type of phosphor used.

these range from a solely blue-emitting phosphor through to green-emitting phosphors, plus combinations of blue and green.

It should be apparent, therefore, that a purely monochromatic film would not respond to the green emissions of a P31 phosphor, for example. In fact, if a monochromatic film is used in this situation an apparently very 'grainy' image is produced. The 'grain' is merely the unresolved green emissions leaving blanks in the image. Figure 8.5A shows the spectral sensitivity curve of a typical imaging film, superimposed onto the emissions of P4, P24, P31, and P11 phosphors. Figure 8.5A clearly shows that a monochromatic film would be unable to respond to the green emissions of the phosphor, and indeed contrast changes significantly with the type of phosphor used (Fig. 8.5B).

The obvious choice, therefore, of emulsion type is orthochromatic. Film of this type will be capable of producing an image from current phosphors in use.

There is yet another decision to be made about the emulsion, i.e. should it be single or double sided?

The main gain of a duplitised emulsion is that the radiation dose can be considerably reduced, whilst there can be a gain in image contrast. At no time can it be said that duplitised emulsions give better resolution.

In monitor photography there is no requirement to reduce the dose to the patient, as this is already decided by other parameters set in the main equipment. There is, however, a requirement for as high a resolution as possible. By this process of elimination the film must be single sided.

A typical resolution for a monitor film would be of the order of 140 lp/mm. It is worth comparing this figure to the typical resolution obtained with screen X-ray film.

Anti-curl, anti-halation layer

If an emulsion is coated onto one side of a polyester base some problems can be created. If the emulsion expands and contracts, as it will do in its journey through the processor, the base will curl in or out depending on the movement of the emulsion. The emulsion could also expand or contract merely by variations in temperature or humidity in storage.

To overcome this unwanted curl, which could lead to problems in transport for example, an anti-curl layer is added to the back of the film. This 'balances' the base and exerts an opposing force to the movement of the emulsion.

Incorporated in the anti-curl layer is the anti-halation layer. If the anti-halation layer were not present, problems would occur from light passing through the emulsion, through the base and then reflecting randomly off nearby objects, causing spurious reflections. The anti-halation layer, which is a dye, absorbs any light passing through the base. See Chapter 1, Film materials.

Identification of emulsion side

Of necessity, imaging film must be loaded with the emulsion facing the lens. With a duplitised emulsion it is not necessary to identify a certain side of the film. With a single-sided emulsion it is vitally important to know which side of the film the emulsion is coated on. If an exposure was made through the back of the film (i.e. the anti-halation layer), it is quite likely that no image would be recorded. To make this identification easy in the darkroom, all imaging film has a notch in the corner of the film. With the notch in the top right hand corner, the emulsion is facing the user.

As the film is coated on one side only, this can lead to a problem which again is peculiar to video imaging. Basically, one side of the film be shiny — the non-emulsion side — and one side will be dulled — the emulsion side.

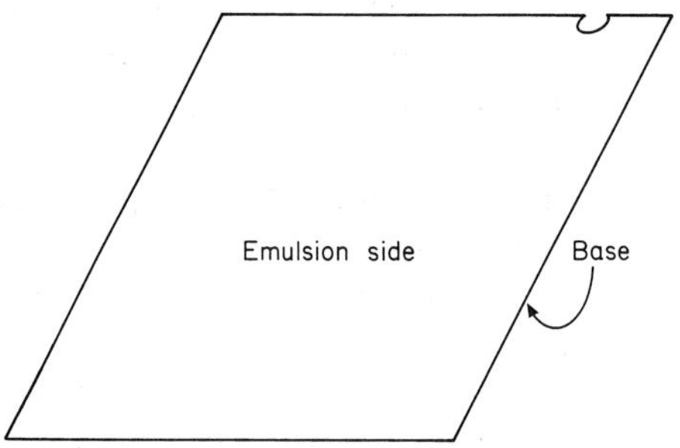

Fig. 8.6 Identifying emulsion side of single-sided emulsion film — if the notch is in the upper right corner, the emulsion is facing the user.

If the film is viewed from the base side, there can be considerable reflection from the base, which can cause problems in reading the film. The easiest way to cure this is to reverse the image in the camera, if this is possible. Reverse, in this case, means a mirror image reversal of the image actually in the camera. This is done electronically. The film can now be viewed from the emulsion side. There will now be fewer reflections and viewing is made much more comfortable.

Emulsion contrast

The final decision to make about the emulsion is the type of contrast. A great deal has been said about what type of contrast should be used in imaging film. The two main schools are divided between high or low contrast. One school of thought insists that a low contrast film must be used for *all* imaging. This is because the raster lines on the monitor image are the highest contrast available on the image, and a high contrast film would merely amplify this high subject contrast.

Historically, imaging film was always high contrast. With the advent of large usage of film in ultrasound, more users began to demand low contrast emulsion. At first, many people felt that this was just a matter of personal preference; however, there is a strictly scientific basis for these decisions.

Low contrast film brings an extended latitude. This would *seem* to mean that the film would cope with fluctuations in the output of the CRT within the camera, and the fluctuations would have much less effect.

This argument seems to be reasonable but the decision about type of contrast really depends on what *type* of image is being displayed. The main difference between CT/MRI images and ultrasound images is the polarity of the image.

A CT/MRI image has a *black* background, hence the original monitor image background is *white*.

An ultrasound image has a *white* background, hence the original monitor image background is *black*.

Anyone who has cleaned an imaging camera, particularly inside, will understand some of the implications of the above statements.

Any dust on the lens or the inside of the camera body, any scratches on the internal paintwork, will cause flare or scattered light inside the camera body. This flare will, in turn, lead to decreased subject contrast. On an already low contrast film, the contrast becomes even lower, because of lower maximum density and higher base fog. The high contrast film will go a long way towards compensating for these losses.

However, a low contrast film is still better for ultrasonographers, because the monitor image background is black and this causes significantly less flare and scatter. Ultrasound also demands a long grey scale, particularly in the toe of the curve (see Clear base, p. 277).

To summarise: the general decision, almost worldwide, is that CT/MRI requires a high contrast film and ultrasound requires a low contrast film.

SENSITOMETRIC CHARACTERISTICS

In monitor photography it is important not to treat the film in isolation but to remember that it is part of a chain of equipment. It is also important to relate the behaviour of the film to certain changes which take place in the imaging equipment.

On most imagers there are usually found three major controls. These are the controls which set *brightness, contrast,* and *exposure time.* The adjustment of any of these controls has a profound effect on the final image quality produced. It is worth considering in some depth what the sensitometric effect is when the controls are adjusted.

Brightness

When the brightness control is adjusted on the monitor, the picture becomes considerably lighter. However, the effect on the film is

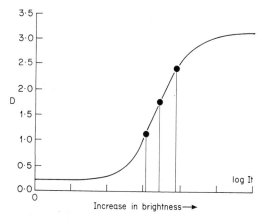

Fig. 8.7 As brightness increases, the maximum density of the final image moves up the slope of the characteristic curve.

noted on the log It axis of the characteristic curve. As the brightness goes up, i.e. moves *right* along the log It axis, so the maximum density of the final image moves up the slope of the characteristic curve (Fig. 8.7).

The converse is also true; as brightness is turned down, i.e. moves *left* along the log It axis, the maximum density obtained on the final image goes down.

Contrast

The movement of the contrast control produces a different effect entirely. The function of this adjustment is to alter the brightness range available on the monitor.

Assuming that brightness (and hence maximum density) has already been set, the density *range* obtainable on the final image will be determined by the setting of the contrast control (Fig. 8.8).

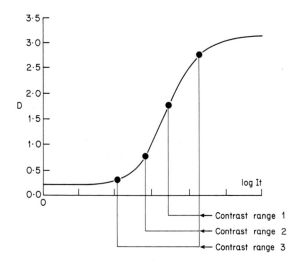

Fig. 8.8 The contrast control determines the density range available on the final image.

Exposure time

If the exposure time is altered, this will have the effect of moving the preset brightness range of the subject up or down the log It axis. Short exposures will produce 'thin' images, long exposures will produce dark images.

Density overall will increase or decrease, but contrast may also increase or decrease if the upper or lower values of the contrast range obtrude into the shoulder or toe of the characteristic curve. In other words, care must be taken to try to keep the parameters of brightness, contrast and exposure time within the region of useful exposure of the characteristic curve of the film (Fig. 8.9).

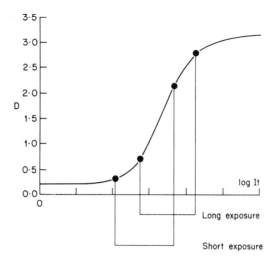

Fig. 8.9 Altering exposure time will shift the preset brightness range up or down the log It axis: short exposures produce 'thin' images, long exposures produce dark images.

Sizing of films

The film sizes for monitor film are many and varied, from conventional sheet film to 75 m roll film.

The list below shows film currently available. It should be stressed that the list below is not comprehensive, but merely illustrative of the formats available.

Sheet film

9 × 10 cm
5 × 4 in
18 × 24 cm
11 × 14 in
10 × 12 in
10 × 10 cm
5 × 7 in
8 × 10 in
14 × 17 in

Roll film

70 mm × 45 m
90 mm × 30 m
105 mm × 45 m
8 in × 75 m

It can be seen from the above list that there is a complete potpourri of sizes obtainable. Initially, imperial sizing was used (with the 5 × 4 in size) and then more and more manufacturers entered the field.

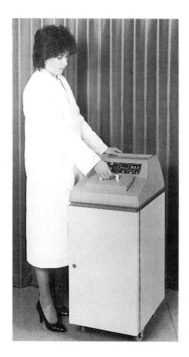

Fig. 8.10 Scopix 300 — imager using roll film (photograph courtesy of D.I.S. Division, Agfa-Gevaert Ltd).

Metric sizes were then introduced as well, meaning that imperial and metric sizes are available, a mixture which is now unique in medical imaging.

It will be noted that roll film is listed above. Imaging cameras are available to handle such roll film. Instead of handling numerous cassettes in a busy session, the department is able to produce large numbers of images (as many as 1300 on one roll) and then sort them out at a later date (Fig. 8.10).

Film or paper images

Another decision to be made when using an imaging camera is whether to use film or paper for making the hard copy.

A simple example will illustrate the problem. Very often, after returning from holiday, a decision is made to get the slides of the holiday snaps copied and have prints made, so that they can be passed round the family or the department. Anyone who has done this will have experienced the disappointment when they realise that the prints are not as good as the slides. This is not the fault of the paper manufacturer or the laboratory, it is merely the intrinsic difference between the two materials.

A slide image is an image designed to be viewed by *transmitted* light; paper prints are to viewed by *reflected* light.

Exactly the same rules apply to monitor photography. A film image is designed for transmitted light, a paper image for reflected light. This simple difference accounts for the different behaviour of these two materials.

Transmitted light image

In chapter 2, Sensitometry, percentage transmission was discussed. It was also pointed out that at density 2.0 only 1% of the incident light actually reaches the eye. The maximum density reached on film depends largely on the amount of silver that the manufacturer is prepared to put in the film. Figures significantly higher than density 2.0 could be reached quite easily, these densities being, for all intents and purposes, totally black (Fig. 8.11).

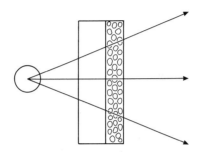

Fig. 8.11 The transmitted light passes straight through the film, generally only its intensity being reduced.

This maximum density on a transmitted light image and the clarity of the base determine the maximum contrast available on the film, i.e. the blackest black and the whitest white. In other words, film can have a maximum density which is determined solely by the silver content and the value of the incident light.

With paper, however, different rules apply. Some incident light will *always* be reflected from the surface of the paper; it can never all be absorbed by the silver in the emulsion. Similarly to film, the

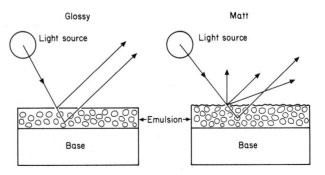

Fig. 8.12 With glossy paper there is reflection from the paper surface, then the light is reflected from the image. Matt paper suffers from multiple reflections from the coarse surface.

maximum density is determined by the incident light, but this maximum density can be changed as it depends on the angle of the viewing light to the viewer and the surface of the paper, which can be glossy or matte (Fig. 8.12).

Because of these effects, film will always have a longer grey scale and a wider dynamic range than paper.

In the case outlined above the discussion was about two similar processes for producing a hard copy of an image; however, there is another type of paper image which uses the *diffusion transfer process*. This should be considered separately.

Diffusion transfer process

The 'instant' picture is often used in ultrasound as a permanent record of the event. It is usually found as a paper image, in which case the same rules apply to this paper image as to conventional paper. It can also be found as a transmission image.

Pros and cons

When using diffusion transfer, some advantages and disadvantages of the system can be noted.

Advantages:

1. No processing facilities required
2. 'Instant' viewing of a finished image
3. High speed (can be approximately 3000 ISO)
4. Useful for museum or history of patient
5. No darkroom or darkroom equipment required.

Disadvantages:

1. High cost per image
2. Low dynamic range (if paper)
3. Poor grey scale (if paper)
4. Can be messy to handle
5. Subject to ambient temperature levels.

None of the above should be taken to mean that diffusion transfer is unsatisfactory. Like many other processes in photography it has its place. It is up to individual users to decide which material suits his/her own particular application.

THE IMAGING CAMERA

As mentioned earlier, imaging cameras were initially simple 'bolt on' cameras linked to a conventional monitor, sometimes even to the diagnostic monitor.

The film was usually carried in a dark slide cassette, usually double-sided. The film is loaded into both sides of the cassette with the emulsion side facing outwards. To expose the emulsion, a slide is removed when the cassette is in the camera. After exposure, the film is covered with the slide and the process is repeated for the second film.

When the matrix size of the diagnostic equipment was small, very few demands were put on the imaging camera; but matrices began to increase in size until it was realised that the definition required was outstripping the performance of simple cameras, and even more importantly, simple monitors. From this point onwards, the dedicated imaging camera was inevitable.

The evolution of the imaging camera

Figure 8.13 shows the development of the imaging camera, from the simple 'bolt on' to the ultra-modern multiformat camera of today.

It can be seen that the cameras have evolved from utilising a simple, usually curved-screen monitor, to sophisticated microprocessor-controlled dedicated cameras.

The second type of camera consisted of a monitor with a flat

A Bolted directly to diagnostic monitor

B Integrated monitor

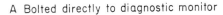

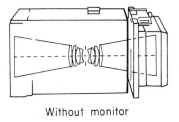

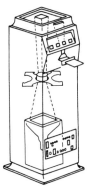

Without monitor

C With monitor plus automatic film transport and processing

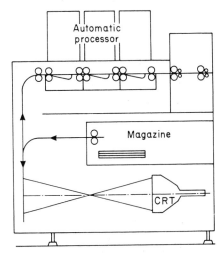

Fig. 8.13 Development of the imaging camera.

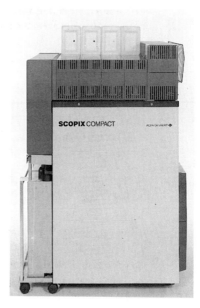

Fig. 8.14 Scopix Compact — modern multi-format imaging system with inbuilt processor.

screen, using only one size of film and giving only one specific format. For example, this could be one image on a 10 × 8 in film, or 4 images on a 10 × 8 in film. This then developed into a multiformat camera, where different numbers of images could be stored on the same 10 × 8 in film. On some types of these cameras there is also the possibility of using different sizes of film as well (e.g. a 10 × 8 in and a 17 × 14 in film).

The line diagrams in Figure 8.13 demonstrate the basic principles of operation of the imagers. In the single format camera the imaging chain is fairly straightforward. In the multiformat camera it becomes more complex. In the latest generation, with an inbuilt processor, the complexity is greatly increased. (Fig. 8.14).

The newest cameras can only be described as 'multiformat, multi-sized' cameras with microprocessor control and an inbuilt processing machine. These cameras allow a single 17 × 14 in film (for example) to image a variety of images from different format sized. Even so, all modern cameras are constrained by certain parameters.

The parameters for an imaging camera

The parameters can be laid down as follows:

1. Type of monitor
2. Stability
3. Exposure
4. Interlacing
5. The lens system.

Each of these will be discussed in turn. These parameters equally apply to a single format or a multiformat camera.

Type of imaging monitor

The monitor must be flat faced, to avoid edge distortion of the image. The phosphors most frequently used in monitors are listed earlier in the chapter.

Stability

It really goes without saying that the raster pattern should be extremely stable, to avoid any loss of resolution of the image. This is sometimes highlighted when changing from a very fast (diffusion transfer, 3000 ISO-type) film, to conventional imaging film. It is sometimes noted that on the slow film the raster lines disappear and this is usually attributed to 'loss of definition'. However, the truth is far from that.

With an extremely fast film, perhaps two or three fields are all that are needed to form an image. Even if the raster lines are slightly unstable, they will clearly be seen on only three fields. With a slow film, perhaps 14 fields will be required. Any raster instability will be clearly demonstrated, as the raster lines will be blurred (or in the worst case absent).

Exposure

In Europe the frequency of the mains supply is 50 hertz. This means that there are 50 fields per second produced on the monitor. The *minimum* exposure possible is 1/25 th of a second, to give one complete frame. An exposure length must guarantee that at least two fields are imaged; any shorter exposure will result in only a partial frame, perhaps only one field. In this case only half the information would be imaged.

An improvement on 'time' exposures would be to translate the exposure time into the number of fields imaged for each exposure. In the more modern imaging cameras, this is exactly what happens. Users merely dial the number of fields they wish to image, and the camera — electronically — does the rest.

An important point arises here which is closely allied to length of exposure. When sensitometric characteristics were discussed earlier in the chapter, it was noted that an increased exposure time could create a change on the characteristic curve of the film similar to the effect of changing the brightness of the monitor. With a monitor image it is extremely important that brightness is not increased to a point at which unsharpness occurs, due to phosphor flare. In other words it is important to use exposure length to determine blackness, rather than increasing the brightness on the CRT to achieve this end.

The intensity of light on the CRT is achieved by the number of electrons hitting a particular spot on the CRT. If the number of electrons is increased (the equivalent of increasing brightness), the spot size at the CRT becomes larger. The result of this is increasing unsharpness for increasing brightness.

This effect is well demonstrated on a viewing monitor, where it will be noted that sharpness is at its best at the black end of the image, sharpness decreasing as the image is whiter.

Interlacing

This was discussed earlier in the chapter. Essentially, the greater the interlacing, the less likelihood there is of raster lines being displayed.

Optical system

There are many problems which have to be overcome in the optical system, some of which are:

1. Vignetting
2. Lens imperfections such as:
   a. spherical aberration
   b. chromatic aberration
   c. curvature of field
   d. astigmatism
3. Density uniformity across the field.

Most of these problems can be overcome or minimised by some of the following techniques.

'In line-optics', whereby the image, lens and film are aligned and used with a flat screen monitor, will help to overcome most of the distortion problems. Vignetting in particular can be reduced by using a CRT larger than the image field: for example, using a 7 in monitor with a 5 in imaging field.

Density uniformity can be more of a problem, as very often there is a fall-off of light to the edge of the film. This can be handled by electronic manipulation of the density profile actually on the monitor. In this case the edge brightness would be higher than the centre brightness.

To maintain the best resolution, the easiest answer would be to use only the centre of the lens system, where resolution is at its highest. This could be achieved by only allowing the user a choice of high f-stop numbers, i.e. f 8, f 16, etc., or even offering no choice at all. Unlike conventional photography, imaging does not need to concern itself with depth of field (associated with low f stop numbers, e. g. f 2.8, and sometimes low resolution) as the 'image' lies on a phosphor which is only microns thick.

Chromatic aberration is not such a serious problem, unless the camera is used for coloured images. In this case great care must be taken in the lens manufacture.

PROCESSING

If the imaging camera does not contain an inbuilt processor, some consideration must be given to the processing of the final film. It should be remembered that an imaging film is single-sided emulsion film, and large quantities of this film going through the department's main processor could lead to gross over-replenishment. In some departments this decision is purely academic, as there may be only the one processor. In the purpose-built department there are a number of decisions to be made.

Automatic processing

The decision will revolve round the choice of low capacity, medium capacity or high capacity processors. Most imaging departments could cope with a low capacity processor, of the order of 30 cm/min running speed as the throughput of film is not as great as a 'normal' department. Nor is there the same demand to see the film as quickly.

Consideration should also be given to darkroom availability, as ideally the darkroom should be nearby and the safelighting must be suitable for orthochromatic emulsions.

Daylight processing

Some manufacturers now offer a cassette compatible with most imaging cameras which can also be used in a their own daylight system. This would obviously offer all the inherent advantages of using a daylight system.

Quality assurance

Monitor photography film is much more susceptible to changes in processing quality than conventional screen film. The image quality will fluctuate quite markedly with chemical changes which would most probably be unnoticed on screen film. It is therefore very important to consider a quality assurance programme as routine. This would of course cover the camera as well as the processor.

Signal generators are now available which produce images suitable for evaluating image quality in cameras. These are extremely useful devices for the quality assurance of imagers.

One useful attribute of monitor photography is that testing of the camera and processor does not involve live patients. There is easy access to the actual patient's images stored on disk, and these can be replayed time after time to assess image quality.

THE FINAL IMAGE

A common complaint is that the final hard copy does not look like the image on the diagnostic console. This can be due to many factors, not least the behaviour of the CRT itself.

The production of this final image is the result of a number of complex factors; the following is a short list of the most important.

Computer algorithms

These are instructions within the complex computer programs which translate the received information (the raw data) into a form usable by the diagnostic apparatus.

Monitor

The image display is a function of the video signal generated by the diagnostic apparatus. This, in turn, is determined by the characteristics of the monitor in use. Of course, some of these characteristics can be modified by the use of the brightness and contrast controls.

Film

This part of the process is determined by the characteristic curve of the film. However, this is inextricably linked with the CRT performance. For example, there are no truly linear relationships in this part of the imaging process. The relationship between log of intensity on the CRT display and the grid voltage means that low grid voltages give better contrast than higher grid voltages. The characteristic curve also is certainly not linear. It should also be remembered that in most cases the film is imaging the reverse polarity of what is seen on the diagnostic monitor. Therefore, the hard copy is essentially a compromise of all these factors.

There is also a disparity between the actual viewing sizes, e.g. a large monitor and a relatively small format image.

The viewer's eye

Perhaps the most complex part of the chain. The eye's response varys from viewer to viewer, as can easily be demonstrated by a Receiver Operating Characteristic Test (see ROC, p. 264). In general, though, the human eye is much better at resolving density differences in the low densities rather than in the high density areas. Windowing can be used to exploit this effect.

COLOUR VS BLACK AND WHITE

Coloured images are used, to a limited extent, in monitor photography. However, they are limited to specialised imaging, for example Positron Emission Tomography (PET)

Part of the reason for the non-acceptance of colour as a universal image may lie in the fact that coloured imaging does not have a standard for colour values. Red may mean high density on one system and low density on another.

However, colour could have a lot of attraction. The eye is capable of resolving about 200 different grey levels, whereas it can discern about 2000 colour levels. These colour levels would be responded to in terms of colour hue and brightness levels.

Again, windowing can play a part in black and white imaging. Because most systems allow considerable windowing, the eye's ability to resolve only 200 grey levels is more than acceptable.

Colour also brings the problem of processing. Generally, the colour process is much more complex than black and white, and this is reflected in the price of the processors and film.

VIEWING CONDITIONS

Perhaps the single most important factor is the actual viewing conditions themselves. The factors involved are discussed in Chapter 6, Quality assurance, but they are worth repeating here.

Glare

This is usually from the surrounding boxes. It can be overcome by the use of masking, either built into the box or using cardboard masks. The mirror image reversal of the image in the camera would also reduce this problem, as reflections would be greatly reduced.

Colour temperature

Vitally important if the film happens to be blue based. Blue base plus a yellow viewing light will considerably lower the visual contrast.

Viewing/ambient light level

Check that the light levels conform to the ANSI specification.

LASER IMAGING

A new type of imager has recently emerged in monitor photography. The laser imager is an optical / electronic / mechanical device which produces hard copy by exposing a film to laser light (see Fig. 8.15). (The principles of laser light and some of the applications of lasers will be discussed in detail in Chapter 9, Holography).

In the laser imager a helium-neon laser can be used, emitting red light. The principle of operation of the laser imager is entirely different from that of a video imager, even though the results obtained look remarkably similar.

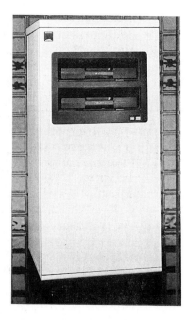

Fig. 8.15 Matrix laser recorder 25 (photograph courtesy of Matrix Instruments Inc.).

Principles of operation

In describing the principles of operation of the laser imager, it is interesting to contrast its image production that of a video imager. The laser imager contains a number of separate modules, all inter-linked, which help in the production of the final image. They are:

1. The laser (usually helium-neon)
2. An interface
3. A large memory store
4. An acoustic-optical modulator
5. An optical system
6. A (mechanical) scanner
7. A (mechanical) film transport system.

The memory store is required because image production on a laser imager is very different from that of a video imager. In a video imager, one image is captured on a CRT and photographed. In a laser imager *all* the digital image information required for one *film* must be put into the memory store, via the interface, before the image recording can start.

The full information from the memory store is now used to modulate the laser beam via an acoustic-optical modulator, in terms of brightness, grey levels, etc. A lens system is now used to focus the laser beam onto a Galvano scanner. This scanner is used to move the laser beam from side to side across the imaging field.

Note another difference between video imagers and laser imagers: in a video imager, writing the lines of information is achieved by the

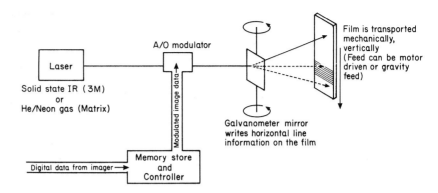

Fig. 8.16 Principles of a laser imager.

continuous deflection of the electron beam. In the laser imager the deflection of the beam in the horizontal plane is achieved by, basically, a mirror. This, of course, leaves vertical movement, which has to be done by moving the *film* in relation to the deflected horizontal beam (Fig. 8.16).

Comparison of video and laser systems

Many departments will be considering the purchase of laser imagers or video imagers over the next few years, and as always in radiography, there are many factors to take into account. At the time of writing (1986) the following pros and cons seem to emerge.

Resolution

In terms of resolution capability there is no comparison between a laser imager and a video imager; the laser imager is far better. The

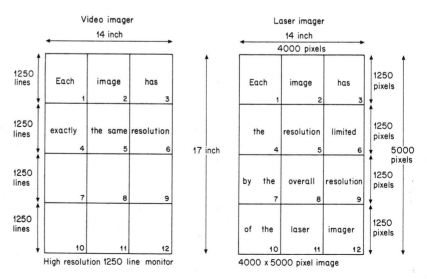

Fig. 8.17 Comparison of laser and video imagers.

laser imager has a resolution of 4000 × 5000 pixel, with 256 grey levels. However, this resolution is always on *one film*, not on *one image*, no matter how many images are on the film. Video imaging has a typical resolution of 1024 × 1024, but this resolution is the same on *every* image. It takes very little simple arithmetic to work out that if both systems have 12 images on a 17 × 14 in film, the resolution of both systems is virtually identical (Fig. 8.17).

Transfer of data

In data transmission terms, the video imager wins: a typical transfer time would be 40 ms. In a laser imager, which relies on digital transmission, a transfer time would be of the order of 3–15 seconds.

Exposure control

Exposure controls on a video imager are straightforward brightness, contrast and time of exposure. With a laser imager, look-up tables have to be used to consider film characteristics, contrast and brightness The actual exposure time of the film in a video imager is between 2–6 seconds. A laser imager requires anything between 25–90 seconds.

Film sizing

At present all major manufacturers seem to be making film for laser imagers. The film sizes available are:

17 × 14 in
10 × 8 in
10 × 14 in.

There is an added complication: 3M have a laser imager using infrared film, whereas all the other manufacturers have opted for a conventional film technology.

Disadvantages/advantages

Video imagers can be affected by strong magnetic fields. In MRI, for example, this can cause problems unless due consideration is given to the siting and shielding of the imager in relation to the MRI apparatus. Also, the phosphor coating on the CRT can sometimes not be uniform, giving rise to areas of low or high intensity on the image.

The laser imager is very susceptible to the ingress of dust and to vibration, particularly as the laser beam transfer is via a mirror. Additionally the vertical movement of the film by mechanical means must remain absolutely in register throughout the whole of the exposure. Any interruption of this travel, caused by vibration or mechanical movement, will produce gross artefacts on the image.

Interfacing a laser imager causes greater problems than interfacing a video imager. This is caused primarily by the need to capture pure digital information, whereas the video imager relies solely on a video signal.

35 mm slide production is at the moment only possible with a video imager.

At present, laser imagers are limited to one film size. The newer generation of mixed size, multiformat cameras give the user an enormous range of size and format capabilities.

Which is best?

To use a phrase which appears a number of times in this book, the choice remains 'horses for courses'. It is indisputable that the laser imager produces superior images when used as a large format single image. However, this image must be produced from a high resolution matrix of 2048 × 2048 or greater. To use a matrix resolution of 512 × 512 on a unit capable of 4000 × 5000 resolution in large format would be patently absurd. However, digital radiography is rapidly requiring just this sort of high resolution area, coupled with the benefit of large grey scale levels.

Video imaging has a large part to play in general imaging, where its resolution capabilities fit in well with the demands of present day systems. The consistent resolution of the image, no matter how many images are on one film, weighs heavily on the side of video imaging. The short wait times for the image to be produced are greatly in favour of video imaging.

It can be fairly safely said that, for very high resolution digital radiography composed of a large single format image, the laser imager is preferred. For conventional imaging, the video imager seems still to be the best.

WHY USE FILM?

It would be very difficult to close this chapter on monitor photography without asking one more question. Why use film? With the proliferation of electronics, it is fair to assume that the answer lies in that area. Well into the future that may be so, but there are a number of facts which should be considered. (At this stage Chapter 10, Computing, may well be considered recommended reading.)

Up until very recently, the ideal detector for X-rays was a photographic emulsion. The main advantages of film can be simply listed.

1. Film has a high emulsion sensitivity to short exposure times.
2. The natural spectral sensitivity of silver halide matches intensifying screen output.
3. Silver halide is capable of a high information density.
4. Silver halide produces a safe and permanent image (we still have images from the 1850s).

Perhaps the two main advantages can be put very simply.

1. Film has extremely high spatial resolution

It has very high resolving power, usually expressed in line pairs per millimetre (lp mm^{-1}). Film resolution can vary tremendously. With X-ray film, a typical figure would be 10 lp mm^{-1}. With a holographic emulsion, 5000 lp mm^{-1} would not be considered exessive.

2. Film has extremely high temporal resolution

It should not be forgotten that the extremely short radiographic exposures of today were only possible through the use of film. Film has the property of being able to freeze fast movement, providing enough energy is available.

It should be noted that to produce a *single* television frame requires 1/25 second. The image produced on the monitor must, of necessity, flicker. Many investigations have been done on the ergonomic design of a viewing station for prolonged reporting sessions, and much consideration has been given to this flicker in particular. Some manufacturers are considering using a monitor phospor with an extended lag, i.e. afterglow, to try and reduce the flicker. Nonetheless, it is at present a problem.

Of course film, or more accurately silver halide, does have some disadvantages.

1. Only about 3–5% of the X-radiation is converted into a visible image.
2. There is poor visualisation of low contrast subjects.
3. Film requires 'offline' three step wet processing.
4. Erratic silver prices tend to destabilise film prices.

Perhaps the worst of these is film's inability to cope with low contrast resolution, the ability to define very small differences in X-ray absorption.

Film versus electronics

One of the major attractions of electronic imaging, be it CT, ultrasound or any other form, is the fact that image processing, or manipulation, is extremely straightforward. Film does not allow this feature, at least not easily. In fact the only real film image manipulation which goes on in the X-ray department is subtraction.

Electronics do not have it all their own way. The main problems are interfacing, i.e. connecting one piece of apparatus to another, and ease of viewing. Film, on the other hand, can be posted, put into albums, or viewed on a viewing box with consummate ease.

Image complexity

The first CTs produced pictures on a square matrix of 80 × 80 pixels.

Compared to today, this image was of very low resolution, using only 6400 pixels.

Matrices have increased in size over the years. First 320×320, then 512×512 and then 1024×1024. These figures give total numbers of pixels as 102 400, 262 144 and a staggering 1 048 576.

Initially magnetic tape, then disk were used to store the data, but it soon became apparent that the floppy disk could not handle the volume of data.

In DSA, with a matrix of 1024×1024, one *10 second* study can generate 262 144 000 pixels at 25 frames a second. This very large number is further modified by the fact that every pixel is not just black or white, it is represented by varying shades of grey.

When computers are considered at their most basic level and ignoring any high level language which enables the user to communicate easily with them, computers use binary arithmetic. They simply count to two and start again.

In binary, 11111111 represents decimal 255; 00000001 represents decimal 1. If 2 is raised from the power 0 to 10, the following decimal numbers are obtained:

1; 2; 4; 8; 16; 32; 64; 128; 256; 512; 1024.

This helps to explain why these decimal numbers constantly recur in computerised imaging technology.

Taking a 512×512 matrix as an example, the matrix is made up of 512 vertical columns and 512 horizontal rows. At each pixel, the brightness level is converted to a binary number. Thus, if the pixel is able to demonstrate 256 brightness levels (2^8) then the pixel is said to be 8 bits deep. Zero will represent black and 255 will represent white.

It is, of course, possible to have a 7 bit deep pixel (128 brightness levels) or a 12 bit deep pixel (4096 brightness levels). Obviously the eye cannot see that number of grey levels, but it enables a very wide range of windowing levels to be used by the operator.

For example, if an image consists of 512×512 pixels, each 8 bits deep, then a total of 262,144 bytes are required.

The numbers required to record dynamic events are astronomical. Take for example a matrix 512×512, 8 bits deep, 25 frames a second and a *one second* event. This requires 6 553 600 bytes: so for dynamic images on this type of matrix, almost 7 megabytes (Mbytes) a second are required.

Image storage

There are a variety of storage methods in use, and it is worth considering the figures for each in turn.

Magnetic disk

A typical 8 in (double density, double sided) disk can hold about 1.2 Mbytes, i.e. four 512×512 images.

Magnetic tape

A 2400 foot tape can hold 180 Mbytes. That represents storage for about:

685 512 × 512 images.
2.3 10 second studies.
11 17 × 14 in film images.

Additionally, it can take nearly 4 minutes to find a specific image on the tape.

Optical disk storage

It is expected that a double sided optical disk can hold about 2.5 gigabytes (Gbytes): that is, 2.5 billion bytes!

For straightforward data storage, i.e. text, that is an incredible amount of storage capacity. To try and put this figure into perspective, a capacity of 600 Mbytes, or only 0.6 Gbytes, would be capable of storing all details, reports, film locations, appointments, X-ray room details, registrations, etc., for about one million patients. That represents the storage of all patient data (in an average hospital) for about 10 years. However, the storage of images is a different matter.

Even 2.5 Gbytes is only capable of handling about 170 17 × 14 chest films. Data compression can be considered at this stage, although it can be difficult to implement. Typical data compression may be able to reduce storage requirements by as much as 50%. Even so, large numbers of optical disks would be required to store all the images archived in a busy general hospital, bearing in mind that statistics say that about 30% of work in a general department is chests.

The main factor in favour of the optical disk is the fact that, *once it is filled*, any image can be found in about a quarter of a second.

The transmission of these large amounts of data to a remote viewing area should also be considered. The transmission of 2.5 Gbytes at even 1 Mbyte a second takes a significant amount of time if the transfer is by hard wire. If optical transmission, by optical fibre, is considered, this transfer time will reduce considerably. However, the installation of optical fibres, even if available, is an expensive exercise.

A 15 MBYTE PROM

This is a solid state, large-scale integrated detection-display device, sensitive to a wide range of the general electromagnetic spectrum. The device is flexible and allows excellent archiveability. The device can be viewed without any electronic display system or computer. It is totally portable and is easily transmitted. The device has a capacity of 15 Mbytes, and a density of 10^9 bits/cm^2. The device is extremely inexpensive.

Reading the above description, the device appears totally revolutionary; however, this inexpensive PROM (Programmable *Read Only Memory*) is a 17 × 14 inch film! (This description assumes that the film is digitised to 0.1 mm pixels).

If X-ray images are recorded onto a 17 × 14 inch film, 15 Mbytes are immediately available to a radiologist, in a form which the eye and brain can easily process and interpret. If these images are microfilmed and 20 of them are recorded onto a 5 × 17 in film, we have the equivalent of 300 Mbytes (0.3 Gbytes).

It seems, from today's viewpoint, that film still has a future in the X-ray department. It is also inevitable that digital equipment will appear in great numbers, although the full implementation of digital equipment will remain costly.

CONCLUSION

Monitor photography has become a mainstay of ultra-modern imaging. The development of this type of imaging is far from over, but monitor photography still uses a technology which is well over 150 years old and, because of the convenience of film, should continue to use it for some years to come. Film technology is developing continually and will continue to develop well into the foreseeable future. Electronic imaging, with its insatiable demand for hard copy, is more than established, yet it seems to have opened even more doors for film.

9
Holography

Introduction

To adapt an old adage, 'Seeing is believing . . . except when viewing a hologram'. This expression may seem trite, unless one has actually seen a hologram; no two dimensional picture can do justice to a hologram.

The very name 'holograph' tells almost the whole story. It is derived from the Greek *holo*, meaning whole and *graphoo* meaning writing. A hologram can only be described as if the viewer is looking through a window at the real object, the image having all the perspective of the original object. So realistic are they that the Russian government have made holograms of priceless works of art so that everyone in that far flung country has an opportunity to see (almost) the real thing.

A fully three dimensional picture floating in space has captured the imagination of science fiction writers for many years. Only a few years ago holography was an unrealisable dream, but in recent years the knowledge and technology associated with the subject have increased in leaps and bounds.

Strangely enough, the concept of holography goes back to 1948 when Dennis Gabor, an engineer physicist, proved that three dimensional pictures could be produced using coherent light.

Gabor, an expatriate Hungarian, was working at the British Thomson Houston Research Laboratories in Rugby. He was trying to improve the resolution of electron microscopes. Unable to use X-ray to prove his ideas he used a heavily filtered mercury vapour light shining through a pinhole one thousandth of an inch in diammeter. Under these conditions the light was extremely dim, but almost coherent, so the 'interferograms' he produced were very small, of the order of millimetres in size. In his article in 'Nature' in 1948 he describes the experiment, and only in passing does he mention that the photographs produced were three dimensional. Incidentally, in 1971 he was awarded the Nobel prize for this achievement.

To understand the concepts of holography, however, the history of the science of light must be investigated.

LIGHT AND THE LASER

The development of holograhy is so interlinked with the development of the laser that it is impossible to separate the two. To this end, it is worth considering how the laser was born from the investigations of the 19th century.

In the 18th and 19th centuries, controversy had raged about the behaviour of light. Was it a particle or did it travel in waves? Dr Thomas Young, a brilliant physician born in Somerset in 1773, had followed this controversy for years. Intrigued as to the answer, in 1803 he passed a beam of light through a narrow slit and found that separate bands of light appeared instead of the expected sharp outline of the slit.

He had also studied the behaviour of sound extensively and, using the analogy of beat frequency, proposed that if light travelled as particles this behaviour would not take place, but if light were a waveform, this was an expected effect. To confirm his predictions he

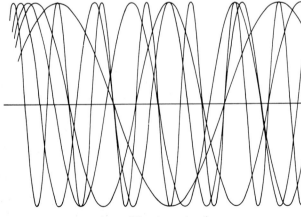

Many different wavelengths

Fig. 9.1 White light — a cacophany in vision.

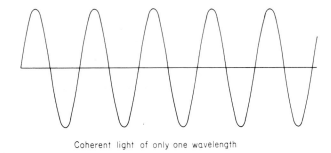

Coherent light of only one wavelength

Fig. 9.2 Laser light — coherent light of only one wavelength.

shone the light through two pinholes. Where the two beams over-
lapped there was a pattern of alternating dark and light areas. The
light areas were caused by waves coinciding with one another and
adding to each other's waveforms. The dark areas were caused by
other peaks cancelling one another out, similar to the behaviour of
waves at sea. It was in this way that the wave theory was finally
confirmed.

It has been long understood that white light is a veritable jumble
of varying wavelengths, ranging from ultraviolet in the short wave,
through visible light, to infrared in the long wavelengths; indeed a
cacophony in vision. Because of the presence of all these wavelengths, white light has very short coherence lengths, due to the
antiphase components cancelling one another out. To produce a
hologram, as Gabor had discovered, a bright source of coherent light
had to be obtained.

With all of this knowledge available, scientists sat back and waited
for a major breakthrough: the development of the laser.

The breakthrough came in a paper in 1958, written by Townes &
Schawlow, called 'Infra Red and Optical Masers'. Maser is an acronym
for Microwave Amplification by Stimulated Emission of Radiation.
They suggested that the techniques used in microwave amplification
could well be used in light amplification. The laser was almost born.

In 1960 Theodore Maiman, working at the Hughes Aircraft Electronic Research Laboratory, built the first laser. His laser was basically
a photographer's electronic flashgun wound around a crystal of
synthetic ruby (aluminium oxide mixed with a small amount of chromium). The synthetic ruby was in the form of a tube with a mirror
at each end of the tube, one mirror being a partial reflector; the
distance between the mirrors was precisely defined, as it was tuned
to make the light produced bounce back and forth in a regular and
reinforcing pattern.

Anyone familiar with Hi-Fi will understand this technique. In a long
narrow room it is almost impossible to produce the correct base
response from a speaker. Either the base response is very weak as the
sound waves cancel one another out, or the bass response is excessive as the waves reinforce one another. The latter technique was

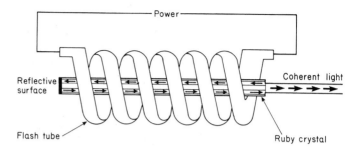

Fig. 9.3 Maiman's original synthetic ruby laser.

used in the ruby rod to create standing waves of light in the rod (Fig. 9.3).

It is difficult to appreciate that the mechanism of operation of a laser was not clearly understood until 1960. In basic terms it is very simple.

If a photon is fired at an atom, the atom can absorb the photon and thus be raised to an excited state. The only way that the atom can return to stability is by releasing this absorbed energy in the form of a photon of light (*spontaneous emission*). (Strangely enough, Albert Einstein had suggested in the early 1900s that atoms could absorb energy and then could possibly be stimulated to release this energy.) However, if a photon is fired at an already excited atom, the atom will release TWO light photons and then return to its stable state. This particular process is known as *stimulated emission*. In a laser, the atoms are stimulated by an external power source (Fig. 9.4).

When a stage is reached whereby half the atoms are in an excited state, a situation known as *population inversion* occurs. If more photons are fired at this stage, stimulated emission takes place. Stimulated emission occurs at this point simply because it is more likely

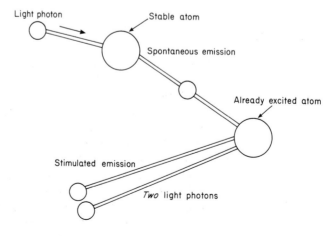

Fig. 9.4 Stimulated emission.

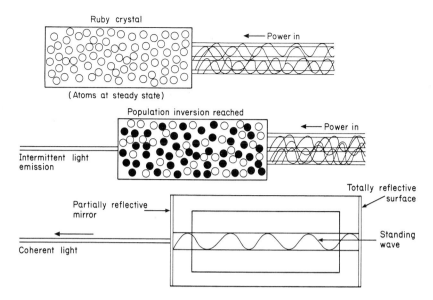

Fig. 9.5 Population inversion.

that the photons will strike an already excited atom rather than a stable atom (Fig. 9.5).

If the events described occur in a tube, the tube can be 'tuned' to encourage the light produced to oscillate in a regular pattern, and to eventually break out as an extremely coherent, parallel beam of light which contains a considerable amount of energy.

All of this work had to be done to develop the laser; then in 1980, for the first time, astronomers identified the light from Mars. The atmosphere of Mars is a natural laser because the unique combination of carbon dioxide and infrared sunlight causes the atmosphere to lase and produce the red laser light of Mars, known to man for many thousands of years.

LASER SOLUTIONS

When the laser first appeared it was referred to as 'the solution looking for a problem to solve'. The laser since then has solved a great many problems.

The National Physical Laboratory has determined that the speed of light is exactly 186 282.397 miles per second, using a laser.

Distance measurements accurate to 1 millionth of a centimetre can be made using a laser.

When the Apollo astronauts left the moon, they left behind a mirror to reflect laser light. When laser light is bounced off this mirror (and even at a distance of some quarter of a million miles the light only spreads about two square miles), the distance of the earth to the moon can be determined to within an accuracy of 1 foot.

Military

Militarily, lasers are used as gun sights (these are infrared lasers) and target designators. There is even a laser Army tank, as well as a projected airborne laser. The United Technology Research Centre in Connecticut has produced a laser which has no power requirements at all. This is a chemical laser, which uses hydrogen and fluorine. When these two gases are combined in the correct quantities, a vigorous reaction takes place which causes the atoms lase immediately. This would enable satellites to be equipped with a laser which has no power requirements. To this extent, the 'Star Wars' speech of President Reagan was really pre-empted many years ago.

Medicine

In medicine, lasers are used in a variety of applications. A few are listed below.

1. They can be used as surgical knives, as they cut and cauterise at the same time.
2. They can be used to kill, very precisely, pre-cancerous cells in the neck of the cervix.
3. They can spot weld the retina back into place.
4. They are used in the treatment of veins in danger of haemorrhaging.

It is at the cellular level, however, that lasers have really come into their own. They can be focussed so precisely (and yet carry such large amounts of power) that they can destroy a single cell, or even part of a cell. In the laboratory at least, lasers have been taught, by computers, to recognise cancerous cells and destroy them.

Perhaps the most interesting observation is that lasers could become a major tool in cancer and genetic research in the future.

Whilst not immediately apparent as a medical use, optical disks will certainly be used extensively in the digital imaging departments of the future. This development would have been impossible without the laser. Optical disks, first seen in the Hi-Fi industry, make extensive use of a laser. In the compact disk, which contains digital musical information, a laser is used to read the digital pits created below the surface of the disk. At the introductory stage these disks were 'read' only, i.e. they could only be played back. The information contained on the disks, however, was of very high quality. The large optical disk then appeared on the scene, capable of playing back images. The modern version of these is capable of 'reading' and 'writing', i.e. the user can now record information on the disk. These disks are capable of very high storage capacity, typically 2.5 Gbytes.

The laser is used in these systems because it can be focussed so accurately below the disk surface. This means that any surface blemish, i.e. scratches, will not be read by the laser. The laser also produces sufficient energy to deform the disk material so as to record the required information.

PULSED OR CONTINUOUS

The laser that Maiman invented was a *pulsed laser*, which had a pulse of about three thousandths of a second.

   The next major step forward was the *continuous wave gas laser* (Fig. 9.6), using helium and neon as the lasing material (see Laser imagers, p. 293). These lasers are extremely coherent and uniform, and can be switched off and on like a simple electric light. In 1961, at the University of Michigan, Leith & Upatnieks repeated Gabor's earlier work. Using a Laser, their work was of course a success. The period of gestation was over; holography was finally born.

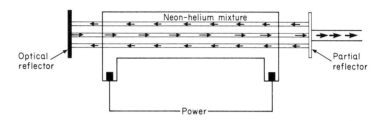

Fig. 9.6 Continuous wave gas laser.

PRODUCTION OF HOLOGRAMS

A conventional photograph relies purely on the intensity and wavelength of light which is reflected from the object. A hologram gains its information from the *amplitude* and *phase* content of the light reflected from the object. To produce a hologram, two beams of light are required. One beam, the reference beam, arrives in the area of the holographic plate uninterfered with. The second beam, the object beam, is reflected off the object and then meets the reference beam in the same area. Where the two beams meet, an interference pattern is produced.

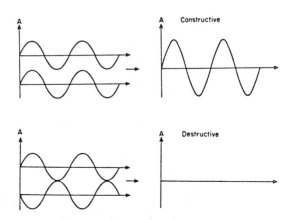

Fig. 9.7 Constructive and destructive interference.

When two beams arrive at the recording medium in phase, they add to each other's amplitude, the wavelength remaining the same. This is referred to as *constructive* interference. If they arrive at antiphase to one another they cancel each other out, i.e. the amplitude is zero. This is *destructive* interference. Obviously, there are degees of in phase and antiphase, which effectively means that the amplitude can vary between zero and twice that of the original amplitude of the beam (Fig. 9.7). The interference pattern is then recorded on the holographic film. When the film is processed and then illuminated with laser light, a three dimensional image is produced.

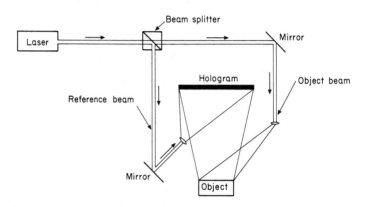

Fig. 9.8 Producing off-axis transmission holograms (after Leith & Upatnieks).

Figure 9.8 shows an arrangement for producing off-axis transmission holograms, as used by Leith & Upatnieks. The reference beam passes through a beam splitter, mirror and lens to be finally focussed onto the film. The object beam passes through a similar arrangement of apparatus to finally be reflected off the object and reach the film. On this film is recorded an interference pattern, which contains all the amplitude and phase content information from the two beams.

When the film is processed and illuminated with laser light, a virtual image is produced behind the film (Fig. 9.9).

However, there are two images available from this transmission hologram. If the viewer moves to the back of the film there is a real image which is in front of the film, but is pseudoscopic (Fig. 9.10).

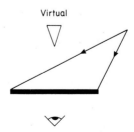

Fig. 9.9 Virtual image seen behind film.

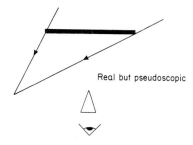

Fig. 9.10 Real, pseudoscopic image: background becomes foreground and perspective is completely distorted.

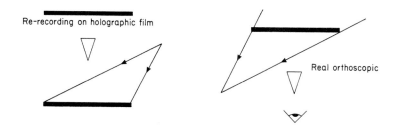

Fig. 9.11 Real, orthoscopic image (correct perspective) produced by re-recording pseudoscopic image onto holographic film.

In other words, the background becomes the foreground and the image perspective is totally distorted.

This real, pseudoscopic image can be the subject of another holographic recording which will produce a real, orthoscopic (correct perspective) image in front of the film (Fig. 9.11).

PROPERTIES OF A HOLOGRAM

Holograms have a number of properties which are difficult to appreciate unless they have actually been seen and handled.

1. The image is totally three dimensional

When a holographic image is viewed, it is exactly as if the real object were there. The image contains full vertical and horizontal parallax, albeit over a limited range of view.

2. Every part of the image contains all the information

If a hologram is broken, and there is sufficient depth of image, every broken piece will contain all the information of the original picture. If it can be imagined that the hologram is like a window, each broken piece will have the information as if it was viewed from that position in the window. In other words, the perspective is seen from that position.

This property can be exploited in data storage, for example. In theory, there is the capability of storing an infinite number of holographic images on one film. This can be achieved by progressively altering the angle of the reference beam.

3. Diffraction causes the image

This means that there is no necessity to develop and fix the image in the acknowledged sense of the words. In fact, the presence of silver in a holographic image presents a problem, as it causes the image to be very dark and the silver has to be bleached out.

Because minute changes produce the image, silverless material can readily be used. For example, dichromated gelatine is often used to produce bright and attractive images. Dichromated gelatine hardens progressively when exposed to light. When placed in water it swells, relative to how hard the gelatine has become. However, as large amounts of energy are needed for this material, this means that the images are usually small.

4. The holographic image is generally monochromatic

The colour of the image is dependent on the type of laser used. Lasers have very precise frequencies. For example:

- Helium-neon gas lasers emit light at 632 nm
- Solid state ruby lasers emit light at 694.3 nm
- The neodymium (rare earth) laser emits infrared radiation at 1060 nm
- The krypton-argon ion laser emits light in the blue, green and red areas of the spectrum.

Not *all* holographic images are monochromatic; these are discussed later in the chapter (see p. 313).

5. A hologram offers precise one-to-one reconstruction

The one proviso to this is that the hologram must be 'played back' with the same wavelength of laser that produced the original. This fact has been exploited by car manufacturers and tyre manufacturers, to name only two branches of engineering. If a transmission hologram is made of a car engine for example, and then played back exactly superimposed over the engine, the object and the image are indistinguishable. It is only when a bolt is tightened that something occurs.

As the bolt is tightened, a series of lines will begin to creep across the surface of the engine. Each line means that the surface has moved by half the wavelength of the laser light illuminating it.

Great care has to be taken in the production of a hologram. Because an interference pattern is being recorded, there must be complete stability of the recording equipment. This means using optical benches of the order of tons of weight, and special care in letting the air temperature in the laboratory, and the temperature of the equipment, stabilise before actually taking the hologram. Unlike a photograph, if a holographic film is moved during exposure the result is not a blurred image, but no image at all.

Finally it should be added that until recently it has always been essential, for recording *and* playback, to use a laser. Lasers are now not always needed for playback due to the advent of white light holograms.

BENTON HOLOGRAMS

The Benton hologram was devised in 1969. This is a hologram which could be viewed in white light or sunlight. The Benton hologram does suffer in that it only has horizontal parallax and also produces a multicoloured image due to achromatic distortion. These holograms have since been achromatised to produce black and white holograms.

A method very similar to Benton's has been used in the Lloyd Cross multiplexed hologram. This is a very attractive and wide-ranging technique for producing three dimensional images from a series of two dimensional pictures. This means that one to one reconstruction is no longer a limitation because of the two stage process in the production stage.

MULTIPLEXING

In this technique a series of pictures is prepared, usually in the form of a cine film. The original film is prepared by rotating the subject on

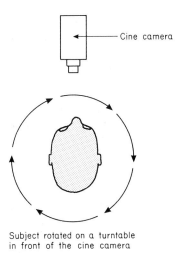

Subject rotated on a turntable
in front of the cine camera

Fig. 9.12 Preparation for multiplexing: the subject is photographed while being rotated on a turntable in front of the cine camera.

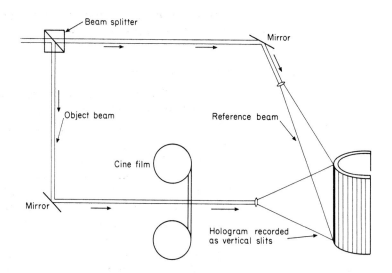

Fig. 9.13 Making the multiplex hologram.

a turntable and photographing this rotation from a fixed camera position (Fig. 9.12).

The information required before processing the multiplexed hologram is essentially the 'space/time' relationships of the camera and subject.

The cine film is then transferred to the curved holographic film in a series of vertical holographic strips, the holographic film being rotated in step with the cine film (Fig. 9.13).

The image is then reconstructed using a white light in the centre of a circle formed by the holographic film. These holograms exist in both 180° and 360° forms.

In the 180° hologram, approximately 1200 images are recorded during the rotation of the film; 800 of these images are used in each vertical holographic strip to produce the final result.

The final result is a three dimensional moving hologram that needs no sophisticated viewing machinery. The hologram has only horizontal parallax and suffers from colour distortion in that, as the viewer moves up and down the hologram, the colours of the spectrum are seen. The applications of this type of holography are great, perhaps even extending to three dimensional television.

A system very like this could be used to produce three dimensional X-ray images, although obviously there are very high dose rates to take into consideration. The images could be taken via an image intensifier and the subject rotated in front of the intensifier.

WHITE LIGHT REFLECTION HOLOGRAMS

This, the most easily viewable and versatile form of holography, was developed in Russia by Professor Denisyuk in the mid-1970s. To gain a basic understanding of this form of holography, we must return to the history of photography.

Lipmann emulsions

In 1891, Professor Gabriel Lippman announced a very unusual method of producing colour photographs using a black and white film. The 'Lipmann' emulsion was an extremely fine grain, panchromatic film.

The photographs were made by placing the emulsion side of the film in contact with a column of mercury. The reflected rays from the mercury interfered with the incident rays from the object and created an image of varying depth within the emulsion. The depth of this latent image was relative to the colour of the incident light.

When the film was processed and viewed in contact with a mirror, a picture could be seen in natural colour. Unfortunately, it was a very difficult to carry out the process, and it has since disappeared from the photographic scene.

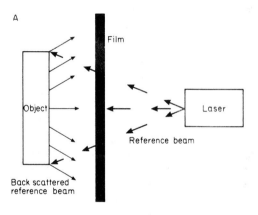

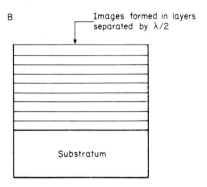

Fig. 9.14 'Denisyuk' holograms. (A) Laser light (reference beam) passes through the film and is reflected from the object towards the back of the film (object beam). (B) Both beams meet in the emulsion, producing image layers separated by half the wavelength of the laser light.

Denisyuk holograms

The Denisyuk method for the production of white light reflection holograms works on a very similar principle. It works extremely well with bright objects, as these will produce a large amount of reflected light. It is the way the incident and reflected light are used which is of particular interest.

The incident light from the laser passes through the film and is then reflected from the object towards the back of the film (Fig. 9.14). This has fulfilled one major need of holography, that there must be a reference beam and an object beam. These two beams meet in the emulsion producing image layers lying parallel to the base of the film and separated by half the wavelength of the laser light, i.e. approximately 300 nm.

Once the film is processed, white light can be reflected off these layers using the wavelength selective Bragg effect, so that the image reflects that part of the white light spectrum that coincides with the wavelength of the laser light used.

PROCESSING

This is a complex subject, necessarily outside the scope of a book such as this. Adequate references are included at the end of this chapter for anyone interested in this part of holography.

It is important to note, however, that the presence of silver in the image is deleterious, causing either very dim pictures or large amounts of scatter within the emulsion, thus worsening the resolution. This means that the silver image should be bleached out to transparency. This is not quite so simple as it sounds; it can cause such problems as collapse of the gelatine or colour shift, which can be a major fault, or at worst no picture at all.

Silverless systems

A conventional medical X-ray film/screen combination has a resolution of the order of 6 lp/mm. In holography a considerably higher resolution must be expected, as now interference patterns have to be recorded. It can be safely assumed that for holographic film the resolution will be of the order of 5000 lp/mm.

It is correct to say that the progress of holography was slowed down until films (and chemistry) were able to take advantage of the very rapid technological advancements occurring in lasers and optical knowledge.

Earlier in the chapter, attention was drawn to the fact that as diffraction causes the image, materials such as dichromated gelatine could be used. Any silverless system in any branch of photography is of interest, for obvious reasons, and holography has spawned many.

Photopolymers have been used as a silverless source. The photopolymer, a metallic acrylate monomer using a dye as a catalyst, is exposed to laser light. The monomer is then polymerised using ultraviolet light. The image is formed in the monomer (which is a gel), and then the film is 'fixed' using a UV light. This hardens the gel and bleaches out the dye which was the catalyst.

An eraseable hologram is a very attractive proposition in areas such as data storage. In this case, the information can be stored (in three dimensions, so the 'sheet' can have a depth of information, i.e. an X,Y and Z axis) until needed, erased and re-used. From the economic point of view the use of such material is obvious.

Photochromic dyes have a peculiar property in that they are capable of light absorption. One particular wavelength will increase the light absorption, whereas another will cause the material to return to its normal state. Using this effect holograms can be produced with one laser and wiped clean with another laser of a different wavelength.

Lithium nobate crystals also have a photochromic effect. In this case, the laser light causes localised excitation of electrons. These excited electrons cause changes in the refractivity of the material, sufficient to be able to reproduce an interference pattern.

Thermoplastics also have a role to play. A charge pattern is formed in the material, and when the material is slightly heated, it deforms in relationship to the charge pattern. This slight deformation is again enough to produce a hologram. To remove the image it is only necessary to reheat the thermoplastic.

Even magnetic films, whose magnetic characteristics can be altered by exposure, have been experimented with.

The Benton holographic technique has been mentioned briefly before. The Benton hologram, also known as the 'rainbow hologram' made available relatively inexpensive holograms. Benton realised that when white light lit a transmission hologram the image was distorted, as the varying colours of white light were bent differently. The result was an indistinct blur. Benton simply produced a hologram which only had a small number of 'views', with no vertical parallax at all, but true three dimensional information in the horizontal plane.

To print a hologram, a transmission hologram has to be prepared first. This hologram is exposed onto a photo-resist. The photo-resist is then processed and produces the interference pattern as a series of fine lines. Nickel is then deposited on the plate by electrolysis, and the result of this process is a printing plate.

This plate is now used to impress the interference pattern onto an easily deformable PVC sheet which is backed with aluminium, acting as a mirror, reflecting light back through the interference pattern. This fact has been exploited in the printed holograms which are now readily, and very cheaply, available.

USES OF HOLOGRAPHY

Holography appears in so many different forms and guises that people are sometimes unaware of it being used. Some of the many and varied applications are listed below.

Industry

Vibrational stress patterns can be made of objects as varied as violins and turbines. In the case of turbines, an exposure is made as the blades are turning. The second exposure is made when the blades are steady. This double amplitude hologram contains information about shock waves, temperature and pressure. Violins can be tested in a very similar way, only in this case the holograms are made when the violin is at rest and when played.

Speckle holography can be carried out in real time. This system does not require any film at all. It merely relies on the laser light producing the typical speckle when shone onto a stationary part of the object and no speckle if the part is moving. This is ideal for identifying vibrational patterns on some objects.

Photogrammetry

Holography in this area allows three dimensional measurements to be made, which means that the operators no longer have to make calculations to allow for error in parallax or magnification.

Optics

If a hologram is made of an optical element, the hologram retains some of the properties of the original element. There are, however, a number of disadvantages to this as, the element will only refract or reflect certain wavelengths. There are some specialised applications of such optics.

Bar code readers

In the latest type of bar code reader, introduced by IBM, there are 21 holographic elements contained in a rotating disc. Each element has different focal length and can be used to deflect a laser beam to illuminate the bar code as it passes over the reader, from almost any angle.

Aviation

'Head up' displays in aircraft now use holographic optical elements to project images from CRT's onto the windscreen of the airliner, so that the pilot has an unobscured view of the airfield, but can have all the vital flight information at eye level.

Security

Major credit cards now have holograms embossed on the surface of the card. This reduces the risk of fraud, since if the card number is interfered with, the hologram will be destroyed or badly distorted.

Medicine

Holograms are made of moulds of castings of a patients' teeth. This is essential in orthodontics where a record must be kept of the patient's development. The resultant hologram is very easy to store, particularly in comparison to a plaster cast, and contains very accurate measurement information (see Photogrammetry, above). The savings in storage space alone is enormous.

Of even more interest is the development pioneered by Keen and Wright of the Royal Sussex County Hospital in Brighton.

First, a series of CT images are recorded in the normal way, i.e. on a conventional imaging film. This series of images is placed in the object beam from the laser, whilst the reference beam enters the face of the emulsion. The holographic film is linked to a motor via a computer, which moves the holographic film forward relative to the slice separation of the original CT scans (Fig. 9.15).

It will be realised that this process uses a technique which is similar to the Denisyuk method, in that the image is formed as parallel layers within the emulsion. The final image can be seen as a white light reflected hologram. The important point to realise is that the images are a total three dimensional view of a series of CT scans, and yet have been produced from a series of two dimensional images.

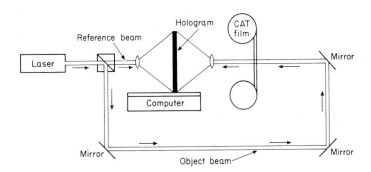

Fig. 9.15 Making a hologram from a series of CT scans recorded on a conventional imaging film (after Keen & Wright).

THE FUTURE

Holography is in many ways connected to the development of better, and more powerful, highly coherent lasers.

With the advent of dye lasers, capable of emitting coherent light over a wide range of wavelengths from ultraviolet to yellow, many possibilities are opened up. In a dye laser, organic dyes are used to re-radiate light of a different wavelength.

Rhodamine 6G was the first dye to be used in a dye laser. Since then methylumbelliferone with hydrochloric acid has been used. With easily tunable lasers such as this, the full, natural colour hologram becomes attainable. Indeed, Professor Denisyuk has already exhibited some examples.

X-ray lasers

Some observers have claimed to have seen coherent X-radiation during laboratory experiments. It is no secret that a number of research groups are working on such a laser, sadly in the military field, closely allied to SDI research. The energy that an X-ray laser could carry is enormous, and as a dynamic, destructive weapon would have no equal.

The peaceful use of an X-ray laser would have tremendous applications in all sorts of areas, indeed it has been said that an X-ray laser would be a 'window on the sub-atomic world'. The X-ray laser, with its extremely short wavelengths, would enable the observer to look at the inside of an atom or molecule. Additionally, if films could be made to record such an interference pattern, holographic images could be made of living cells or microscopic particles. Whether the X-ray laser will ever appear in the X-ray department as a diagnostic tool is a point for conjecture. If it did, three dimensional radiographs would be an exciting possibility.

Acoustic holography

It is very easy to obtain a coherent source of sound by coupling an oscillator to an amplifier and loudspeaker. Researchers are now working on the production of acoustic holograms, using frequencies up to 10 MHz.

Whilst still in their infancy, successful acoustic holograms have been produced. The transmitters for this technique are immersed in a liquid and the interference pattern forms on the surface. This is obviously not a permanent hologram, unless the image is recorded on something like heat sensitive thermoplastic (mentioned earlier in the chapter).

CONCLUSION

Holography, although still in the early stages of its development, has opened up new areas of imaging in a vast number of fields. It would seem highly unlikely that it will remain a static science; it can only continue to develop.

REFERENCES

Agfa-Gevaert Technical Information Sheet, NDT/Holography
Boraiko A A 1984 A splendid light: lasers. National Geographic 165 (3): 335–363
Caulfield H J 1980 Handbook of optical holography. Academic Press, London
Caulfield H U 1984 The wonder of holography. National Geographic 165 (8): 365–377

Chen F S, La Macchia T, Fraser D B 1968 Letter. Applied Physics 13: 223–225
Close D H et al 1969 Letter. Applied Physics 14: 159–160
Denisyuk YuN, Soskin S 1971 Optics and spectroscopy (from the Russian) 31: 992
Dowbenko G 1978 Homegrown holography. Amphoto, New York
Gabor D 1948 Nature 161: 777
Gabor D 1949 Proceedings of the Royal Society (Series A) 197: 454–487
Gates J W C 1968 Journal of Scientific Instruments (Series 2) 1: 989–994
Leith E N, Upatnieks J 1962 Journal of the Optical Society of America 52: 1123–1130
Leith E N, Upatnieks J 1964 Journal of the Optical Society of America 54: 1295–1301
Lin L H 1969 Applied Optics 8: 963–965
Ostrovsky YuI 1977 Holography and its applications. Mir Publishers, Moscow
Phillips N J 1979 Wireless World May: 63–67
Phillips N J, Porter D 1976 Journal of Physics E. Scientific Instruments 9: 631–634
Roberts D P 1979 Holography. Radiography 46: 118–124
Wenyon M 1978 Understanding holography. David and Charles, Newton Abbot

10

Computing

Introduction

In the past few years computers have arrived in the X-ray department. Computers have appeared on items as diverse as CT scanners and ultrasound units, to a computer to cope with the day-to-day running of patient records in Reception.

With so many developments in information exchange it has become very obvious that the computer is to become an important item in the department. Since the announcement of the Korner Report and the knowledge that this will require many more statistics to be derived, a computer that will help in the management of the X-ray department has become almost a necessity.

In many subjects, a knowledge of the development of a technology provides an insight into why things are as they are. In computing, history provides a great deal of information. To this end, this chapter is first of all devoted to a brief history of the development of the computer. Many buzzwords have arisen in computing science and a short glossary of buzzwords (Appendix A) is also included.

Computers have to be programmed in a language which they understand. A brief description of programming language is included in the chapter, as is the ASCII code (Appendix B).

The final part of the chapter relates to a management system for a modern imaging department. Whilst a chapter such as this can never hope to be comprehensive, it will serve as an introduction to what can be a bewildering array of technology.

HISTORY

The abacus must be the first 'computer', in the literal sense. Still in use thousands of years after its initial discovery, it is outstanding proof that the simplest can sometimes be the best. However, over three centuries many people and many ideas have contributed to make the computer we know today. Whilst the following list is by no means comprehensive, it is interesting to look at some of the more important names and their ideas and see how each played its part in the evolution of computing.

Blaise *Pascal* (1623–1662) must rank as a founding father. He made one of the first gear-driven 'calculating machines'. It was he who laid down the ground rules of modern probability theory in cooperation with an Italian, Fermat. Pascal's name was honoured over 300 years later, when a computer language was named after him.

John *Napier* (1550–1617) realised that all numbers could be expressed as exponents, i.e. 2 to the power 2 was 4, 2 to the power 3 was 8, etc. He also worked out that other numbers could be arrived at by having fractional exponents. If these exponents were added, the numbers were being multiplied; if they were subtracted, the numbers were divided. In 1614, he published his 'log tables'. These were to prove indispensable to thousands of mathematicians.

Leibniz (1646–1716) was a contemporary of Isaac Newton. He invented a gear-driven machine that could multiply and divide. He also mentioned the use of binary arithmetic, although Francis *Bacon* first made the reference to binary in 1623.

Charles *Babbage* (1792–1871) had an idea in 1812. This was to build a Difference Engine which could calculate, amongst other things, the exact position of the moon, so that accurate nautical tables could be produced. The machine was advanced but, because it was gear-driven, was unable to be made accurately enough. It should be remembered that in the middle of the 19th century, high tolerance gear-cutting machinery, such as that required by Babbage, simply did not exist. The project failed and he carried on with another machine, the Analytical Engine, which more closely resembled a modern computer in operation but not in construction. The gear-driven machine was programmable and gave a printed output.

It is often claimed that the world's first computer programmer was his assistant, Countess Ada *Lovelace*, the daughter of Lord Byron. It was she who helped Babbage in the complex task of trying to programme the complicated machinery to perform the routines demanded of it.

Babbage's work failed, primarily due to the fact that he required sophisticated machinery which was years ahead of its time. However, in the 1850s a much less sophisticated version of Babbage's machine was made and used in Sweden to calculate life insurance and astronomical tables.

George *Boole* (1815–1864) was a great mathematician who developed what is now known as Boolean algebra, the logic of calculators and computers of today. He was the first to recognise the '*and*' and '*or*' mathematical operations.

Herman *Hollerith* (1860–1929) was originally a clerk in the United States National Census Office. He was amazed that when the time came round for the next census, 10 years later, the original census had not been finished. He was convinced that there must be a device that was capable of analysing results quickly.

He left the Census Office and joined the Patent Office, with the intention of becoming an inventor. His main aim at that time was to invent an analysing device. He succeeded, and invented the punched card as an input for machines to read. This type of card is still used as a computer input device today.

Many other types of machines were produced in the early 20th century, mainly in the field of calculating. They were usually very large, mechanically-driven devices which worked reasonably well but very slowly.

In the 1930s IBM, who were to become the world leader in business computers, made electromechanical office machines which used punched cards as programmable inputs. By 1947, IBM made its first computer. This had 800 000 (mostly mechanical) parts and took *ten seconds* to divide two numbers.

However, it was the World War Two which pushed computer development and led companies such as IBM to develop the knowledge for the construction of the new generation of computers.

World War Two

In the early part of World War Two, it was quickly realised that the Germans were using a sophisticated form of cryptography, the codes being generated by a typewriter-like machine known as *Enigma*. It became imperative for the codes to be broken and the problem was handed over to the former GCHQ at Bletchley. The machine developed to crack the codes was *Colossus*.

Colossus and after

Colossus was an unsophisticated, valve-driven computer. It eventually cracked the Enigma codes, but more importantly, the pioneering work done at Bletchley led to the world's first programmable computer at Manchester.

The research team at Manchester combined a great deal of wartime experience. Professor Max Newman had worked on Colossus, F. C. Williams had experience in radar and Tom Kilburn was also in radar research during the war. This team eventually produced a world first: the first programmable computer.

The Royal Society had been persuaded to invest £35 000 in the Calculating Machine Laboratory at Manchester University. In June 1948, the investment paid off and the first program was run.

The Mancester Mk.1 could execute an instruction in 1.2 milliseconds.

The government were so impressed with this computer that they asked a local company, *Ferranti*, to build a commercial unit. The Ferranti Mk.1 became the world's first commercially available computer.

A little prior to the Manchester development, a computer known by the acronym Eniac had been developed in the USA. Eniac stood for *E*lectrical *N*umerical *I*ntegrator *a*nd *C*alculator. It had been a project which had been initiated at the request of a US Army colonel who wanted a machine to calculate trajectory for shells. The statistics for ENIAC are quite enormous.

It had 18 000 valves and 1500 relays. It had the capability of storing only 20 ten-digit numbers. If it was to be reprogrammed, the wiring had to be re-arranged. It consumed almost 200 kW.

The world's first business computer was Leo, again an acronym, this time for *L*yons *E*lectronic *O*ffice. It was prepared for Lyons Coffee Houses, to speed up their business transactions.

Lyons gave a grant of £3000 to Cambridge University to help in the production of Edsac, *E*lectronic *D*elay *S*torage *A*utomatic *C*omputer. The grant was used by Cambridge to buy war surplus valves. By 1949 Edsac completed its first job: calculating a table of prime numbers.

Leo became operational in 1954 and was used to calculate the company's weekly payroll. What had taken a clerk eight minutes was done by Leo in one and a half *seconds*.

The transistor

The device which changed the face of computing, however, was the transistor.

In 1938 an electrical engineer, Claude *Shannon*, proved that a relay could act as part of a logic circuit. At first, valves or mechanical relays were used to perform this logic task.

In 1947, *Shockley*, *Bardeen* and *Brittain* invented the transistor; in 1954, they were given the Nobel Prize for this work.

In Manchester University, the research team had been joined by Alan *Turing*, a mathematician, who had gained a great deal of experience during World War Two. Turing later invented the Turing Test, a test for assessing machine intelligence. A complicated test, it was basically a means of assessing whether an individual could determine if he was conversing with a machine or a human being. Armed with the knowledge of transistor development, Manchester University produced the world's first transistor computer in 1953.

It can be safely said that from this point on, the computer as we know it today was established. There are more obvious milestones on the way, mostly due to pressure for microcomponents in the 'space race'.

In the late 1960s, Russia had obviously gained considerable experience in lifting heavy objects into space. The USA did not have the expertise for such heavy rockets and therefore pushed research to new levels to produce microcomponents for flight control, etc. This equipment obviously lightened the payload considerably and gave the added benefit of smaller, lighter microcircuitry.

When the evolution of the computer is talked about, the first reference must always be the early valve computer. The characteristics of this were:

Large

The initial machines like Colossus, Eniac and Leo are outstanding proof of this.

Slow

Most of the early machines had a maximum capacity of 20 ten-digit numbers. Any complex calculation meant reprogramming and consequently considerable time.

Large power consumption

Eniac required about 200 kW. The average calculator today, with infinitely more calculating power, will operate from a 1.5 volt battery.

Limited memory

The Eniac had a memory of 250 bytes. A typical home computer of today has about 256 *kilobytes* of memory which is readily accessible.

High cost

Table 10.1 shows how, in 1950, a 350-word page of memory would cost about £1 000 000, whereas in 1983 the typical price was £30.

All of these values were affected by the development of the transistor, and even more by the development of the integrated circuit.

The integrated circuit

Jack *Kilby*, of Texas Instruments, invented the integrated circuit in 1958. He constructed a package which was half an inch by a quarter of an inch. It is difficult to appreciate today what a revolution this was.

In 1959, only one component could be made into an integrated circuit. By 1978, large scale integrated circuits (LSIs) could have over 250 000 components.

The future development of the computer seems to be heading for smaller, faster computers using very large scale integrated circuits, or even light, as the transfer medium, rather than electrons. There is even research into a biological chip, leading to a computer that in theory could be grown from organic material.

THE FUTURE OF THE CHIP

Silicon has been the basis of the chip for a long time. It is interesting to note that the relative price of silicon is the same now as it was in 1973, but many more thousands of chips can now be put onto a 4-inch disc.

Satellite television, however, has placed extreme demands on silicon; for this purpose, gallium arsenide is replacing silicon. Gallium arsenide is much faster than silicon, which is a big advantage in computing.

Printing the chip

Microchips are basically printed, using a form of photography, through a photo-resist and directly onto the chip material. Naturally the final resolution of this process is all important, as the final result is basically produced by reducing a large negative to a microscopically small size. The printing of the circuitry originally used ultraviolet light as the printing light: this gives a typical final resolution of 1/1000 of a millimeter. If beams of electrons are used to print, instead of UV, the resolution is about twice that of UV.

However, both of these media suffer from scatter within the photographic medium, and experimentation has suggested that *heavy ion* imaging would produce finer detail and permit 'ballistic transfer' of electrons, as the chip would be very small indeed. Ballistic transfer simply means that the distances within the chip are so small that the electrons travel like bullets to their destination, without even atoms intervening their path.

In one research laboratory, it has been proven that 100 000 000 single transistors can be printed per square *millimetre*, or 20 bibles could be printed on a pinhead!

The implication of this development is enormous, as the final microchip would be miniscule. This means much faster, as well as smaller, computers in the very near future.

The computer has evolved very rapidly indeed, perhaps more rapidly than any other comparative technology. Table 10.1, culled from the Sunday Times Business News, shows in graphic detail the growth of the computer and its memory and the parallel dramatic reduction in costs.

Table 10.1 Evolution of the computer. *Source: Sunday Times Business News 8.7.84*

Size
The approximate size of a computer with the same computing power as a human brain:

1950	London
1960	Albert Hall
1970	Double decker bus
1980	London taxi
1990	Television set
2000	Same size as brain

Cost of memory
Cost of storing 350-word page of memory:

Valve/transistor/chip	Year	Back up memory: tape/disk
£1 Million	1950	Non-available
£30 000	1960	£5000
£1000	1970	£100
£100	1980	£6
£30	1983	£1
£3	1985	30p
50p	1990	5p

Cost of computing power
Per 1 million instructions/second:

1969	$200 000
1973	$150 000
1981	$50 000
1984	$25 000
1985/6	$2500

The table does not tell the whole story. In 1984, many meetings were held which refer to the 'fifth generation' computer or the 'metacomputer', a word coined by Sir Clive Sinclair to describe a computer which will have a kind of intelligence similar to the human brain. Most probably this computer will communicate in an entirely different way to computers as we know them today.

It is envisaged by many people that, by the end of the century, computers could be self-reproducing devices, not even needing a human designer or builder any more.

BUZZWORDS

In every trade and profession there are always words in common use which are meaningless to outsiders. The computer industry has generated more than its fair share of these so-called *buzzwords*.

The word 'buzzword' was itself an invented word. The word first appeared in the early 1960s from the publicity department of Honeywell, who had prepared a 'buzzword generator'. This was a three column table of words. Words were then taken from each column, to make a three-word, usually meaningless phrase, such as 'Homogenised Image producer'.

However, there are numerous words and phrases in computing which pepper everyday conversation, and whilst to the uninitiated they appear to be meaningless, they in fact have a great deal of meaning. The glossary found in Appendix A is by no means comprehensive, but it contains many of the buzzwords in current use.

COMPUTER LANGUAGES

Machine code

When computers first arrived on the scene, the inputs and outputs were on paper tape and involved laborious calculations whereby the instructions were turned into binary arithmetic (machine code), the *only* language that a computer understands.

It became very obvious to everyone that unless there were a great many mathematical geniuses around, computers would stay in universities and laboratories and would remain inaccessible to the general public.

High level languages

This led to the development of a 'high level language' for computers.

A high level language can be defined as a language in which each instruction or statement (in almost plain English) corresponds to several machine code instructions.

The most common of the high level languages has become *BASIC*, initiated by *Microsoft*, a leading company in America.

Unfortunately, BASIC has many dialects and this generally means that a program written in one dialect of BASIC will not run on another dialect of BASIC.

BASIC reserved words

To enable any computer to RUN it must have some form of language for it to be able to LOAD a program. You may wish to SAVE the program onto disc or tape. It may also be necessary in the program for the computer to READ a set of DATA and, from time to time, GOTO various sections of the program to be able to LIST certain variables which have been turned into STRING$.

You may also have to WAIT WHILE the computer WENDS its way through very long CHAINs of numbers before it can RESTORE itself and RETURN to the program and allow you to INPUT more information before it will PRINT out the name you wanted to DELETE. Eventually the program will STOP, END and finally CLOSE.

Admittedly, the above two paragraphs are contrived, but all of the words in capitals are 'reserved words' in BASIC; they give a computer specific instructions as to what to do. BASIC is, of course, an almost universal language amongst home computers, mainly due to the simplicity of programming in the BASIC language.

Exactly the same constraints are put on all high level languages. It is impossible to use these words within a program without the computer translating them into a piece of specific instruction.

Unfortunately, BASIC is unsuitable for large scale programming as, in computer terms, it is very slow. This is due to the fact that all the instructions given in BASIC have to be translated into machine code by the computer.

Portability

Simple programs can be written on most of the popular computers in a fairly standard BASIC, using the same reserved words. However, these programs, even though they use the same notations, are not *portable*, i.e. the recorded program will *not* run on a different machine.

However, once the realm of BASIC is left behind, this situation changes quite considerably. For example, CP/M is a fairly standard 'business' computer language. Any computer capable of running CP/M is capable of running any program written in that language.

Syntax

The BASIC language, which most people have some knowedge of, provides an excellent example of the use of syntax.

Just as in any foreign language, the BASIC language has its own syntax which differs from English. In some dialects of BASIC for example, the word GOTO can only be entered as GOTO, not GO TO. The computer may reject one or the other version as incorrect. Similarly, a comma (,) or a colon (:) or double quotes (") all have their own parts to play. Without the correct insertion of specific punctuation and words, the program will simply refuse to run.

The keyboard

First of all, when approaching a computer it is essential to familiarise oneself with the computer keyboard. Most people approaching a computer for the first time recognise the keyboard as being similar to a typewriter, but with several extra keys which are totally unrecognisable.

Return

The most important key to recognise immediately is the <Return> key. This key is the 'carriage return' key and performs exactly the same function as on a typewriter. This key can appear in many forms but is usually marked 'carriage return' or 'return'. This means that after every line in the program has been entered, or after a single instruction has been entered, <Return> must be pressed. There is another key seen on computers, namely the <Enter> key, which has a similar use to the <Return> key.

Cursor

The other keys which are significantly different from a typewriter are the cursor control keys. These can move the cursor in four directions — up, down, left and right — enabling the accurate positioning of the cursor.

Tab

In some cases this performs a function similar to the 'tab' key on a typewriter. In some instances, however, the key is used within a program for entirely different purposes.

There are obviously many other keys which may seem unfamiliar. Some keys are used to insert or delete letters or words when editing text or programs. Many keys are 'dedicated' to, i.e. used only for, a special function connected with a particular make of computer. Most programs can be used without a specialised knowledge of the function of these keys, although their use can be extremely advantageous.

Binary

The words 'bit' and 'byte' frequently crop up in talk of computers. This is simply because this is the language that is 'spoken' by the computer. The words are a description of how the computer stores and manipulates numbers.

From childhood, we are taught to manipulate numbers in base 10, i.e. '2 × 5 = 10'. Computers, being simplistic devices, can only handle a 0 or a 1. Binary arithmetic is thus ideal for computers, because it counts to the base 2 instead of 10; '01 plus 10' = 3. This enables very large numbers to be represented by a series of ones and zeros, e.g. 01110111 is the binary equivalent of 119.

The smallest piece of information that a computer can handle is called a 'bit', supposedly derived from BInary digiT. This bit is represented by a simple electrical signal. Very simply, an electrical signal can either be ON or OFF; the 'bit' can therefore be represented by an 'ON' or 'OFF' signal.

Consider a row of two simple switches, each of which can be ON or OFF. There can only be the following four possible states:

OFF OFF or 0 0 (decimal 0)
       [or]
OFF ON or 0 1 (decimal 1)
       [or]
ON OFF or 1 0 (decimal 2)
       [or]
ON ON or 1 1 (decimal 3)

Four different states is a very small range of numbers. In binary this could only represent the (decimal) numbers from 0 to 3.

If 8 switches are used, the higher decimal numbers could be displayed. If all the switches were on they would represent the following decimal total:

ON ON ON ON ON ON ON ON
128 64 32 16 8   4   2   1

The values add up to 255.

Now consider the same row of switches, some switches ON and some OFF, in the positions illustrated.

ON OFF ON OFF ON OFF OFF ON

Now substitute binary numbers in place of the switching states, and the row becomes:

ON OFF ON OFF ON OFF OFF ON
1   0   1   0   1   0   0   1

Translating the binary numbers into their decimal equivalents, the values are:

ON OFF ON OFF ON OFF OFF ON
1   0   1   0   1   0   0   1
128 0   32 0   8   0   0   1

Thus the decimal equivalent of:

1 0 1 0 1 0 0 1

is the sum of the 'ON' switches, or the binary 1s, i.e. 128 + 32 + 8 + 1, or 169.

In other words, in binary, these eight switches can now show all the numbers between 0 and 255 inclusive, or 256 separate states.

When eight of these 'bits' are grouped together they are known as a 'byte' and each byte is a unique combination of zeros and ones.

When a computer stores this byte, it effectively means that a number between 0 and 255 is stored, in binary form, in a specific location within the computer's memory.

In certain computers, e.g. if sophisticted graphics are used, they are created using binary code and then used as data by the computer.

However, the main use of the numbers 0 to 255 is in the ASCII code to designate numbers, characters and symbols used on the computer keyboard. In Appendix B may be found the decimal value, the binary equivalent and the ASCII character for each number.

Hexadecimal

Another type of numbering is favoured in computing: this is the hexadecimal system, which uses base 16. Hexadecimal is unusual in that it uses numbers and letters in the notation. Decimal numbers from 0 to 20 are listed in Table 10.2 to illustrate the big differences between hexadecimal and decimal.

Table 10.2 Comparison of decimal and hexadecimal number systems: 0–20

Decimal	Hexadecimal
0	0
1	1
2	2
3	3
4	4
5	5
6	6
7	7
8	8
9	9
10	A
11	B
12	C
13	D
14	E
15	F
16	10
17	11
18	12
19	13
20	14

DEPARTMENTAL MANAGEMENT WITH A COMPUTER

Generally, most radiographers meet a computer for the first time in a working environment in CT or ultrasound. However, it is now becoming more and more common for them to also use a computer which is used in the actual management of the department.

A senior consultant radiologist listed the requirements for a computer system for an imaging department. The main points are listed below.

Reduce repetitive tasks

With a computer installed in the department, the routine, repetitive form-filling should become a thing of the past. For example, once a patient's name has been entered, it should not be necessary to have to re-enter it.

Reduce paper handling and filing

Whilst the paperless department will not be with us for many years to come, a considerable reduction can be expected in jobs such as filing or storage of (paper) details of patients, etc.

Improve intra-departmental communications

Ready access is assured, with the proviso of password protection, to all the necessary details which enable the department to run smoothly.

Improve efficiency

A computer system can increase the overall efficiency of the department considerably.

Improve confidentiality and security

Files, reports and patient details can be very secure. To try and retrieve details without a password, or knowledge of the system, would be made very difficult.

Automate data collection

With a computer system, retrieval of all data can be accomplished 'at the touch of a button'. With the arrival of Korner statistics and the need to collect considerable amounts of data for these, a computer is now almost essential. Clinical budgeting can be very successfully helped by a computer.

A management computer installed in an X-ray department should also be able to supply the following ancillary functions.

Research and museum

Patient details and their films could be retrieved easily, using some simple identifying procedure. This would prove invaluable for research purposes or for the compilation of a museum.

Spreadsheet

The increasing demands of clinical budgeting could be well-supported using a Spreadsheet, an electronic accounting ledger, which could project 'what if' calculations easily.

Word processing

Most people who have used a word processor would never go back to a conventional typewriter. Routine letters, requests, etc., could be stored for immediate printout.

Space invaders

Not quite as unusual as it sounds! Games on any computer system can increase the keyboard skills of the players, as well as encouraging the use of the computer for more mundane applications.

The use of a computer for departmental management can bring many benefits. It is worth looking in detail at some aspects which can bring considerable improvements to a modern X-ray department.

Patient enquiries

In a major London teaching hospital, a survey was conducted into the number of patient enquiries passing through the department per day. These were enquiries such as:

'Have you the report on . . .?'
'Has he arrived . . .?'
'Can we have the films for . . .?'
'Have you got the films for . . .?'
'Can we make an appointment for . . .?'

The enquiries were broken down as follows:

Phone	90
Appointments	65
Arrival	300
Report request	36
Film request	450
Total	940

At the end of the day, 940 patient enquiries had been made. The average response time to answer these queries was 55 seconds.

940 queries at an average of 55 seconds adds up to a staggering 14.36 man hours per day!

Using a computer, which should have an average response time of significantly less than five seconds, the 940 queries can be tackled in about 2 man hours per day. This represents a saving of more than 12 man hours per day.

It has been said many times that a computer system should never ask the user to do something which they have already done before, or something which is not required in the manual system. If the system does put extra pressures on the user, it is almost guaranteed that the staff will be very much against using the system.

In this context, consider the number of times in a manual system where the patient details have to be repeatedly recorded. Take the case of a patient request arriving from a GP.

Table 10.3 Comparison of manual and computer systems: processing a patient request from a GP

	Manual system	Computer system
Request from GP	YES	YES
Registered in department	YES	YES
Appointment book	YES	NO
Appointment slip	YES	NO
Envelope	?YES	NO
Patient attends	YES	NO
Film marker	?YES	NO
Film envelope	YES	NO
Report form	YES	NO
Envelope to GP	YES	NO
Opportunities for error	?10	2

A computerised film store

Of interest to a great many people is how a computer can help in film store management, which can be a major problem in many departments.

The use of a computer would enable sequential filing to take place. This means that at the end of a day's session, the films are filed sequentially and placed in the file in that particular day's slot. Eventually a 'hot' area will be created at the end of the file, where the most frequent attenders will be found, and a 'cold' area where all of the 'dead' films will eventually arrive.

Apart from being extremely simple and quick to use, sequential filing offers a very high degree of security, as the films are filed under days rather than under a hospital or computer number. No longer can films be removed furtively. Unless the location is known, the films are virtually impossible to find. Sequential filing, which is used by many large companies with vast indexes, is only really manageable with a fast computer which is able to store and retrieve locations quickly.

It is interesting to compare a manual and a computer-controlled film store system (see Table 10.4).

Table 10.4 Comparison of manual and computer-controlled film storage systems

	Manual system	Computer-controlled system
Patient attends	*Search* for old films: If found, fill in tracer and exchange If not found, make a new packet	Computer confirms presence or absence of films If they exist, current film location shown
Examination completed	*Search* for tracer and exchange	Place film at end of file
Patient attends clinic	*Search* for packet: If found, fill in tracer and exchange	Computer indicates film location *Search* file for films
Films returned to store	*Search* for tracer and exchange	Place films at *end* of file
Patient never seen again	*Search* for 'dead' films and remove	'Dead' films at *beginning* of files

[Summary]

Manual system	Computer-controlled system
5+ *Searches* for film packet	All films in sequence of acquisition
Misfiles easy = *total loss*	A computer can record date (even bin number)
Search essential to determine presence/absence of films	'Hot' store for films most likely to be pulled
Requires tracer cards	Refiles *always* at end of file
No immediately available record of outstanding films and their destinations and durations	A computer can give file date, or location and date if film is out of the files

The above examples merely illustrates some of the benefits that management computers can bring into an X-ray department. The systems currently on offer vary tremendously in size and therefore capacity, and in the functions they are able to undertake. Some systems are capable of using and generating bar codes, which enable much quicker entry into the computer and reduce the keyboard skills required by the users (they also considerably reduce the opportunities for error).

Larger systems are capable of storing vast amounts of data, some indeed capable of storing all patient reports and film details for one million patients.

CONCLUSION

It seems inevitable that computers, in many forms and guises, will occupy a major place within the imaging department of the future, not simply in management, but also in imaging technology. It is very difficult to determine where their future influence may lie: they have obviously already made an impact on imaging in general, and other uses for them may well arise.

REFERENCES

Asimov I 1975 Biographical encyclopaedia of science and technology. Pan Books, London
Meire H B 1986 Private communication

Appendix 1

Glossary of computer buzzwords

The following glossary is by no means comprehensive, but it contains many of the buzzwords in current use.

Access time The time taken for the computer to get information from a storage device, e.g. disk or tape.

Address A number which designates a particular storage area in the memory of the computer.

Algorithm Logical steps which define how a problem can be solved.

Analogue Represents a quantity changing in steps which are continuous, as opposed to *digital*, which is in discrete steps.
   A voltmeter with a needle pointer is an *analogue* device. It can record an infinitely variable number of readings. A voltmeter with a digital display is limited to the number of steps it is allowed to display, i.e. is a *digital* device.

Analogue to digital convertor A device which converts analogue signals into digital signals which can be understood by the computer.

ASCII The American Standard Code for Information Interchange.
   This code defines the decimal and binary code of all the characters stored in the computer.
   For example:

[Decimal]	[Binary]	[Character]
115	01110011	s
34	00100010	"
68	01000100	D

For a list of standard ASCII codes, see Appendix B.

BASIC A high level language for computers and almost universally used for home computers. It is an acronym of Beginners All-purpose Symbolic Instruction Code.

Baud This is the unit for measuring the rate at which data is transmitted or received.

It was named after Emile Baudot, the inventor of a telegraphic code similar to the Morse code.

Binary A system of counting to base two, i.e. generating figures with only 1 or 0 (see Appendix B).

Bit The smallest unit of data in a computer. It is a contraction of BInary digiT.

Booting Starting up the computer by loading it with its starting instructions.

Buffer An area which stores information at one rate and releases it at a slower rate to another device.

For example, a buffer can be sited between a computer (fast) and a printer (which is significantly slower). Data can then be passed at a fast rate and stored in the buffer until the printer can print the data. The computer is thus freed for further work much more rapidly.

Bug A problem in the computer or (usually) in the program.

Bus A semi-standard connector to the computer through which all data is passed to an external device.

Byte The number of bits which are needed to form a single character. This is usually 8.

It is interesting to note that 1 kilobyte (1K) is not 1000 bits but 1024 bits! This is because of binary arithmetic; one kilobyte is $2\times2\times2\times2\times2\times2\times2\times2\times2\times2$ bits, or 2 to the power 10.

Centronics A type of standard interface between computer and peripheral.

The standard defines the plug and socket sizes and how the data is transmitted between the computer and peripheral.

CP/M One of the most common 'universal' languages.

A number of computers speak BASIC but, as in all languages, there are many dialects. This means that there are very few computers on which it is possible to use a program from another computer of a different make.

CP/M is a disk-based language which tries to rectify this. Most computers running CP/M can interchange programs quite easily.

CPU Central Processing Unit: the core of the computer.

Chip A piece of silicon which contains the microcircuitry which operates the computer. Gallium arsenide is also used.

Cursor A flashing marker on the screen which indicates where the next character is to be inserted.

Daisy wheel printer A high-quality printer, in which the printing head consists of characters arranged on a series of 'petals' arranged in a circle. This device, the 'daisy wheel', has replaced the 'golf ball' (q.v.) as a printing head in many instances.

Database Software designed to store information in a systematic way, and at the same time to allow easy retrieval and manipulation of all data.

Debugging The correction and, much more importantly, the finding of errors or bugs in a program.

Digital See *analogue*.

Disk A circular plastic disc coated with magnetic material used for storing data. Disks are usually high speed devices.

Dongle Any device used to protect software from piracy.

Download To transfer information from one computer to another.

DOS Disk Operating System. This is the software which controls the disk drive.

Dot matrix A square or rectangle of dots which, given instructions by the computer, forms a character. Usually refers to a printing head, but could refer (for example) to the construction of a character on the screen.

Editing Altering the text or program.

EPROM Eraseable Programmable Read Only Memory. A memory store which can be programmed but erased, if wished, by UV light.

File Information stored on disk or cassette.

Firmware Software, but stored on a chip.

Floppy disk A flexible disk (see disk) usually $5\frac{1}{4}$ inches in diameter.

Flowchart A diagrammatic representation of a computer program.

Forth A programming language which is between BASIC and machine code in difficulty.

Gate A gate performs a single logical operation when subjected to a number of inputs. It is the basis of all computer operations.

Golf ball A printing head usually found on electronic typewriters. Shaped like a golf ball, with printing characters arranged around its surface, the ball rotates very rapidly to present different characters to the typewriter ribbon.

Graphics This can refer to a number of things.

  1. Computerised 'drawing', known as CAD (Computer Aided Drawing).
  2. The ability of the computer to produce pre-programmed graphic characters.
  3. The mode the computer has to be placed in prior to drawing graphics.

Graphics tablet A piece of equipment that can digitise drawings or graphs ready for input into the computer.

Handshake An electronic signal which indicates the end of the passage of data from the computer.

Hard copy The paper printout of the program or screen display.

Hardware The mechanical and electronic part of the equipment.

Heuristic A 'trial and error' method of trying to solve a problem.

Hexadecimal A mathematical system which employs 16 digits from 0 to 9 plus A, B, C, D, E, F. For example, hexadecimal 24A is equal to decimal 570.

Icon A relatively new move in computers to make them more 'user friendly'.
  An icon is displayed on the screen, e.g. a waste basket. This indicates that, if this icon is selected, the software is programmed to dump the data, as if it were a real waste basket.

Initialise At the beginning of computation all variables are given specific values in the program.
  For example: A=l, B=7, C=4.
  In this example, A, B and C are the variables initialised at those values.

Intelligent peripheral A keypad linked to a computer that can act as a computer in its own right.

Interface The connection from the computer to other hardware, allowing free communication between the two.

Iteration To repeatedly execute an instruction in a program.
  For example:

100 FOR X = 1 TO 200: NEXT X

  In line 100, the routine has been iterated 200 times.

Keyboard The computer interface with a human being. Usually very similar to a typewriter.

Light pen A device, shaped like a pen, which interfaces with a computer screen and enables the computer to know which part of the screen is being pointed to.

LISP LISt Processor language. A language used a great deal in Artificial Intelligence research. It is a high level language.

LOGO A high level language usually used in schools to introduce primary school children to computers.

LSI Large Scale Integration. A means of packing large numbers of electronic circuits into small chips.

Soon to be followed by VLSI, or Very Large Scale Integration.

Machine code The language the computer can understand directly.

In a high level language, commands are simplified into pure English. In machine code, all instructions are written in binary.

Mainframe A large computer, usually the centre of a system. Intelligent peripherals can then be attached to this.

Menu A set of choices presented in a program.

For example:

1. New patient
2. Alter patient details
3. Next appointment
4. Report details
ENTER NUMBER OF CHOICE.

Microprocessor A very complex integrated circuit that can be pre-programmed to perform a variety of tasks.

Modem MOdulator-DEModulator. A device, also known as an acoustic coupler, which allows the computer to transmit data down a conventional telephone line.

Monitor A device very similar to a television, but which receives video signals directly from the computer, rather than RF-modulated signals, giving much more accurate resolution.

Mouse Again, a device for making the computer more 'user friendly'. Instead of accessing the computer via a keypad, the mouse is used by rolling the device across a desk top. This, in turn, moves a cursor to icon displays on the screen.

MSX A new standard for home computers based on Microsoft Extended Basic.

This standard specifies minimum capacity, graphic display size and fittings for peripherals. Hopefully the MSX standard means that any program written for one MSX computer will be interchangeable with another make of MSX computer.

Network A system, usually connected by telephone line, which interconnects a number of computers enabling multi-way communication within the network.

OCR Optical Character Recognition. A means of the computer directly reading printed or written characters.

OCR was meant originally to be used with post codes, but it constantly runs into a classic computer problem known as the 'B8 problem'. In other words, the computer has great difficulty in recognising the difference between B and 8, apart from problems of handwriting differences.

Output Data and information leaving a computer. This data can then be sent to a display screen, printer or another computer.

PASCAL A high level language for computers.

Peripheral Any device attached to a computer, e.g. a printer or modem.

Pixel PICture cELl. A pixel is the smallest number of dots which can be used by a character on the display screen.

It can also be used to define the resolution of a system by describing the resolution of a matrix in pixels, i.e. 1200×1200 gives a resolution of 1200 separate points horizontally and vertically.

Program A set of written instructions for the computer. (Note how many of the buzzwords are Americanised in their spelling.)

PROM Programmable Read Only Memory. A specially-prepared chip which can be programmed, turning it into a Read Only Memory.

RAM Random Access Memory. This is the part of the memory of the computer which can be accessed by the user.

The amount of RAM available determines how much data can be stored by the user. It is usually shown as 16K, 32K, 48K or 64K in the smaller home computers.

In the bigger business type computers, many hundreds if not thousands of kilobytes may be quoted.

Real time Usually defined as a computer controlling, or recording, events as they are actually happening.

Remark Usually seen in a program as REM. This instruction is ignored by the computer, but enables the user to add comments in plain English.

RGB input This refers to a colour input on a monitor (q.v.). The signal from the computer or video apparatus is taken by the monitor as a basic Red, Green and Blue input, thus bypassing any RF device.

ROM Read Only Memory: the pre-programmed part of the computer which enables it to run programs. Whilst it may be accessible to the user, it cannot be altered.

RS 232 A type of standard interface between computer and peripheral. The standard defines the plug and socket sizes and how the data is transmitted between the computer and peripheral.

Scrolling The movement of text or data on the display screen. Scrolling can be upwards, downwards or even sideways.

Software The programs run by the computer.

Speech recognition A software development allowing computers to be operated by human voice commands.

Speech synthesis A software development allowing the computer to 'talk' to the user.

Spreadsheet A program which allows forecasting and financial planning. It can be thought of as a massive financial ledger in which, if any variable is altered, the effects throughout the ledger can be demonstrated and the figures changed throughout the ledger without further input from the user.

Sprite A user-generated character, much used in game playing. The sprite can be kept moving at a certain speed by the computer, independent of any other movement on the screen.

Statement An instruction in a program.

Subroutine A self-contained part of a program which can be returned to time and time again within a program.

Syntax error Two words which are shown on the display when an incorrect input or statement has been made.
   Very familiar to any computer user!

Teletex The sending of documents at high speed electronically.

Teletext The non-interactive public information service on television. The BBC transmits Ceefax, the ITA transmits Oracle. See also *videotext*.

Time bomb A device used by some software suppliers to prevent piracy of programmes, which is a growing menace in the computer world. The software is protected by a certain phrase or code which can be removed by the legitimate supplier. If it is not, after a period of use the software is so arranged that it will wipe itself out and erase all the company records.

Turnkey A term used to denote a company which will provide all the necessary software and hardware plus back-up support to enable the user to *'turn a key'* and use the equipment.

Turtle A wheeled mechanical device, used for graphics, attached to a computer via cables. Initially associated with LOGO (q.v.) where the Turtle would draw its path (the Turtle Trail) across paper.

VDU Video Display Unit.

Videotext The interactive public information service broadcast on television. The public Viewdata channel is known as Prestel.

VOXEL A pixel (q.v.) but in three dimensions.

Winchester disk A very large capacity *hard* disk, as opposed to *floppy*. The disk is housed in an hermetically sealed container, as any ingress of dust or dirt, no matter how microscopic, could possibly destroy very large amounts of data.

Word processor A combination of computer, software and printer enabling the user to produce high quality text which can be manipulated electronically before being committed to paper.

Zap! Usually found when playing Space Invaders.

More seriously, it is sometimes used to mean a small alteration to a program.

Appendix 2
List of ASCII Codes

The following is a list of standard ASCII codes, comparing the decimal and binary values with their ASCII equivalents.

It should be noted that codes between 0 and 32 are usually reserved for special printer control codes.

Up to the decimal number 122, the ASCII range is adopted by most manufacturers. Like so many 'standards', however, the numbers after 122 have been freely adopted by various manufacturers for their own purposes.

[Decimal]	[Binary]	[ASCII]	[Decimal]	[Binary]	[ASCII]
0	00000000		26	00011010	
1	00000001		27	00011011	ESCape
2	00000010		28	00011100	
3	00000011		29	00011101	
4	00000100		30	00011110	
5	00000101		31	00011111	
6	00000110		32	00100000	SPACE
7	00000111		33	00100001	!
8	00001000		34	00100010	"
9	00001001		35	00100011	£
10	00001010		36	00100100	$
11	00001011		37	00100101	%
12	00001100		38	00100110	&
13	00001101		39	00100111	'
14	00001110		40	00101000	(
15	00001111		41	00101001	)
16	00010000		42	00101010	*
17	00010001		43	00101011	+
18	00010010		44	00101100	,
19	00010011		45	00101101	-
20	00010100		46	00101110	.
21	00010101		47	00101111	/
22	00010110		48	00110000	0
23	00010111		49	00110001	1
24	00011000		50	00110010	2
25	00011001		51	00110011	3
			52	00110100	4

Dec	Binary	Char	Dec	Binary	Char
53	00110101	5	88	01011000	X
54	00110110	6	89	01011001	Y
55	00110111	7	90	01011010	Z
56	00111000	8	91	01011011	[
57	00111001	9	92	01011100	\
58	00111010	:	93	01011101	]
59	00111011	;	94	01011110	^
60	00111100	<	95	01011111	_
61	00111101	=	96	01100000	`
62	00111110	>	97	01100001	a
63	00111111	?	98	01100010	b
64	01000000	@	99	01100011	c
65	01000001	A	100	01100100	d
66	01000010	B	101	01100101	e
67	01000011	C	102	01100110	f
68	01000100	D	103	01100111	g
69	01000101	E	104	01101000	h
70	01000110	F	105	01101001	i
71	01000111	G	106	01101010	j
72	01001000	H	107	01101011	k
73	01001001	I	108	01101100	l
74	01001010	J	109	01101101	m
75	01001011	K	110	01101110	n
76	01001100	L	111	01101111	o
77	01001101	M	112	01110000	p
78	01001110	N	113	01110001	q
79	01001111	O	114	01110010	r
80	01010000	P	115	01110011	s
81	01010001	Q	116	01110100	t
82	01010010	R	117	01110101	u
83	01010011	S	118	01110110	v
84	01010100	T	119	01110111	w
85	01010101	U	120	01111000	x
86	01010110	V	121	01111001	y
87	01010111	W	122	01111010	z

Index